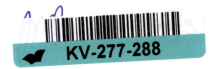

KV-277-288

BRITISH MEDICAL BULLETIN   1993   VOL. 49   No. 4

BRITISH MEDICAL BULLETIN

British Medical Bulletin is published four times each year, in January, April, July and October.

Subscriptions and single-copy orders should be sent to: Longman Group UK Ltd, PO Box 77, Harlow, Essex CM19 5BQ. Tel: 0279 623760

Subscription rates for 1994 are: £126 (UK, £6 postage), £126 (Europe, £8 postage), $207 (USA, $15 postage) or £126 (RoW, £11 postage)

NEXT ISSUE

BRITISH
MEDICAL BULLETIN

VOLUME FORTY-NINE
1993

CHURCHILL LIVINGSTONE
EDINBURGH, LONDON, MADRID, MELBOURNE,
NEW YORK AND TOKYO

CHURCHILL LIVINGSTONE
Medical Division of Longman Group UK Limited

Distributed in the United States of America by Churchill
Livingstone Inc., 650 Avenue of the Americas, New York,
NY10011, and by associated companies, branches and
representatives throughout the world.

ISSN 0007-1420
ISBN 0-443-04928-9

Produced by Longman Singapore Publishers (Pte) Ltd.
Printed in Singapore.

This journal is indexed, abstracted and/or published online in the following media:
Current Contents, Scientific Serials Review, Excerpta Medica, USSR Academy of
Science, Biological Abstracts, UMI (Microform), BRS Colleague (full text), Index
Medicus, BIOSIS, NMLUIS, Adonis

Notes to users in the USA: Authorisation to photocopy items for internal or personal use
is granted by Longman Group UK Ltd provided that the appropriate fees are paid directly
to Copyright Clearance Center, 27 Congress Street, Salem, MA 01970, USA. For more
information, please contact CCC. For territories outside North America, permission should
be sought direct from the copyright holder. This consent does not extend to other kinds of
copying, such as copying for general distribution, for advertising and promotional purposes,
for creating new collective works, or for resale.

British Medical Bulletin is published quarterly in January, April, July and October by
Churchill Livingstone c/o Mercury Airfreight International Ltd Inc, 2323 Randolph
Avenue, Avenel, New Jersey 07001. Subscription price is $222.00 per annum. Second Class
Postage paid at Rahway NJ. Postmaster: Send address corrections to British Medical Bulletin
c/o Mercury Airfreight International Ltd Inc, 2323 Randolph Avenue, Avenel, New Jersey
07001.

Spongiform Encephalopathies

Scientific Editor: *I V Allen*

1993 Vol. 49 No. 4

Professor Sir K Murray chaired the committee which included Dr Skehal and Professor Raff which planned this number of the British Medical Bulletin. We are grateful to them for their help and particularly to Professor Allen for her work as Scientific Editor.

British Medical Bulletin is published by Churchill Livingstone for The British Council, 10 Spring Gardens, London SW1A 2BN

British Medical Bulletin (1993) Vol. 49, No. 4, pp(i)–(ii)
©The British Council 1993

Preface

The spongiform encephalopathies or prion-associated diseases are an excellent example of rapid development of a scientific field from a position of relative obscurity to one of prominence in mainstream neurobiology. This change is reflected, perhaps somewhat unusually, not only in terms of scientific achievement, but also by increased media attention and public awareness in general. A few years ago scrapie, Creutzfeldt-Jakob disease and other associated conditions, while intriguing pathogenic puzzles to specialists in the field, had little wider biological impact and were largely unrecognised by the general public. All this has changed and, in acknowledging the advances, recognition must be given to the interaction of molecular biology with classical epidemiological, transmission and neuropathological studies. This is not to say however that we have all the answers, rather the questions are better defined.

In this Bulletin the key issues are addressed, including the nature of the infectious agent, the genetic control of host susceptibility, and salient pathogenetic mechanisms. It is therefore appropriate that the first series of papers give an overview of the transmissible spongiform encephalopathies and their infectious agents. In these papers detailed descriptions of the naturally-occurring diseases (familial and sporadic) are amplified by descriptions of experimental models, including transgenic mouse models. The latter indicate the importance of mutations in the host PrP gene in genetic forms of transmissible encephalopathies. They also indicate the importance of the structure of PrP in host response. These same experiments however raise the question of the significance of specific strains of the infectious agent. Transmissions to mice from natural scrapie and BSE suggests that strain variation exists and that interactions of different strains of agent with hosts of varying PrP genotype determine the outcome of transmission.

The second group of papers within the Bulletin is concerned with the nature of the prion protein. This sialoglycoprotein, the produce of a single host gene, is a normal constituent of the nervous system, as yet of unknown function. In this section, therefore, issues related to the genetics, synthesis, structure, processing and function of this protein are reviewed and compared with that of other amyloidogenic proteins.

Bovine spongiform encephalopathy (BSE), a form of spongiform encephalopathy, only recognised relatively recently, has both basic scientific and practical importance. The epidemiology of the condition is reviewed in detail and these studies indicate the importance of ruminant-derived feed in the form of meat and bone meal, in the present epidemic. They also indicate how the epidemic may be controlled by appropriate legislature and other measures.

This Bulletin aims to give detailed scientific reviews of the key issues in the field of spongiform encephalopathies, written by those actively involved in this research; as such it is of interest to all scientists and to those involved in medical and veterinary practice.

Ingrid V. Allen
September 1993

British Medical Bulletin (1993) Vol. 49, No. 4, 725–737
© The British Council 1993

Overview of the transmissible spongiform encephalopathies: Prion protein disorders

S J DeArmond
Department of Pathology (Neuropathology), University of California, San Francisco, USA

The subacute transmissible spongiform encephalopathies (TSE) are a complex group of neurodegenerative disorders which includes genetic, infectious and sporadic forms exemplified by scrapie in animals and Creutzfeldt-Jakob disease in humans. An extensive mass of data indicate that the infectious agents which transmit these diseases as well as the pathogenic mechanisms leading to clinical signs are related to abnormalities of a single cellular protein, designated the prion protein (PrP). The goals of this overview are to summarize the characteristics of TSEs and of their infectious agents and to indicate how the prion hypothesis is consistent with and provides an explanation for them. Transgenic mouse studies are emphasized which verify that genetic forms of TSEs are linked to mutations in the host PrP gene and that the host species barrier to scrapie infection, scrapie incubation time and the distribution of neuropathology, which define scrapie prion isolates ('strains'), are determined by the structure of PrP.

From today's perspective, the aetiology and pathogenesis of the transmissible spongiform encephalopathies (TSE), while uniquely complex among neurodegenerative disorders, appear to be related to abnormalities of a single cellular glycolipoprotein designated the prion protein (PrP).[1] Scepticism about the pre-eminent role of PrP was originally based on the absence of a precedent for a proteinaceous infectious agent, designated a 'prion' by Prusiner[2] to distinguish it from viruses and viroids, and because each publication leading to the prion protein hypothesis could be subjected to multiple interpretations. However, to-day our understanding of the TSEs is based on a large mass of varied and consistent data with no objective evidence for a viral aetiology. Recent studies with transgenic (Tg) mice expressing different forms of PrP have provided convincing corroborative evidence for the central role of PrP. These have verified that genetic forms of these diseases are related to mutations of the PrP gene; that the 'host species barrier' and different clinical-neuropathological subtypes of scrapie are determined by the structure of PrP; and that the parameters which define different scrapie prion isolates ('strains'), including scrapie incubation time and the distribution of vacuolation in the brain, can be manipulated by changing the amino acid sequence of the prion protein. The goal of this overview is to summarize the key features of the TSEs and how the prion hypothesis is consistent with them.

CHARACTERISTICS OF TSE SYNDROMES

Complexity of TSEs
The TSEs comprise a complex group of human and animal syndromes exemplified historically by scrapie in animals and kuru, Creutzfeldt-Jakob disease (CJD) and Gerstmann-Sträussler-Scheinker syndrome (GSS) in humans (Tables 1 and 2). Consequent to clinical experience and recent molecular genetic studies, we now recognize that this group of disorders comprise multiple clinical syndromes in both humans and animals which include sporadic, familial and infectious forms. Sporadic cases are defined by the failure to find either an infectious or genetic ae-tiology. These disorders share in common spongiform (vacuolar) degen-eration of neurons and variable amyloid plaque formation. However, the unique characteristic which distinguishes this group, whether sporadic, dominantly inherited or acquired by infection, is that all of them can be transmitted to experimental animals. Incubation times are typically prolonged ranging from months to years. The pattern of inheritance in cases of familial CJD and GSS argued for a single gene.

Host species barrier to scrapie
Several notable characteristics of scrapie were discovered largely by investigators in the United Kingdom. In a large scale unpublished study of scrapie transmission among sheep undertaken by WS Gordon[3] at the Moredun Institute beginning in 1939, it was found that 78% of Herd-wicks but 0% Dorset Downs developed disease following inoculation with scrapie from infected sheep. While the percent of sheep which developed scrapie was quite variable with an average of about 25%, 100% of goats developed disease after inoculation with sheep scrapie.[4]

Table 1 Human prion diseases

Etiologic categories	Traditional name*
Infectious prion diseases	Kuru
	Iatrogenic CJD
Inherited prion diseases	
Inherited Prion Disease (PrP leucine 102)	GSS[40–42]
Inherited Prion Disease (PrP valine 117)	GSS[44,45]
Inherited Prion Disease (PrP asparagine 178)	Familial CJD[58], FFI[56]
Inherited Prion Disease (PrP serine 198)	GSS-nft[52]
Inherited Prion Disease (PrP lysine 200)	Familial CJD[46–49]
Inherited Prion Disease (PrP arginine 217)	GSS-nft[53]
Inherited Prion Disease (PrP 96 bp insertion)	Familial CJD[50,51]
Inherited Prion Disease (PrP 120 bp insertion)	Familial CJD[50,51]
Inherited Prion Disease (PrP 144 bp insertion)	Familial CJD[50,51]
Inherited Prion Disease (PrP 168 bp insertion)	Familial CJD[50,51]
Inherited Prion Disease (PrP 192 bp insertion)	Familial CJD[50,51]
Inherited Prion Disease (PrP 216 bp insertion)	Familial CJD[50,51]
Sporadic prion disease	CJD

*Creutzfeldt-Jakob disease (CJD), Gerstmann-Straussler-Scheinker syndrome (GSS), GSS with neurofibrillary tangles (GSS-nft), fatal familial insomnia (FFI)

Table 2 Animal prion diseases

Infectious prion diseases
 Bovine spongiform encephalopathy
 Feline spongiform encephalopathy
 Transmissible mink encephalopathy
 Chronic wasting disease
 Exotic ungulate encephalopathy
 Experimental scrapie
Inherited prion disease
 Transgenic mice expressing GSSMoPrP102L[43]
 Natural scrapie?
Sporadic prion disease
 Natural scrapie?

This suggested that there is a genetically determined susceptibility to infectious scrapie. The failure to transmit scrapie to some animal strains was designated the 'host species barrier'.

Scrapie isolates ('strains')
Pattison and Millson[5] were the first to recognize that there are distinct clinical patterns of scrapie in goats. Moreover, they found that '. . . the type of clinical syndrome produced by experimental inoculation will resemble the syndrome exhibited by the animal from which the material for inoculation was obtained.' This was the first evidence that there are

different scrapie isolates and that each encodes different information. Subsequently, more than 15 scrapie isolates were identified in rodents[6] which could be distinguished by scrapie incubation time, the distribution and intensity of spongiform degeneration[7] and whether or not cerebral amyloid plaques formed.[8] These characteristics were preserved during multiple sequential passages of a given prion isolate within a single inbred mouse strain or hamster species but varied markedly or even failed to appear when transferred to a different animal species (host species barrier). Thus, the transmissible agent carries information which influences incubation time, distribution of neuropathology, amyloidogenesis and the host species barrier.

CJD isolates

CJD also consists of multiple clinical subtypes which correlate with different distributions of neuropathology. Transmission of CJD and kuru from many patients into a variety of subhuman primates, cats and rodents have shown that the host range, incubation time, duration of illness and type of clinical disease vary considerably among isolates.[9] Once a CJD isolate was transmitted to a rodent, such as an inbred hamster strain, other rodents strains which had previously been resistant to primary infection from a human CJD case could now be infected with the CJD isolate passaged in hamster.

The results of CJD and scrapie transmission studies indicate that the properties of the transmissible agents were modified by the animals through which they were successfully passaged. And, furthermore, the properties of the isolate remained constant as long as the isolate was passaged in the same animal strain.

Scrapie incubation time gene

From their classical genetic studies of scrapie, Dickinson and his colleagues proposed that a single host gene is the main determinant of susceptibility to scrapie infection.[10] Mouse strains with short and long scrapie incubation times were found. VM mice had a particularly prolonged incubation time of greater than 280 days following inoculation with the Me7 isolate whereas incubation times were shorter with other isolates, varying between 100 and 180 days. Incubation times in F2 and backcross populations argued for a single autosomal gene which was designated *sinc* (scrapie incubation).

These results plus others described above support the view that a single host gene plays an unusually important role in determining the properties of the transmissible agents of these diseases.

PROPERTIES OF THE SCRAPIE AND CJD AGENTS

The properties of the scrapie agent are atypical for a virus

In 1968, Alper[11] found that UV irradiation of the scrapie agent occurs at wavelengths below 240 nm where nucleic acids show a reduced level of inactivation whereas a broad spectrum of viruses, but not the scrapie agent, are inactivated at wavelengths greater than 250 nm, with a peak of inactivation between 260 and 270 nm where nucleic acids absorb energy. This argued that the scrapie agent was not a virus. In a review of the physical and chemical characteristics of the scrapie agent, Millson et al.[12] outlined results from several laboratories which indicated that infectivity was selectively decreased by treatment with proteases but not with nucleases, carbohydrases or lipases which also argued against a virus and that a protein is critical for infectivity; however, it could not be ruled out that the effects of enzymes were attenuated by crude preparations of the scrapie agent.

PURIFICATION OF THE SCRAPIE AGENT: THE PRION HYPOTHESIS

By the end of the 1970s, the main characteristics of the transmissible spongiform encephalopathies had been determined. It was clear that hypotheses about the transmissible agents of these disorders would have to account for infectious, genetic and sporadic forms of the diseases; that the properties of the infectious agent are influenced significantly by the host; and that the agent has unusual properties.

Purification of the scrapie agent: The discovery of PrPSc

Stanley Prusiner's laboratory achieved a 100-fold purification of the scrapie agent from Syrian hamster brains and for the first time showed that infectivity of the agent depended upon protein.[13] To obtain enriched fractions, crude homogenates were subjected to prolonged centrifugation to sediment the scrapie agent in microsomal membrane fractions followed by limited proteolysis with proteinase K and micrococcal nuclease and then by preparative agarose gel electrophoresis to obtain select populations of proteins. Scrapie infectivity titre in enriched protein fractions, but not the crude preparations, was attenuated by prolonged treatment with proteinases but unaffected by nucleases or UV irradiation, eliminating many of the concerns about the ineffectiveness of inactivation procedures with crude tissue homogenates. A search for proteins which resisted limited proteolysis and were unique to fractions enriched in the scrapie agent was begun using a new purification protocol which yielded a 3000-fold enrichment of the scrapie agent with respect to protein. This led to the discovery of a 27 000 to 30 000 molecular weight protein which was found in all purified scrapie fractions

but not in control preparations.[14] Scrapie infectivity in these preparations was also resistant to physical and chemical treatments which
denature nucleic acids but not to treatments which denatured protein.
For these reasons, Prusiner proposed the term 'prion', meaning proteinaceous infectious agent, to distinguish the scrapie agent from viruses
and viroids; the 27–30 kD protein was designated the prion protein (PrP
27–30).[2] Very rapidly, a partial sequence of PrP 27–30 was determined
in Leroy Hood's laboratory, a synthetic oligonucleotide probe was made
in Charles Weissmann's laboratory, and a cDNA library derived from
scrapie infected Syrian hamster brain was screened.[15] This led to the
discovery that PrP 27–30 is the proteinase K digestion product of a
larger 33–35 kD protein found in scrapie-infected brain, designated
PrP^{Sc} and that there is a normal, constituitivley expressed and protease
K sensitive cellular form of PrP, designated PrP^{C}. Both PrP^{Sc} and PrP^{C}
are synthesized by a single copy cellular gene in which the entire open
reading frame is in a single exon.[16] They are distinguished by their
physical properties. PrP^{C} is completely digested by limited hydrolysis
with proteinase K whereas it only removes the N-terminal 67 amino
acid residues from PrP^{Sc} to yield PrP 27–30 without loss of infectivity.
PrP 27–30 forms into rod-like particles in vitro whereas PrP^{C} does
not.[17] These rods resemble the structures purified from amyloids and,
like them, bind Congo red dye which displays green birefringence in
polarized light. Immunogold studies using prion protein specific antibodies indicate that the rods are composed of PrP 27–30.[18] Antibodies
made to PrP 27–30 revealed that the amyloid plaques which develop
in scrapie-infected brains also contain protease resistant PrP[19, 20] as do
the amyloid plaques in cases of CJD, GSS and kuru.[21–24]

In 1981, Wisniewski and Iqbal's laboratories reported that abnormal fibrillary particles, designated 'scrapie associated fibrils' (SAF),
are found in subfractions from multiple host animal strains infected
with different scrapie isolates regardless of whether amyloid plaques
were formed in the brain.[25] While this was a potentially important and
relevant finding, SAFs were never completely characterized including
the failure to demonstrate binding of Congo red dye and the failure to
specify their composition.

Purified scrapie prion preparations do not contain viral nucleic acid
The hypothesis that the scrapie agent is not a virus is supported by
sensitive physico-chemical methods to detect nucleic acids in highly
purified prion preparations.[26,27] These studies have failed to reveal a
viral-like polynucleotide; however, heterogeneous populations of small
nucleic acid fragments of less than 100 nucleotides in length were
found. Whether these nucleic acids are contaminants or are essential

for infectivity remains uncertain. It has been proposed that an accessory cellular RNA designated a 'co-prion' can modify the properties of PrP^{Sc} to account for the different clinical-neuropathological characteristics which distinguish different prion isolates.[28] While the co-prion hypothesis presents an intriguing mechanism to explain multiple distinct prion isolates, the failure to modify scrapie agent behavior by chemical or physical methods which denature nucleic acids argues against it.

The alternative hypothesis is that prions are devoid of functional nucleic acids and that prion replication and the specific clinical-neuropathological characteristics of different prion isolates are determined solely by PrP^{Sc}. The challenge of this hypothesis is to explain how PrP^{Sc} can exist in multiple, stable configurations since multiple prion isolates can be prepared from a single host animal. Furthermore, it assumes that structural information in PrP^{Sc} of the infecting prion can be transferred to PrP^{C}. There is considerable evidence that the synthesis of nascent PrP^{Sc} by a host animal involves post-translational conversion of pre-existing PrP^{C}.[29–31] It is believed that PrP^{Sc} in the infecting prion as well as nascent PrP^{Sc} form a transient complex with PrP^{C} molecules and that this interaction initiates the conversion of PrP^{C} to PrP^{Sc}.

Two recent studies with transgenic (Tg) mice support the hypothesis that PrP^{Sc} is the sole component of the scrapie prion by suggesting a plausible mechanism for the origin of prion diversity and for the differential selective vulnerability of neurons which must underlie the multiple clinical-neuropathological scrapie syndromes caused by different prion isolates.

Selective targeting of neurons by prion isolates
The patterns of PrP^{Sc} accumulation in the brain are unique for and determined by the scrapie prion isolate and are not a function of incubation time.[32–34] Thus, in Tg(SHaPrP)-7 mice which express high levels of Syrian hamster PrP^{C},[35–36] scrapie incubation times with the Sc237 and 139H prion isolates were similar, about 50 days; however, with the Sc237 isolate, PrP^{Sc} accumulation was largely confined to selected nuclei in the thalamus, septum and brainstem whereas it was widely distributed throughout the CNS with 139H.[34] When the Me7H prion isolate was inoculated into Tg(SHaPrP)-7 mice, PrP^{Sc} deposition was even more restricted than with Sc237 since the thalamus showed no accumulation while the densest accumulations occurred in the hypothalamus, zona incerta, nucleus accumbens septi and periaqueductal grey of the midbrain.[33] Scrapie incubation time with the Me7H isolate in these mice was about 185 days and, therefore, the highly restricted distribution of PrP^{Sc} could not be attributed to insufficient time for prions to spread in the CNS.

Prion isolates bind to homologous PrP^C molecules
Tg mouse studies have suggested a potential mechanism for the differential targeting of neuron populations. In Tg mice expressing both SHaPrP^C and mouse (Mo) PrP^C, it was found that hamster adapted Sc237 prion selectively interacted with homologous SHaPrP^C to form nascent SHaPrP^Sc and new Sc237 prions and that mouse adapted RML prions interacted exclusively with MoPrP^C.[35] The distribution and type of neuropathological changes caused by Sc237 prions were virtually identical to those caused by this isolate in the Syrian hamster including the development of amyloid plaques containing SHaPrP^Sc. No plaques formed with RML and the distribution of vacuolation in both grey and white matter was identical to that caused by RML in the non-Tg parent mouse strain. Because the non-Tg parent mouse strain is resistant to the Sc237 prion isolate, production of scrapie in Tg(SHaPrP) mice with Sc237 prions indicated that the host species barrier was breached and that the host animal barrier is determined by the structure of PrP^C.[36]

Prion isolates are determined by neurons
Finding that prion isolates target homologous forms of PrP^C and that they target selected populations of neurons raises a new testable hypotheses about the origin of prion isolate diversity. Specifically, the possibility is raised that each subset of neurons as well as other cell types synthesize a different isoform of PrP^C, each with the same amino acid sequence but with different secondary structures. Prion stimulated conversion of PrP^C into nascent PrP^Sc would occur only in those neurons which synthesize an isoform of PrP^C compatible with the PrP^Sc of the infecting prion.

These data and this hypothesis link the origin of different prion isolates with mechanisms underlying different clinical-neuropathological syndromes of scrapie. With regard to the latter, there are now multiple reasons to believe that local accumulation of PrP^Sc in the brain is pathogenic. Spongiform degeneration and reactive astrocytic gliosis follow the accumulation of PrP^Sc in each brain region.[37] Spongiform degeneration and reactive astrocytic gliosis colocalize precisely with the distribution of PrP^Sc.[20,32–34] Moreover, the rate and pattern of PrP^Sc accumulation, and therefore, the rate and pattern of formation of neuropathology, has also been found to correlate with scrapie incubation time.[34] Direct evidence for a cause-effect relationship comes from transgenic mouse studies described above which indicate that the pattern of neuropathology and whether amyloid plaques form are dependent on the amino acid structure of PrP^C. However, the strongest supporting evidence comes from molecular genetic studies which link familial prion disorders to mutations in the human prion protein (PRNP) gene.

Familial CJD and GSS are linked to mutations in the PRNP gene
Until recently, only two forms of inherited human prion diseases were recognized, familial CJD[38] and GSS.[39] However, recent molecular genetic studies indicate that multiple PRNP gene mutations and multiple clinical characteristics comprise cases classified as CJD and GSS by neuropathological criteria.[1] GSS cases in which ataxia predominates have been genetically linked to a mutation in PRNP codon 102 which leads to a proline to leucine substitution.[40–42] The cause-effect relationship between the codon 102 mutation and prion disease was verified in Tg mice expressing a mouse PrP transgene mimicking the human codon 102 mutation, Tg(GSSMoPrP102L) mice.[43] The founder and its offspring expressing the transgene developed a spontaneous neurodegenerative disorder with the neuropathological features of scrapie. The primarily dementing form of GSS has been linked to a PRNP gene codon 117 mutation.[44–45] A PRNP gene codon 200 mutation has been identified in some familial CJD pedigrees including familial CJD among Libyan Jews[46–49] while octapeptide-repeat insertions at codon 53 have been identified in others.[50,51] In addition, molecular genetics has led to the discovery of new prion disorders. PRNP gene codon 198 and 217 mutations[52,53] have been found in a unique form of GSS in which Alzheimer's disease-like neuropathological changes, including neuritic plaques and neurofibrillary tangles, are associated with deposition of PrP amyloid and not the βA4 peptide.[54,55] A codon 178 mutation[56] has been found in families with fatal familial insomnia (FFI), a unique disorder in which nerve cell loss is highly localized to the mediodorsal and anterior ventral nuclei of the thalamus.[57] The codon 178 mutation has also been described in some familial CJD pedigrees.[58] Whether GSS with neurofibrillary tangles and FFI are transmissible, that is form prions, is not known.

The scrapie incubation time gene and the PrP gene are tightly linked
Classical genetic studies of the short incubation time allele in NZW mice and long incubation time allele in I/LnJ mice of the scrapie incubation time gene coupled with restriction fragment polymorphism analysis which distinguished the NZW and I/LnJ open reading frames of their PrP genes showed that the scrapie incubation time gene and the PrP gene are so tightly linked that appear to be one and the same.[59] Thus both inherited and infectious forms of prion disease are linked to the prion protein gene.

The PrP null mouse

The final argument for the primacy of PrP in the aetiology and pathogenesis of scrapie comes from mice in which the PrP gene has been deleted.[60] These animals live into adulthood without obvious anatomical or behavioral abnormalities. Furthermore, they have been disease free for more than 300 days following inoculation with a variety of scrapie prion isolates (Prusiner & Weissmann, personal communication).

THE TRANSMISSIBLE SPONGIFORM ENCEPHALOPATHIES ARE PRION PROTEIN DISORDERS

Although the diseases comprising the TSEs were originally grouped together because of similar clinical-neuropathological features, including cerebral amyloidosis, and because of transmissibility, the more fundamental unifying characteristic now appears to be the presence of abnormal prion protein. Today, abnormal PrP appears to include both protease resistant and mutated isoforms. Mutated PrP in some genetic prion syndromes may not be protease resistant based on the experience with Tg(GSSMoPrP102L) mice.[43] Indeed, protease resistance may not be the most important pathogenic determinant. With infectious forms of prion disease, the most fundamental interaction appears to be that between PrP^{Sc} of the infecting prion and PrP^{C} synthesized by the host. That interaction triggers the conversion of PrP^{C} into nascent PrP^{Sc} which amplifies the conversion cycle. The host species barrier appears to represent an incompatibility of PrP^{Sc} of the prion with host PrP^{C}. The diversity of prion isolates and the diversity of clinical-neuropathological syndromes characteristic of human and animal prion diseases appear to be determined largely by the PrP gene and the structure of the prion protein. If indeed the prion protein hypothesis is true, as it seems to be, its present form predicts that sporadic CJD, which accounts for 85% or more of human prion diseases, may be the result of an age-related somatic mutation of the PRNP gene. This prediction is based on the facts that multiple PRNP mutations are pathogenic and that a single focus of abnormal PrP introduced into the body can trigger a cascade of pathogenic PrP formation.

Although the prion protein hypothesis is compatible with all of the main characteristics of TSEs, multiple new questions and issues have arisen because of it such as, the chemical and/or structural differences between PrP^{C} and PrP^{Sc}, whether PrP^{C}-PrP^{Sc} dimer formation is the first step in the conversion of PrP^{C}, the structure and composition of the smallest prion particle, the mechanisms by which PrP^{Sc} and mutated forms of PrP cause clinically relevant pathology, the nature of the neuronal dysfunction which causes clinical signs and spongiform degeneration, whether each neuron population synthesizes a different PrP^C isoform, and whether or not all abnormal forms of PrP are associated with infection. The prion hypothesis and the data which support it have revolutionized our understanding of the TSEs and have introduced a new disease mechanism. The validity of the hypothesis will in part reside in resolving these new issues.

ACKNOWLEDGEMENTS

This work was supported by research grants from the National Institutes of Health (AG02132, AG08967, NS14069), the American Health Assistance Foundation, as well as by gifts from the Sherman Fairchild Foundation and National Medical Enterprises.

REFERENCES

1 Prusiner SB. Molecular biology of prion diseases. Science 1991; 252: 1515-1522.
2 Prusiner SB. Novel proteinaceous infectious particles cause scrapie. Science 1982; 216: 136-144.
3 Pattison IH. A sideways look at the scrapie saga: 1732-1991. In: Prusiner SB, Collinge J, Powell J, Anderton B, eds. Prions diseases of humans and animals. London: Ellis Horwood, 1992: pp 15-22.
4 Pattison IH, Gordon WS, Millson GC. Experimental production of scrapie in goats. J Comp Pathol Ther 1959; 69: 300-312.
5 Pattison IH, Millson GC. Scrapie produced experimentally in goats with special reference to the clinical syndrome. J Comp Path 1961; 7: 101-110.
6 Bruce ME, Fraser H. Scrapie strain variation and its implications. Curr Top Microbiol Immunol 1991; 172: 125-138.
7 Fraser H, Dickinson AG. Scrapie in mice. Agent-strain differences in the distribution and intensity of grey matter vacuolation. J Comp Pathol 1973; 83: 29-40.
8 Bruce ME, Dickinson AG, Fraser H. Cerebral amyloidosis in scrapie in mouse: effect of agent strain and mouse genotype. Neuropathol Appl Neurobiol 1976; 2: 471-478.
9 Gibbs CJ Jr, Gajdusek DC, Amyx H. Strain variation in the viruses of Creutzfeldt-Jakob disease and kuru. In: Prusiner SB, Hadlow WJ, eds. Slow transmissible diseases of the nervous system, Volume 2. New York, NY: Academic Press, 1979: pp 87-110.
10 Dickinson AG, Meikle VMH. Host-genotype and agent effects in scrapie incubation: change in allelic interaction with different strains of agent. Mol Gen Genet 1971; 112: 73-79.
11 Alper T, Cramp W A, Clarke MC. Does the agent of scrapie replicate without nucleic acid? Nature 1967; 214: 764-766.
12 Millson GC, Hunter GD, Kimberlin RH. The physico-chemical nature of the scrapie agent. In: Kimberlin RH, ed. Slow virus diseases of animals and man. Amsterdam: North-Holland, 1976: pp 243-266.
13 Prusiner SB, McKinley MP, Groth DF, et al. Scrapie agent contains a hydrophobic protein. Proc Natl Acad Sci USA 1981; 78: 6675-6679.
14 Prusiner SB, Bolton DC, Groth DF, Bowman KA, Cochran SP, McKinley MP. Further purification and characterization of scrapie prions. Biochemistry 1982; 21: 6942-6950.
15 Oesch B, Westaway D, Wälchli M, et al. A cellular gene encodes scrapie PrP 27-30 protein. Cell 1985; 40: 735-746.
16 Basler K, Oesch B, Scott M, et al. Scrapie and cellular PrP isoforms are encoded by the same chromosomal gene. Cell 1986; 46: 417-428.
17 Prusiner SB, McKinley MP, Bowman KA, et al. Scrapie prions aggregate to form amyloid-like birefringent rods. Cell 1983; 35: 349-358.

18 DeArmond SJ, McKinley MP, Barry RA, Braunfeld MB, McCulloch JR, Prusiner SB. Identification of prion amyloid filaments in scrapie-infected brain. Cell 1985; 41: 221-235.
19 Bendheim PE, Barry RA, DeArmond SJ, Stites DP, Prusiner SB. Antibodies to a scrapie prion protein. Nature 1984; 310: 418-421.
20 DeArmond SJ, Mobley WC, DeMott DL, Barry RA, Beckstead JH, Prusiner SB. Changes in the localization of brain prion proteins during scrapie infection. Neurology 1987; 37: 1271-1280.
21 Prusiner SB, DeArmond SJ. Prions causing nervous system degeneration. Lab Invest 1987; 56: 349-363.
22 Kitamoto T, Tateishi J, Tashima T, et al. Amyloid plaques in Creutzfeldt-Jakob disease stain with prion protein antibodies. Ann Neurol 1986; 20: 204-208.
23 Roberts GW, Lofthouse R, Allsop D, et al. CNS amyloid proteins in neurodegenerative diseases. Neurology 1988; 38: 1534-1540.
24 Snow AD, Kisilevsky R, Wilmer J, Prusiner SB, DeArmond SJ. Sulfated glycosaminoglycans in amyloid plaques of prion diseases. Acta Neuropathol (Berlin) 1989; 77: 337-342.
25 Merz PA, Somerville RA, Wisniewski HM, Iqbal K. Abnormal fibrils from scrapie-infected brain. Acta Neuropathol (Berlin) 1981; 54: 61-74.
26 Kellings K, Meyer N, Mirenda C, Prusiner SB, Riesner D. Further analysis of nucleic acids in purified scrapie prion preparations by improved return refocussing gel electrophoresis (RRGE). J Gen Virol 1992; 73: 1025-1029.
27 Meyer N, Rosenbaum V, Schmidt B, Gilles K, Mirenda C, Groth D, Prusiner SB, Riesner D. Search for a putative scrapie genome in purified prion fractions reveals a paucity of nucleic acids. J Gen Virol 1991; 72: 37-49.
28 Weissmann C. A 'unified theory' of prion propagation. Nature 1991; 352: 679-683.
29 Borchelt DR, Scott M, Taraboulos A, Stahl N, Prusiner SB. Scrapie and cellular prion proteins differ in their kinetics of synthesis and topology in cultured cells. J Cell Biol 1990; 110: 743-752
30 Borchelt DR, Taraboulos A, Prusiner SB. Evidence for synthesis of scrapie prion proteins in the endocytic pathway. J Biol Chem 1992; 267: 6188-6199.
31 Caughey B, Raymond GJ. The scrapie-associated form of PrP is made from a cell surface precursor that is both protease- and phospholipase-sensitive. J Biol Chem 1991; 266: 18217-18223.
32 Bruce ME, McBride PA, Farquhar CF. Precise targeting of the pathology of the sialoglycoprotein, PrP, and vacuolar degeneration in mouse scrapie. Neurosci Lett 1989; 102: 1-6.
33 DeArmond SJ, Yang S-L, Lee A, Bowler R, Taraboulos A, Groth D, Prusiner SB. Three distinct scrapie prion isolates exhibit different patterns of PrP^{Sc} accumulation. Proc Natl Acad Sci USA (in press).
34 Hecker R, Taraboulos A, Scott M, et al. Replication of distinct prion isolates is region specific in brains of transgenic mice and hamsters. Genes Dev 1992; 6: 1213-1228.
35 Prusiner SB, Scott M, Foster D, et al. Transgenic studies implicate interactions between homologous PrP isoforms in scrapie prion replication. Cell 1990; 63: 673-686.
36 Scott M, Foster D, Mirenda C, et al. Transgenic mice expressing hamster prion protein produce species-specific scrapie infectivity and amyloid plaques. Cell 1989; 59: 847-857.
37 Jendroska K, Heinzel FP, Torchia M, et al. Proteinase-resistant prion protein accumulation in Syrian hamster brain correlates with regional pathology and scrapie infectivity. Neurology 1991; 41: 1482-1490.
38 Masters CL, Gajdusek DC, Gibbs CJ Jr. The familial occurrence of Creutzfeldt-Jakob disease and Alzheimer's disease. Brain 1981; 104: 535-558.
39 Masters CL, Gajdusek DC, Gibbs CJ Jr. Creutzfeldt-Jakob disease virus isolations from the Gerstmann-Sträussler syndrome with an analysis of the various forms of amyloid plaque deposition in the virus-induced spongiform encephalopathies. Brain 1981; 104: 559-588.

40 Hsiao K, Baker HF, Crow TJ, et al. Linkage of a prion protein missense variant to Gerstmann-Sträussler syndrome. Nature 1989; 338: 342-345.

41 Hsiao KK, Doh-ura K, Kitamoto T, Tateishi J, Prusiner SB. A prion protein amino acid substitution in ataxic Gerstmann-Sträussler syndrome. Ann Neurol 1989; 26: 137.

42 Kretzschmar HA, Kufer P, Riethmuller G, DeArmond SJ, Prusiner SB, Schiffer D. Prion protein mutation at codon 102 in an Italian family with Gerstmann-Sträussler-Scheinker syndrome. Neurology 1991; 42: 809-810.

43 Hsiao KK, Scott M, Foster D, Groth DF, DeArmond SJ, Prusiner SB. Spontaneous neurodegeneration in transgenic mice with mutant prion protein of Gerstmann-Sträussler syndrome. Science 1990; 250: 1587-1590.

44 Doh-ura K, Tateishi J, Sasaki H, Kitamoto T, Sakaki Y. Pro-Leu change at position 102 of prion protein is the most common but not the sole mutation related to Gerstmann-Sträussler syndrome. Biochem Biophys Res Commun 1989; 163: 974-979.

45 Hsiao KK, Cass C, Schellenberg GD, Bird T, Devine-Gage E, Prusiner SB. A prion protein variant in a family with the telencephalic form of Gerstmann-Sträussler-Scheinker syndrome. Neurology 1991; 41: 681-684.

46 Goldfarb L, Korczyn A, Brown P, Chapman J, Gajdusek DC. Mutation in codon 200 of scrapie amyloid precursor gene linked to Creutzfeldt-Jakob disease in Sephardic Jews of Libyan and non-Libyan origin. Lancet 1990; 336: 637-638.

47 Goldfarb LG, Mitrova E, Brown P, Toh BH, Gajdusek DC. Mutation in codon 200 of scrapie amyloid protein gene in two clusters of Creutzfeldt-Jakob disease in Slovakia. Lancet 1990; 336: 514-515.

48 Goldfarb LG, Brown P, Mitrova E, et al. Creutzfeldt-Jacob disease associated with the PRNP codon 200Lys mutation: an analysis of 45 families. Eur J Epidemiol 1991; 7: 477-486.

49 Hsiao K, Meiner Z, Kahana E, et al. Mutation of the prion protein in Libyan Jews with Creutzfeldt-Jakob disease. N Engl J Med 1991; 324: 1091-1097.

50 Goldfarb LG, Brown P, McCombie WR, et al. Transmissible familial Creutzfeldt-Jakob disease associated with five, seven, and eight extra ocatapeptide coding repeats in the PRNP gene. Proc Natl Acad Sci (USA) 1991; 88: 10926-10930.

51 Owen F, Poulter M, Collinge J, et al. Insertions in the prion protein gene in atypical dementias. Exp Neurol 1991; 112: 240-242.

52 Dlouhy SR, Hsiao K, Farlow MR, et al. Linkage of the Indiana kindred of Gerstmann-Sträussler-Scheinker disease with neurofibrillary tangles. Nature Genetics 1992; 1: 68-71.

53 Hsiao K, Dloughy S, Ghetti B, et al. Mutant prion proteins in Gerstmann-Sträussler-Scheinker disease with neurofibrillary tangles. Nature Genet 1992; 1: 68-71.

54 Ghetti B, Tagliavini F, Masters CL, et al. Gerstmann-Sträussler-Scheinker syndrome. II. Neurofibrillary tangles and plaques with PrP-amyloid coexist in an affected family. Neurology 1989; 39: 1453-1461.

55 Tagialvini F, Prelli F, Ghisto J, et al. Amyloid protein of Gerstmann-Sträussler-Scheinker disease (Indiana kindred) is an 11-kd fragment of prion protein with an N-terminal glycine at codon 58. EMBO J 1991; 10: 513-519.

56 Medori R, Tritschler H-J, LeBlanc A, et al. Fatal familial insomnia, a prion disease with a mutation at codon 178 of the prion protein gene. N Engl J Med 1992; 326: 444-449.

57 Manetto V, Medori R, Cortelli P, et al. Fatal familial insomnia: Clinical and pathological study of five new cases. Neurology 1992; 42: 312-319.

58 Brown P, Goldfarb LG, Kovanen J, et al. Phenotypic characteristics of familial Creutzfeldt-Jakob disease associated with the codon 178Asn PRNP mutation. Ann Neurol 1992; 31: 282-285.

59 Carlson GA, Kingsbury DT, Goodman PA, et al. Linkage of prion protein and scrapie incubation time genes. Cell 1986; 46: 503-511.

60 Büeler H, Fischer M, Lang Y, et al. The neuronal cell surface protein PrP is not essential for normal development and behavior in the mouse. Nature 1992; 356: 577-582.

British Medical Bulletin (1993) Vol. 49, No. 4, pp. 738–777
©The British Council 1993

Neuropathology of spongiform encephalopathies in humans

J E Bell
J W Ironside
Department of Pathology (Neuropathology), University of Edinburgh, UK

The historical aspects and classification of human spongiform encephalopathies are reviewed and the newer concept of 'prion dementias' is explored. Guidelines for safe laboratory and autopsy handling of spongiform encephalopathy tissues are outlined: this includes an update on strategies which are currently thought to be effective in decontamination. A wide ranging review of the pathology of the various human spongiform encephalopathies includes newly emerging data on microglia, and cell-specific and neurodegenerative proteins. A large section of this chapter is devoted to the methodology of immunocytochemical demonstration of PrP in tissue sections, and the dilemmas inherent in interpretation. Clinicopathological correlations are provided for classical cases of spongiform encephalopathy, together with the newly recognised atypical dementias associated with PrP gene mutations. The pathology of iatrogenic cases of CJD is described. The chapter concludes with problems in differential diagnosis, and discussion of the histopathological features which help to resolve diagnostic dilemmas.

HISTORICAL ASPECTS

The history of human spongiform encephalopathies began in 1920, when Creutzfeldt described a case of progressive fatal dementia in a 22-year-old female which was accompanied by multiple neurological abnormalities including spasticity and myoclonus.[1] In the following years, Jakob described 5 similar cases with progressive fatal dementia accompanied by evidence of extrapyramidal and pyramidal signs and symptoms.[2] Afterwards, there was considerable debate on the clinical and pathological features of Creutzfeldt-Jakob disease (CJD), leading to a proliferation of synonyms.[3,4] In 1960, the term 'subacute spongiform encephalopathy' was proposed, and more recently spongiform change in the central nervous system (CNS) has been accepted as the major pathological criterion for the diagnosis of Creutzfeldt-Jakob disease.[5,6,7] Subsequent review of the original cases reported in the 1920's indicates that Creutzfeldt's case does not fulfil the major histological criteria for the diagnosis of CJD.[3,7] However, at least 2 of Jakob's cases show convincing evidence of spongiform change in the CNS, and CJD has remained the generally accepted term for cases of sporadic spongiform encephalopathy in humans.

In 1936, Gerstmann, Sträussler and Scheinker described a familial disorder characterised clinically by cerebellar signs and symptoms accompanied by other abnormalities including pseudobulbar symptoms, speech difficulties and limb weakness.[8] The most striking histological abnormality in this disorder was the accumulation of amyloid plaques throughout the cerebrum and cerebellum, along with variable spongiform change. Several other families with a similar illness have been reported, and the disorder now bears the name of the authors of the original report, usually abbreviated to GSS disease. Subsequent studies on the pathology of this disorder revealed similarities to other human spongiform encephalopathies including kuru and CJD.[9,10,11] A variation in the histological features of this disease within various affected families has been reported, although amyloid plaque formation is the predominant feature in all cases.

In 1957, Gajdusek and Zigas described kuru, an unusual progressive neurological disorder in the Fore tribe in Papua New Guinea.[12] The name kuru means shivering or trembling, and the disease was characterised clinically by cerebellar ataxia and tremor progressing to death within one year from onset. Spongiform change and neuronal loss were evident on histology throughout the CNS and around 70% of cases contained amyloid plaques, particularly in the cerebellum.[5,13] The similarity of these histological appearances to those of scrapie, the transmissible spongiform encephalopathy in sheep, led to a successful attempt at transmission of the disease from human kuru brain to chimpanzees,[14] the recipient animals showing a similar range of histological abnormalities to those in humans. The recognised similarity in histopathology between kuru, CJD and GSS led to successful transmission experiments for CJD in 1968,[15] and GSS in 1981.[16] These experiments confirm the close relationship between CJD, kuru and GSS as transmissible neurodegenerative diseases characterised pathologically by spongiform change, neuronal loss, reactive gliosis and amyloid plaque formation. Even at this stage, it was recognised that a spectrum of histopathological changes occurred within each disease entity, and a wide range of sub-groups of CJD has been proposed, relating to both clinical and pathological features of the disease and including those cases with atypical features.[3,4,13] Since the first animal transmission experiments, cases of iatrogenic CJD following human-human transmission have been reported involving inadequately sterilised intracerebral electrodes, dura mater grafts, corneal grafts and inoculation of human pituitary-derived growth hormone and gonadotrophin.[17] In the latter category, multiple cases have been reported from across the world.[18]

CLASSIFICATION

The historical classification of human spongiform encephalopathies recognised three entities: CJD, kuru and GSS.[5,6] It was also recognised that CJD could occur as a familial disorder, and cases of accidental transmission of CJD to humans were subsequently recorded.[17] Since then, the enormous advances in our understanding of the protein chemistry and molecular biology of this group of diseases has added other potential criteria for the classification of human spongiform encephalopathies[10,19,20] (see Table 1). Although no consensus has yet been reached regarding the nature of the infectious agent in this group of disorders,[19,21] it seems that the abnormal isoform of the human prion protein (PrP) is associated with the infectious agent, and accumulates within the CNS in cases of human spongiform encephalopathy, most strikingly as a major constituent of the amyloid plaques.[22] The identification and sequencing of the human PrP gene on chromosome 20 has led to the identification of several genetic abnormalities occurring at this site in some human spongiform encephalopathies.[11,20] Abnormalities in the PrP gene have not been confined to classical cases of CJD, GSS or kuru, and cases of atypical dementia with PrP gene abnormalities have been reported in the apparent absence of spongiform change, amyloid plaque formation or any other characteristic histological feature of human spongiform encephalopathies.[23] Furthermore, PrP gene mutations have been identified in other rare inherited disorders, eg the fatal familial insomnia syndrome.[24,25] Many cases of sporadic CJD do not appear to be associated with PrP gene mutations.[26,27,28]

Several criteria have been proposed for the diagnosis of spongiform encephalopathies in humans; these are summarised in Table 1. To date, the main morphological criterion for diagnostic purposes is the pres-

Table 1 Diagnostic criteria for human spongiform encephalopathies

1	Clinical history
2	EEG abnormalities
3	Spongiform change
4	Transmissibility
5	PrP accumulation
6	SAF/PrP rods
7	PrP gene abnormalities

ence of spongiform change within the CNS,[3,6] to which may now be added the accumulation of PrP in the CNS either in the form of amyloid plaques, discrete areas of accumulation in the CNS particularly in relation to spongiform change, or intracellular accumulations[5] (vide infra). Although some authors lay great emphasis on the presence of spongiform change as a requirement for diagnosis, early observations on the pathology of GSS disease and kuru recognised that spongiform change was not an invariable histological feature of these disorders. Consequently, it is apparent that within each of the three historical entities – GSS, kuru and CJD – a spectrum of pathological abnormalities have been recognised, few (if any) of which are within themselves specific for human spongiform encephalopathies. Accordingly, most classifications are now concerned with clinical, pathological and molecular genetic abnormalities in these illnesses[29]; this has resulted in the coinage of terms for 'new' entities, eg prion dementia without characteristic pathology.[23] The relationship of such entities to the three historical categories of human disease still awaits clarification.

Table 2 Pathological classification of human spongiform encephalopathies

1	CJD sporadic
	familial
	iatrogenic
2	Kuru
3	GSS
4	Fatal familial insomnia
5	Atypical dementias requiring further investigation

A classification for human spongiform encephalopathies cannot therefore be based on pathological features alone, particularly as new clinical entities continue to be recognised. In current diagnostic neuropathological practice, it is convenient to retain the main historical categories for the classification of human spongiform encephalopathies, with appropriate modifications to accommodate recently-described entities (*see* Table 2). A fourth entity, fatal familial insomnia is now accepted as a category of human spongiform encephalopathy on grounds of clinical features, neuropathology and molecular genetic abnormalities.[24,25] To this may be added a final category of diseases whose relationship to other groups is uncertain, or requires further investigation. This includes prion dementias without characteristic pathology, and other atypical dementias which may exhibit some of the clinical or histological features of human spongiform encephalopathies.

LABORATORY AND AUTOPSY HANDLING OF HUMAN SPONGIFORM ENCEPHALOPATHIES

Safe handling of CJD tissues in the laboratory, and at autopsy, is influenced by several important factors including:

A. The disease is transmissible between humans and therefore represents a hazard to workers.[5,30]
B. All the evidence suggests that the infective agent is concentrated in nervous tissues, cerebrospinal fluid and lymphoid tissues.[31–34]
C. The agent is resistant to the usual cleansing and disinfecting agents.[35–38]
D. The agent is remarkably persistent in the environment.[39]

For these reasons, exposure to CJD infective tissue should be minimised to a level consistent with confirming the diagnosis.[31] During life, no hazard is entailed in routine clinical care of the patient or in analysis of samples outwith the CNS or lymphoid systems. Blood from CJD patients is not thought to represent a hazard.[40] There is no place for attempting to confirm a diagnosis of CJD by cerebral biopsy since this may well be negative if the focal lesions of CJD are not sampled, and also raises the problem of having to dispose of neurosurgical instruments unless CJD can be excluded.[41] Little is known of possible infectivity during the 'incubation' period for the disease, which may pose a problem if neurosurgical procedures are undertaken in a patient who is diagnosed subsequently as having CJD.

Much of the information regarding decontamination of spongiform tissues is derived from animal work but it is assumed that the sensitivities of the human agent are similar.[42] It is known that the infectivity of the agent is reduced but certainly not abolished by boiling water, formalin, alcohol, phenol, gluteraldehyde, hydrogen peroxide, ionising or UV radiation, or dry heat up to 360°C. Enzymes such as nucleases and proteases are also ineffective.[42] The agents which are thought to be effective include 96% formic acid, 2N sodium hydroxide, steam autoclaving at 134°C (18 min in porous load, 60 min in gravity displacement), sodium hypochlorite (20 000 ppm available chlorine) and incineration.[42,43]

Because recommended procedures for decontamination have varied in the past it is important to realise that prior fixation in formalin appears to preserve the agent's infectivity through subsequent autoclaving,[44] and that post-formalin autoclave cycles, or post-formalin exposure to phenol[43] does not decontaminate spongiform encephalopathy tissues.

The principles governing laboratory or necropsy procedure are firstly, to contain the infected tissue and secondly, to decontaminate any exposed surfaces or instruments, and the tissue itself. A summary of the appropriate decontamination and disposal protocols is listed in Table 3. So far as autopsy procedures are concerned, we have recently published guidelines which permit safe removal of the brain from human spongiform encephalopathy cases.[45] In the laboratory, the aim would be to use either a dedicated room, or more likely a limited area of laboratory where tissues could be examined on disposable, water resistant material and using disposable instruments. Immersion of formalin fixed spongiform tissues in 96% formic acid for 60 min reduces infectivity to undetectable levels so that subsequent handling during processing and more importantly, in section cutting, is without hazard.[43] Formic acid immersion has the added advantage that it enhances subsequent immunocytochemical techniques,[46] although sections of treated tissue tend to wash off more frequently than normal during staining procedures (vide infra). The guidelines listed in Table 3 represent a counsel of perfection and are appropriate to laboratories which handle considerable quantities of spongiform encephalopathy tissue. All neuropathology laboratories handle occasional cases of CJD including cases in which the diagnosis is made only at histological examination: it is unlikely that such an occasional contamination of the environment represents a significant hazard. When such a case is discovered, it may be possible to identify the equipment which was used and to employ decontamination or incineration procedures as appropriate. Similarly, although spongiform encephalopathy is not transmitted by inhalation, laboratory workers may feel more comfortable handling tissues within a class 1 cabinet.[36]

PATHOLOGY

Autopsy examination in human spongiform encephalopathy has demonstrated no specific abnormalities outwith the CNS at either macroscopic or microscopic examination.[5,6] General autopsy findings usually include cachexia with widespread muscle wasting, particularly in cases with a lengthy clinical history. As with other progressive neu-

Table 3 Decontamination and disposal procedures

A.	Formalin fixed tissues	Immersion in 96% formic acid for 60 min (unless tissue has previously been exposed to phenol which interacts deleteriously with formic acid)
B.	Disposable clothing, instruments etc	Double bag and incinerate as for clinical waste
C.	Disposable sharps	Collect in suitable container (eg sharpsafe) and incinerate
D.	Non-disposable metal instruments	Steam autoclave at: 134°C for 60 min (gravity displacement) or 134°C for 18 min (porous load)
E.	Glassware	Immerse for 60 min in hypochlorite: 20 000 ppm free chlorine (eg 7 Presept tabs in 500 ml water freshly made up)
F.	Work surfaces	Flood with 2N NaOH for 60 min (except on aluminium)
G.	Class 1 cabinets	Wash liberally with 2N NaOH for 60 min. Dispose of filters by incineration
H.	Laboratory chemicals (formalin, xylene, alcohol)	Absorb on sawdust in stout container, then incinerate
I.	Paraffin wax	Incinerate

rodegenerative disorders, bronchopneumonia and pulmonary embolism are common immediate causes of death. Recent reports of PrP accumulation in the lymphoreticular system in scrapie-infected animals[34] have not yet been matched by comparable investigations in humans. On routine microscopy, the reticuloendothelial system in most cases of human spongiform encephalopathy appears unremarkable, as does the peripheral nervous system.

CJD

Macroscopic examination of the brain in CJD may reveal no significant abnormality, particularly in cases with a relatively short clinical history.[6,13] In most cases, however, there is evidence of cortical atrophy on external inspection which may be global (Fig. 1) or focal, with selective involvement of the frontal, temporal or occipital lobes. In extreme cases, the brain weight is substantially reduced to below 1000g, and in such cases the deep grey matter structures appear atrophied. No consistent pattern of atrophy in the basal ganglia, thalamus

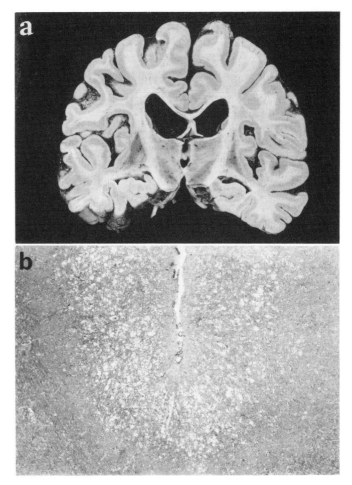

Fig. 1 (a) The cerebrum in CJD often shows mild non-specific cortical atrophy with accompanying ventricular dilatation, as in this case. The deep grey matter structures appear unremarkable. (b) Low-power histology of the superior temporal gyrus shows vacuolation affecting the full thickness of the cortical ribbon. The underlying white matter is spared. H&E x 40.

or hypothalamus has been reported in relation to cortical atrophy. In extreme cases, inspection of the cut surfaces of the cerebrum may suggest a resemblance to Pick's disease, particularly if focal cortical atrophy is accompanied by basal ganglia atrophy. However, no unique pattern of macroscopic abnormalities in the cerebrum has been recorded for

CJD.[5,6,13] Cerebellar atrophy is not an uncommon finding, particularly in the region of the superior vermis; in iatrogenic CJD following growth hormone inoculation, cerebellar atrophy may be the single most striking macroscopic abnormality.[47,48] Predominant cerebellar involvement has also been recorded in the ataxic variant of sporadic CJD.[49,50] Macroscopic examination of the brainstem and spinal cord in CJD usually shows no significant abnormality.

The characteristic histological findings in CJD comprise spongiform change, neuronal loss, astrocytosis and amyloid plaque formation in the grey matter.[5,6] As might be anticipated in relation to the range of macroscopic pathology, these histological abnormalities are not consistently present throughout the CNS and vary enormously from case to case (Figs 1 and 7). The most characteristic abnormality is spongiform change (Fig. 2) which consists of a fine vacuolation of the neuropil of the grey matter which is often unrelated to neurones and glial cells.[4] The vacuoles vary in size from around 2–20μm, the larger spaces appearing to become confluent to form larger cystic cavities.[6,13] Neuronal vacuolation may also occur, occasionally with marked distortion of the cellular architecture. Extensive neuropil cavitation, usually accompanied by neuronal loss, is a characteristic feature of status spongiosus (Fig. 2) where the collapse of the cortical cytoarchitecture resembles that seen in the end stages of other severe neurodegenerative disorders, particularly Alzheimer's disease.

As with spongiform change, neuronal loss is variable in distribution and severity from case to case. Neuronal loss tends to be most severe in cases with a prolonged clinical history,[13] where the cerebral cortex may be reduced in areas to a narrow band of gliotic tissue with few residual nerve cells (Fig. 2). Surviving cortical neurones may exhibit a range of structural abnormalities, with marked abnormalities in the dendritic pattern.[51] Other neuronal abnormalities have occasionally been described, including Hirano bodies and neurofibrillary tangles of the type usually found in Alzheimer's disease. Ballooned neurones are occasionally present in the cerebrum and cerebellum,[52] many of which give a strong staining reaction with antibodies to αB crystallin[53] (Fig. 3). Abnormal neuronal processes can be detected around PrP amyloid plaques in the cerebellum and cerebrum;[54] many of these neurones contain ubiquitinated proteins as revealed by immunocytochemistry. Ubiquitin immunocytochemistry has also demonstrated small intraneuronal inclusions,[55] similar to those seen in the murine experimental scrapie models.[56] In the areas of confluent spongiform change immunocytochemical studies have revealed granular deposition of ubiquitinated proteins and lysosomal enzymes, eg cathepsin D[55] (Fig. 4). These appear to

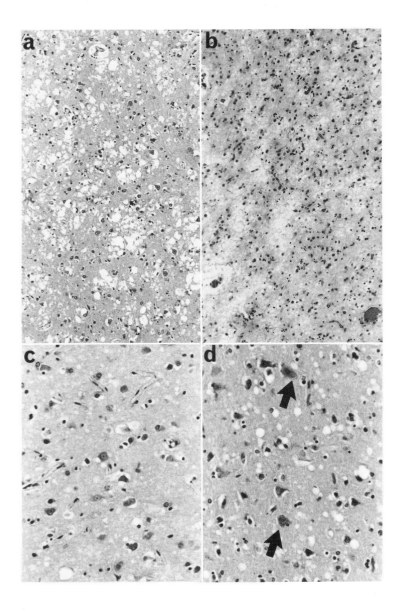

occur in relation to granular accumulations of PrP, suggesting lysosomal processing of this abnormal protein.[57]

Fig. 2 (a) In a typical case of CJD, spongiform change with fine background vacuolation in the neuropil is evident, with coalescence into larger vacuoles. Perineuronal vacuolation is also evident although neuronal loss is not a prominent feature. H&E x 100. **(b)** In status spongiosus, there is widespread neuronal loss and reactive gliosis, with rarefaction of the neuropil and coarse background vacuolation. Perineuronal vacuolation is not evident. H&E x 100. **(c)** Spongiform change can be a subtle feature which is easily overlooked in initial inspection. A patchy fine background vacuolation is evident in this case, with occasional perineuronal vacuolation. Nerve cell loss and reactive gliosis are not evident. H&E x 200. **(d)** Spongiform-like change can occur within the neuropil in diffuse Lewy body disease. In this disorder, affected neurons contain ill-defined cytoplasmic inclusions (arrows) and the neuropil may exhibit irregular vacuolation, which may undergo coalescence. H&E x 200.

Previous studies of CJD have emphasized the fine vacuolation characteristic of spongiform change in the neuropil.[4,7] However, the occurrence of neuronal and perineuronal vacuolation has not consistently been reported.[6] This form of vacuolation is not always evident, particularly on thick paraffin or celloidin sections, but thin paraffin sections are suitable for demonstrating the presence and distribution of this abnormality (Fig. 2). Neuronal vacuolation is characteristic of spongiform encephalopathies occurring in other species, particularly bovine spongiform encephalopathy,[58] where vacuolation in brainstem neurones is a consistent abnormality. Spongiform change has also been reported in the cerebral white matter, occasionally accompanied by ill-defined myelin loss and reactive gliosis.[6,13] These changes are usually most evident in the subcortical white matter, and are rarely seen in the white matter of the brainstem and spinal cord. Other white matter abnormalities occurring in CJD include amyloid plaques, usually accompanied by plaque formation in the cerebellum, cerebral cortex and other grey matter structures (Fig. 3). Reports from Japan have described necrotising lesions in the white matter in several patients with other characteristic features of CJD, including amyloid plaque formation.[6,59] This type of change appears to be exceptional in cases occurring in Western countries, but the detailed description in the Japanese cases suggests that this form of necrosis appears to be part of the disease process, and not related to any co-existing vascular pathology or any other pre-existing abnormality. The nature and evolution of these abnormalities as yet remain poorly understood. Reactive gliosis is often a prominent feature in CJD (Fig. 4), particularly in cases with extensive neuronal loss and established status spongiosus.[5,6] Previous authors have tended to dwell exclusively on reactive astrocytosis;[13] astrocytic hypertrophy and hyperplasia is usually most conspicuous in affected regions of the grey matter, where astrocytic processes may be seen to extend around spongiform vacuoles. Astrocytic processes are also seen in the peripheral region of PrP

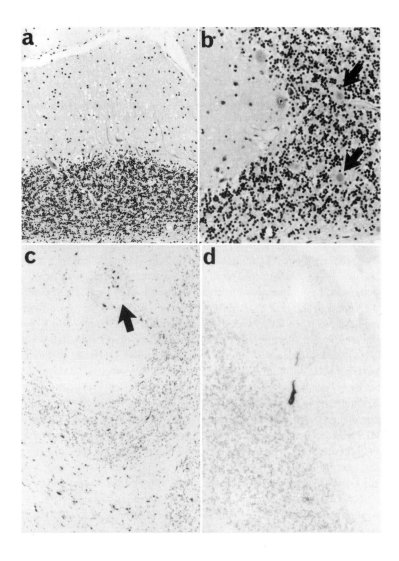

plaques in the cortex and in the white matter. Reactive astrocytosis is usually a less conspicuous feature in the white matter in CJD, but has been reported around areas of spongiform change and around necrotising lesions.[59] The nature and distribution of the astrocytic changes indicates that they are reactive phenomena; the question of PrP accu-

Fig. 3 (a) The cerebellum in CJD is frequently involved, although often in a patchy distribution. In this case, spongiform change in the molecular layer is accompanied by patchy neuronal loss involving Purkinje cells and reactive gliosis. H&E x 100. **(b)** Around 10% of sporadic CJD cases contain PrP amyloid plaques in the CNS. In this case, two 'kuru' plaques consist of a rounded eosinophilic core surrounded by a pale halo (arrows). H&E x 200. **(c)** Microglial cells expressing the CD68 epitope are present in increased numbers in human spongiform encephalopathy. In this case of GSS, increased numbers of microglia are present around cerebellar PrP plaques (arrow) and within the white matter. Immunoperoxidase using PGM1 antibody (Dako Ltd) x100. **(d)** Occasional ballooned nerve cells in CJD contain increased quantities of αB crystallin, as in this cerebellar Purkinje cell. The underlying basis for this reactive change is not yet fully understood. Immunoperoxidase x100. Antibody to αB crystallin kindly supplied by Prof. R J Mayer, Nottingham.

mulation in astrocytes as a possible primary abnormality is discussed below.

In addition to astrocytic reactions, microglial reactions have recently been recognised in CJD.[60] Although earlier reports indicate that microglial reactions were not a striking or common feature in this disease,[13] the relative ease with which microglial cells can now be recognised by immunocytochemistry[61] has allowed a fuller assessment of the role of this cell type in human and experimental spongiform encephalopathies. In CJD, widespread microglial hypertrophy and hyperplasia is noted, particularly in involved areas of grey matter where microglial cell processes may be seen extending around areas of spongiform change, in a similar manner to astrocytic processes. Microglial cells also participate in reactions at the periphery of PrP plaques, and are increased in number and size throughout the white matter in affected cases (Fig. 3). Microglial activation is demonstrable by up-regulation of MHC class II antigen and increased expression of lysosomal enzymes, eg cathepsin D.[60] The widespread microglial proliferation and activation occurring in CJD is not accompanied by a classical inflammatory reaction. Although previous descriptions of a chronic inflammatory reaction (predominantly lymphocytic) exist,[6] most reports now agree that no significant inflammatory reaction occurs in CJD, as with spongiform encephalopathies in other species.

Numerous ultrastructural abnormalities in CJD have been described, particularly in relation to the spongiform change, which has been attributed to a dilatation of membrane-bound structures in perikarya and dendritic synaptic processes (probably originating in the endoplasmic reticulum).[3,6] A variety of ultrastructural inclusions have been described in nerve cells in CJD,[62,63] some of which appear to have been artifacts, but recently attention has focused on tubulovesicular structures.[64] These structures are found in distended pre-and post-synaptic terminals, measuring approximately 35 mm in diameter and of greater electron density

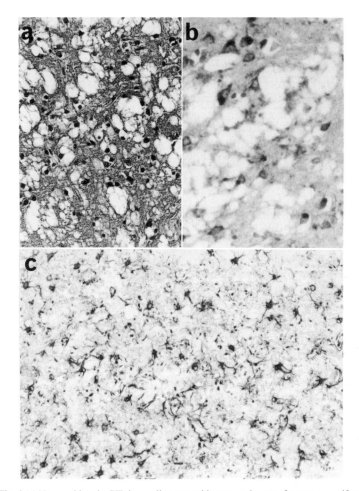

Fig. 4 (**a**) Neuronal loss in CJD is usually most evident around areas of severe spongiform change, accompanied by reactive gliosis which is not always conspicuous on routine stains. LFB/CV x 200. (**b**) The neuropil within and around areas of spongiform change in CJD contains increased quantities of the lysosomal enzyme cathepsin D, usually in a granular distribution. Surviving nerve cells also express this enzyme. Immunoperoxidase x 400. Antibody to cathepsin D kindly supplied by Dr W A Reid (Leeds). (**c**) Reactive astrocytosis in CJD is best demonstrated using immunocytochemistry for glial fibrillary acidic protein. Astrocytic hypertrophy and hyperplasia are evident, with elongated cell processes often extending around areas of spongiform change. Immunoperoxidase x 100 (Dako Ltd).

than synaptic vesicles. Similar structures have previously been reported in naturally-occurring animal spongiform encephalopathies and in the murine scrapie model. It has been suggested that their occurrence in all types of transmissible spongiform encephalopathies irrespective of the host and agent strain implies a fundamental biological significance.[64] The relationship of this structure to the agent responsible for this group of diseases is unclear, but it seems that these structures may serve as ultrastructural markers for this group of disorders.

Other structures reported to be involved in CJD include the retina and trigeminal ganglia,[6] both of which may exhibit neuronal cell loss, vacuolation and reactive gliosis. The distribution of PrP in these sites has not yet been thoroughly studied and the relationship of retinal abnormalities to other abnormalities in the optic nerve and more distal parts of the visual system is still unclear. The visual cortex in the occipital lobe is frequently affected by spongiform change in CJD, but as yet no evidence for selective visual pathway involvement has been demonstrated. The distribution of the CNS pathology of CJD in relation to clinical features is discussed below. In most cases of sporadic CJD previous studies have indicated that cerebral cortical involvement occurs in a variable distribution which is not always symmetrical.'[3,4,6] Any region of the cortex may be involved but hippocampal involvement is relatively rare, apart from the later stages in cases with a prolonged clinical course.[4] In the deep grey matter structures, the caudate nucleus and putamen are involved more often than the globus pallidus, and in the thalamus the dorsomedial nucleus is more severely affected than the anterior and ventrolateral nuclear groups.[4] Cerebellar cortical involvement is also common, but in an uneven distribution throughout the hemispheres (Fig. 3). The midbrain is involved more often than the other regions of the brainstem, which frequently exhibit no evidence of spongiform change, neuronal loss or gliosis. The spinal cord has not been studied extensively in CJD; experience in the Edinburgh CJD Surveillance Unit suggests that spongiform change is uncommon, although grey matter involvement can occur, particularly in the amyotrophic variant.

A detailed neuropathological examination of the brain in CJD may demonstrate other co-existing pathology, particularly in elderly patients who exhibit age-related changes involving nerve cell loss in the cerebral cortex and hippocampus accompanied by formation of neurofibrillary tangles and senile (Alzheimer-type) plaques. Although the degree and distribution of neuronal loss within the cortex is variable in relation to age, these background changes must be taken into consideration when assessing nerve cell loss attributable to CJD. Cerebrovascular disease is common in elderly individuals in Western countries and in most cases is clearly distinguishable from the pathology of CJD. Occasional patients have been reported to show features of both Alzheimer's disease and

CJD;[65] the precise classification of amyloid deposits by immunocytochemistry should enable a more detailed study of these fascinating cases, particularly in relation to plaque type and distribution.

CJD variants

Although in clinical terms a number of variants of sporadic CJD have been described, eg the ataxic variant and the amyotrophic variant,[3,6] the neuropathology of these conditions is generally characteristic, although the distribution of spongiform change may vary in a pattern corresponding to the predominant clinical manifestations. However, other varieties of CJD have demonstrated unusual neuropathology, particularly in familial cases. Even within families, the spectrum of neuropathology is variable with individual cases corresponding in neuropathological terms to GSS, while others show the characteristic features of CJD.[11] In some families molecular genetic studies have identified PrP gene abnormalities, but these do not in themselves correspond precisely with the clinical features or neuropathology in individual cases.[11,66,67] Other molecular genetic studies on sporadic CJD have suggested that a methionine to valine change at codon 129 is associated with a prolonged clinical course in which ataxia is a prominent early feature, with characteristic neuropathological findings, including unicentric PrP plaques.[68] Amyloid angiopathy has been reported in CJD but the vascular amyloid deposit stained positively with antibodies to the A4 protein, rather than PrP, suggesting a similarity to other forms of CNS congophilic angiopathy.[69]

The term 'prion dementia' has been used by some authors to replace spongiform encephalopathy, and to denote cases of dementia occurring in families with PrP gene mutations,[23,70] in which no characteristic spongiform change has been identified. Such cases require extensive neuropathological investigations in order to investigate the possibility of subtle or focal neuropathology, with PrP deposition investigated by a range of appropriate antibodies. The transmissibility of such cases is not proven; it has been recently concluded that cases of prion dementia without characteristic pathology are exceptional, apart from in a few well-documented families.[71]

The neuropathology of the recently described fatal familial insomnia includes spongiform change,[24,72] which in some affected family members was widespread, while in others it seemed to predominantly involve the dorsomedial nucleus of the thalamus, with evidence of neuronal loss and reactive gliosis elsewhere. This disorder appears to represent another instance where a PrP gene abnormality is accompanied by striking clinical features and neuropathology which, although characteristic of spongiform encephalopathy, is notable for its unusual distribution.[24,25]

Although most cases of iatrogenic CJD have characteristic neuropathology, recent observations on cases associated with pituitary-derived growth hormone inoculations have demonstrated unusual clinical and pathological features.[47,48] Cerebellar involvement is particularly striking, and in affected individuals there is a disproportionately severe loss of neurones in the cerebellar cortex, Purkinje cell layer and granular layer. This is accompanied by spongiform change, reactive gliosis and PrP plaque formation, with axonal loss in the cerebellar white matter and associated brainstem pathways. Spongiform change is not confined to the cerebellum in these cases, and cortical involvement can occur in a widespread distribution. Cerebral PrP plaque formation has been reported in one recent case, in which molecular genetic studies revealed valine homozygosity at codon 129 in the PrP gene.[73]

Kuru

In the earliest reports on the neuropathology of this now virtually extinct disorder the presence and distribution of spongiform change was not clearly recorded. Subsequent reviews have indicated that spongiform change is present in all cases involving the cerebral cortex and deep grey matter structures in addition to the cerebellum.[5,6,13] The spongiform change seen in this disorder is identical to that occurring in sporadic CJD. One of the most striking neuropathological features of kuru is the presence of amyloid plaques, which occurred in around 70% of all cases. These plaques were particularly conspicuous in the cerebellum, where a variety of plaque morphologies was described.[6,13] The significance of these morphological variations is now perhaps overshadowed by the recognition that these plaques are all composed of PrP. The characteristic kuru plaque comprised a homogeneous centre with a fibrillary structure radiating away from the centre, and surrounded by a pale peripheral region or halo. Transmission electronmicroscopy has confirmed the amyloid nature of these radiating fibrils, similar to those identified in PrP plaques in GSS and CJD.[3] It has been suggested that kuru plaques occurred most frequently in cases with a prolonged clinical history,[16] but no extensive molecular genetic studies have been performed to identify PrP gene mutations in this disorder.

GSS

In this disorder, PrP amyloid plaques are present throughout the cerebrum and cerebellum. Various plaque morphologies have been described in GSS and there is considerable overlap with the neuropathology of kuru and sporadic CJD.[9,16] Spongiform change has been described in some (but not all) cases, particularly in the cerebral cortex. In the Indiana GSS kindred, patients have a mutation at codon 198 of the PrP gene, and in the CNS neurofibrillary tangles and abnormal neuritic processes may be accompanied by deposition of the Alzheimer precursor A4 protein around PrP amyloid plaques.[74] Most cases of GSS are associated with a proline-leucine change at codon 102,[66] and in these cases neurofibrillary tangle formation is not usually evident. The neuropathology in the Indiana kindred is not unique and other cases of GSS with neurofibrillary tangles have been recently described.[75] Similar cases may in the past have been reported as familial Alzheimer's disease,[76,77] before PrP immunocytochemistry and molecular analysis of the PrP gene were available as investigative techniques.

PrP IMMUNOSTAINING

Current thinking suggests that a disorder of the normal cellular protein, PrP^C, is central to the aetiology and/or pathogenesis of the classical human spongiform encephalopathies.[78,79] It is known that in CJD and in GSS there is an accumulation of the disease-specific form of PrP (PrP^{CJD}).[80] Biochemical assay can identify those areas of the brain in which PrP^{CJD} is accumulating but does not identify the cellular components involved. This highlights the need for immunocytochemical studies which will localise PrP^{CJD} at the cellular level and which will reliably and consistently distinguish between PrP^C and PrP^{CJD}. Because of the close similarity between these two forms of the protein,[79] and despite the fact that the latter is protease resistant, it has not been possible thus far to develop antibodies which clearly distinguish between the two.[81] Therefore, on theoretical grounds, it is likely that immunocytochemical staining will localise both the normal and the abnormal form. Since the function of the normal form is not understood, there might be some interest and value in demonstrating PrP^C, but in a disease related study, it is PrP^{CJD} which is usually the focus of interest. Various factors might influence the critical distinction between the two forms in tissue sections.

1. PrP^C may be expressed transiently or at too low a level to be detectable by immunocytochemical techniques, in a manner similar to p53 protein in non-neoplastic cells,[82] whereas PrP^{CJD} is persistent and cumulative.[80]
2. It is possible that post mortem delay or exposure of tissue to fixative and the chemicals of processing removes all or most of the more soluble PrP^C and leaves a residuum of PrP^{CJD} so that positive staining is obtained only in diseased cases.

3. A variety of pretreatments may be applied to tissue sections in the expectation that they will reduce the likelihood of positivity for PrP^C. The most logical example of such pretreatment might be the use of protease predigestion of tissue sections.[83] Unfortunately the cellular and tissue structure is often destroyed if protease treatment is rigorous. An alternative pretreatment strategy would be to enhance PrP^{CJD} staining thereby allowing use of antibody at such a high dilution as to reduce even further the chances of staining PrP^C and also to reduce non specific staining.[84]

4. The accumulation of PrP^{CJD} in spongiform tissue may be accompanied by an actual decrease in PrP^C since the interrelationship between the two forms in CJD brain tissue is not understood at present.[78]

5. Conformational differences may exist between the two forms which affect the exposure of critical epitopes.[85,86]

A number of studies of PrP immunostaining patterns in human disease have now been published[65,87–93] and these show some differences from those reported in animals.[94] While some patterns of staining seem to be consistent, and disease-related, others have been more controversial especially in cases of atypical dementia which have PrP gene mutations but which lack the characteristic pathological features of spongiform encephalopathies.[95] Not all of these studies have debated the issues which might influence the staining results and their interpretations. Most rely on the clear demonstration of immunopositivity for PrP in cases of spongiform encephalopathy, contrasted with lack of staining in the 'control' population. This comparison may be valid for clear cut cases of spongiform encephalopathy but becomes more difficult in atypical cases. It is probable that cases vary considerably not only in the distribution and type of pathology but also in the distribution and amount of PrP^{CJD}. For these reasons, it is important to establish a protocol for PrP immunostaining which is reliable and consistent in cases of classical CJD and then to extend the study to include less typical cases, including those with PrP gene abnormalities. All staining results should be interpreted most carefully in light of what has been said above.

The PrP antibodies that are currently available are of two kinds. First, a number of different antibodies have been raised against varieties of so-called prion rods or scrapie fibrils,[87–89,96] and second, antibodies to synthetic peptide fragments of the PrP molecule have recently been developed.[5,87,88] As stated above, the antibodies against prion material, whether polyclonal or monoclonal, do not clearly discriminate between normal and abnormal forms of PrP, but they have been used widely in

Western blotting techniques for quantitation of abnormal protein,[80,85,97] as well as in immunocytochemical studies. Experience with the antibodies against synthetic peptides is more limited.[5,87,88]

Table 4 Pretreatment schedules in immunocytochemical demonstration of PrP[CJD]

Pretreatment	Reference
80–100% Formic acid 5–60 min	Kitamoto et al 1987[46] Kitamoto and Tateishi 1988[88] Powers et al 1991[65] Lantos et al 1992[5] Bugiani et al 1993[74]
4M Guanidine thiocyanate 2 h	Serban et al 1990[97] Doi-Yi et al 1991[84]
Proteinase K 10 µg/ml, 15 min, 37°C	DeArmond et al 1987[83] Piccardo et al 1990[87]
Pepsin 10%, 30 min, 37°C	Guiroy et at 1991[89]
Hydrolytic autoclaving 2.5 mM HCl, 10 min, 121°C	Kitamoto et al 1991[34]
30% Formic acid 1 min in microwave oven	Hashimoto et al 1992[92]
96% Formic acid 60 min folloed by 4M guanidine thiocyanate, 2 h, 4°C	Ironside et al 1993[55]

The path to finding a reliable protocol for PrP immunostaining in our own laboratory has been influenced in several important ways. First, we have been guided by experience in the published literature and have visited other laboratories which specialise in PrP immunostaining. Second, we have compared PrP immunostaining results using a variety of antibodies from different sources (Table 5) and in the large majority of the 150 plus cases retained in the Edinburgh CJD Unit. Third, we have employed a variety of pretreatments which on theoretical grounds might be expected to eliminate most, if not all, PrP[C], or, more commonly, to enhance staining of PrP[CJD] (Table 4). Fourth, we expect that the results of staining with antibodies to synthetic peptide should reproduce the staining patterns which result with polyclonal antibodies, and that these should be abolished when immune serum is pre-absorbed with excess peptide antigen. Fifth, and as for any other immunocytochemical study, there should be complete absence of positivity in age-matched, non-demented control cases.

Table 5 PrP antibodies in use in Edinburgh CJD laboratory

Antibody	Source	Antigen	Clonality	Dilution
ME7	Dr J Hope	Scrapie	Polyclonal	1 in 500, 30 min
IB4	Edinburgh	Fibrils	Polyclonal	1 in 500, 30 min
IB3			Polyclonal	1 in 1000, overnight
IA8			Polyclonal	1 in 1800, overnight (with pretreatment)
RO73	Dr S Prusiner	Hamster	Polyclonal	1 in 400, 30 min
611	California	Prion	Monoclonal	1 in 2000, overnight (with pretreatment)
1755	Dr H Diringer Berlin	Synthetic peptide (partial sequence sheep SAF protein)	Polyclonal	1 in 1500, overnight (with pretreatment)
SP30	Prof B Anderton	Synthetic	Polyclonal	1 in 1500, overnight
SP40	London	peptide (partial sequence sheep PrP)	Polyclonal	1 in 1500, overnight

Experience in the Edinburgh CJD laboratory has shown that the following protocol yields reliable results for PrP immunostaining in our human SE cases. All brain tissue blocks are decontaminated after formalin fixation by immersion in 96% formic acid for 60 min.[43] The tissue is then routinely processed to paraffin wax. While this pretreatment effectively sterilises the tissue, it also causes problems in section adherence to glass slides and the sections tend to wash off during prolonged immunocytochemical procedures. For this reason the sections are floated onto slides coated with 20% poly-L-lysine. The antibodies to PrP, or to synthetic peptide, that have been used in our laboratory are listed in Table 5 together with their working dilutions. Tissue sections are routinely prepared for PrP immunostaining by immersion in 96% formic acid for 10 min (this is additional to the 1 h pre-processing immersion), washed in water and then immersed in 4M guanidine thiocyanate for 2 h at 4 °C. The sections are then immunostained in the usual fashion using an avidin-biotin complex method. In our experience this pretreatment schedule with the polyclonal PrP antibodies generated by the Edinburgh Neuropathogenesis Unit produces consistent patterns of staining in almost all CJD cases which show classical spongiform encephalopathy. The staining patterns and localisation are described below. Pretreatment with 0.1% proteinase K in our cases, with or without a second pretreatment with formic acid, increases non-specific staining to an unacceptable level, and the use of stronger concentrations of proteinase K destroys all or part of the tissue sections. We have also experimented with hydrolytic and hydrated autoclaving using 2.5 mM HCl for 10 min at 121 °C, with or without the formic acid and guanidine thiocyanate pretreatments, and it is interesting to note that this sometimes yields positive results in cases which have been stubbornly negative for PrP immunostaining despite the presence of spongiform changes. Recent work also suggests that exposure to microwave treatment may be helpful (Table 4).[92] The enhancing effects of formic acid and guanidine thiocyanate are additive and when used in combination are likely to lead to the strongest possible positivity for PrP in tissue sections.

Theoretical implications of these pretreatments suggests that the majority are staining enhancers or that they have a role in unmasking previously hidden epitopes. The only theoretically 'correct' pretreatment, proteinase K, proves unsatisfactory in use in paraffin sections of human tissue in our experience. Most other recent reports have employed formic acid alone as a pretreatment and it is clear from the published illustrations that this does not cause problems with background staining. The only caveat would be that formic acid alone may be insufficient to reveal all PrP^{CJD} deposits in a particular section, or the different forms of staining in an individual case, or indeed any positivity at all in equivocal cases. It is certainly our experience that the addition of guanidine thiocyanate intensifies staining results with particular PrP antibodies, and increases the range and type of staining patterns in an individual case. The techniques need to be evaluated in individual laboratories and the increasing corporate experience of PrP immunostaining lends increasing credibility to the results.

PrP immunostaining has the potential of adding considerably to our understanding of human spongiform encephalopathies.[5] Even in classical cases of CJD spongiform encephalopathy, these techniques are beginning to show discrepancies between the topography of spongiform change and the localisation of PrP deposits. Since PrP has an intimate association with the infective agent, the lack of total concordance between PrP immunostaining and classical pathology is of great interest. In our experience all cases of CJD with classical spongiform changes show positive PrP immunostaining, which is of several different patterns. Where the cortical grey matter shows severe spongiform change, particularly where the vacuoles form confluent, multiloculated deficits in the neuropil, then this pattern is always associated with strongly positive PrP^{CJD} deposits within and around the vacuolated areas (Fig. 5a). If the cortex shows only microcystic vacuolar change with small circular vacuoles scattered evenly through the cortex, this pattern seldom co-localises with positive PrP^{CJD} immunostaining. We may call these

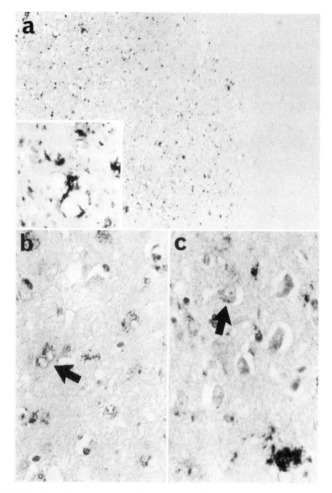

Fig. 5 (a) Section of temporal cortex showing spongiform change and focal positivity for
PrP(1A8, Table 5) confined to the grey matter. No positivity is seen in the white matter.
x 40. Inset – vacuolar pattern of PrP immunopositivity in spongiform change of grey
matter. x 200. (b) Granular pattern of PrP(1A8, Table 5) immunostaining in astrocytes
in CJD. x 400. (c) Granular pattern of PrP(1A8, Table 5) immunopositivity in neuronal
perikarya, together with vacuolar pattern of PrP positivity, in grey matter from a case of
CJD. x 400.

the vacuolar pattern of PrP immunostaining. The molecular layer of
the cerebellum does not display a vacuolar pattern of PrP staining even
when spongiform change and PrP-positive plaques are present, possibly

because confluent multiloculated vacuoles are not found at this site. Second, classical 'kuru' plaques (vide supra) are PrP positive, mostly in the cerebellar cortex and, to a lesser extent, in the cerebellar white matter. This plaque pattern of staining is at its most conspicuous in cases of GSS (Fig. 6), where the molecular layer of the cerebellum may be largely occupied by irregular, intensely positive and confluent plaques of PrP^{CJD}. It is noteworthy that the Purkinje cells are always negative for PrP^{CJD}, both in cases of CJD and in GSS (Fig. 6c,d). PrP immuno-staining techniques also reveal compact and diffuse plaques distributed much more widely through the brain and they may be present not only in the cortical grey matter but also in the basal ganglia, thalamus and hypothalamus. These areas of deep grey matter are often spongiform in CJD, but we have found that PrP^{CJD} positive plaques also occur in these sites in the absence of significant spongiform change. Plaques are found in the brain stem in some cases, whereas spongiform change is not a prominent feature of the brain stem in human cases, in contrast to the pathology findings in bovine spongiform encephalopathy.[98]

Positivity for PrP^{CJD} is not confined to the vacuolar and plaque patterns, both of which appear to be in the neuropil. In addition, intracellular deposits of immunostained PrP are also seen in some cases. We have observed definite granular staining of astrocytic cytoplasm similar to that reported in animals,[99] and particularly in the cortex of those cases which show very prominent astrocytosis with rather minimal spongiform change (Fig. 5b). Occasional evidence of a similar pattern of staining is also seen in unequivocal neurones (Fig. 5c) but this is rather infrequent. Enhancing pretreatments, particularly autoclaving, result in more neuronal staining and the neuronal positivity has been linked with a pattern of synaptophysin deposition.[93] In some cases there is quite widespread granular staining of the grey matter neuropil, apparently in cell processes but the exact location of deposits is hard to determine at the light microscope level. A few cases display apparent positive staining reactions in microglia and/or oligodendrocytes but validation of these observations requires further study using cell specific antibodies in combination with PrP immunocytochemistry.

How do we judge if these staining reactions represent genuine deposition of disease-related PrP? The fact that this pattern of staining is never seen in non-demented, age-matched controls, and, indeed, that there is no positive staining whatsoever in such cases, offers some grounds for optimism. More importantly, the staining patterns are reproducible time after time, not only in the same case but also in different cases (although the topographical distribution, and the positively stained features ie. vacuolar, plaque, astrocytic etc., vary from case to case) and that the same results are produced by more than one antibody, although not

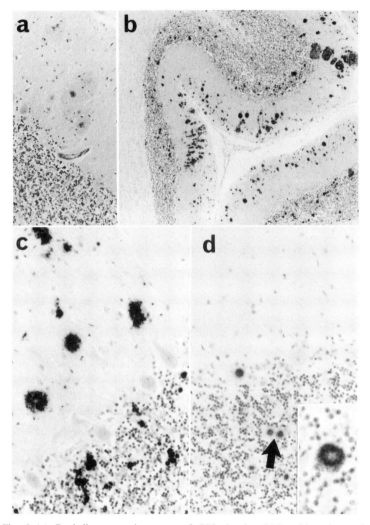

Fig. 6 (a) Cerebellar cortex in a case of GSS showing PAS-positive plaques in
the molecular layer. x 100. (b) Cerebellum from a GSS case showing PrP-positive
plaques(611, Table 5) in the molecular and granular layers. x 40. (c) Higher power view of
GSS cerebellum showing PrP-positive plaques, and Purkinje cells of normal appearance
which lack immunopositivity. x 200. (d) Similar view of cerebellum from a case of CJD
showing smaller and less numerous PrP-positive plaques in the Purkinje and granular
layers. x 200. Inset higher power view of PrP-positive plaque showing pale centre. x 400

always with the same intensity of staining. The panel of antibodies
includes polyclonal and monoclonal antibodies raised against prion pro-

tein and against synthetic peptides. When these latter antibodies were pre-absorbed against the synthetic peptides, the typical staining patterns were entirely abolished and sections from CJD cases were negative throughout. The patterns of staining reactions reported here concur with experience elsewhere, but the complete topographic distribution of PrP positivity in human SE cases has not been reported previously.

Having established a body of experience with PrP^{CJD} immunostaining in cases of classical human spongiform encephalopathy including GSS and CJD it is imperative to examine also cases of atypical dementia which do not show classical spongiform changes. It will be particularly necessary to examine cases with PrP gene mutations in view of the claim that 'prion diseases' may have been underdiagnosed previously.[5,70] In such cases it would be desirable to try all recommended pretreatments which are alleged to enhance PrP immunostaining in order to detect possible low level PrP^{CJD} expression especially if initial results appeared to be negative. Trials of this kind in our laboratory show that neither non-demented control cases nor Alzheimer's disease cases show PrP^{CJD} immunopositivity even after autoclaving in the recommended fashion. Recent reports suggest that PrP^{CJD} immunostaining patterns are somewhat different in atypical cases from those seen in CJD.[5] In the small number of cases of atypical dementia in the Edinburgh collection, which lack spongiform change, we find consistent PrP^{CJD} staining of many glial cells but convincing PrP-positive plaques are not a conspicuous feature. Some caution must be employed in the interpretation of plaque-like structures which appear to be PrP positive. A recent study has shown that at least some of these may be fungal contaminants.[100]

CLINICOPATHOLOGICAL CORRELATIONS

Sporadic cases

Classically, cases of CJD have been sub-divided as subacute, intermediate and amyotrophic.[101] In the subacute cases, vague prodromal symptoms are rapidly followed by neurological disturbance, ataxia and dizziness and impaired mental function. Myoclonus is present in a high proportion of cases and all proceed rapidly to a stage of akinetic mutism and cortical blindness, the majority being dead within 6 to 8 months. In cases described as intermediate, the clinical course is slower and death may ensue up to 2 years after the onset of symptoms. A poorly defined category of patients is described as having the amyotrophic form of CJD in which slowly progressive dementia is combined with muscle weakness and wasting but without myoclonus. These cases probably represent a form of motor neurone disease and most of them lack spongiform change at autopsy.

Before the advent of PrP immunostaining it was clear that sporadic cases of CJD varied in their pathological picture even though the characteristic feature of spongiform encephalopathy was focally present.[4] Examination of multiple areas from any individual case allows mapping of the most affected grey matter and differences in the extent and severity of the spongiform change soon become evident between cases. Abrupt transition zones are sometimes seen between grossly spongiform zones and much more nearly normal zones of grey matter, particularly in the cortical ribbon and in the hippocampus. The degree to which the basal ganglia are involved varies from case to case and the individual nuclei may also vary. Although the diagnosis may be established positively by one section from an affected area, the focality of the lesions means that some areas may appear virtually normal and certainly lack spongiform change. This highlights the potential pitfalls in examination of a single block from an individual case, and clearly illustrates the possibility of missing the diagnosis in a surgical biopsy from a suspected CJD case.

The clinical history may give some clues as to the location of likely spongiform pathology within the brain. Those patients with a cerebellar syndrome and ataxia usually show cerebellar cortical involvement and the cerebral cortical changes may be rather minimal or not very widespread. Conversely, an initial presentation of dementia is more likely to have cortical or deep grey matter involvement and may or may not have cerebellar spongiform change. The relatively rapid clinical progress to a near vegetative state in which neurological status is hard to fully assess, may mask those cerebellar signs which have their onset after the cortical signs. Topographical mapping of the lesions in CJD reveals the variety of patterns and these do not always seem to fit well with the clinical story (Fig. 7). The varying distribution of spongiform change has been described above. However there is some evidence that the nature and distribution of the pathological changes may vary with the duration of illness.[4] Spongiform change may be a comparatively early phenomenon and may well disappear in patients with a long duration of illness, being replaced by a pathological picture of neuronal loss and severe gliosis with terminal status spongiosus in advanced cases (*vide supra*).

Animal studies suggest that accumulation of PrP^CJD in astrocytes is a very early phenomenon[99] and precedes the astrocytosis and loss of neurones, raising the possibility that this is a primary, rather than reactive, event. Whether this is also true in humans remains to be seen. Simple observation of the cortex shows that there is very considerable

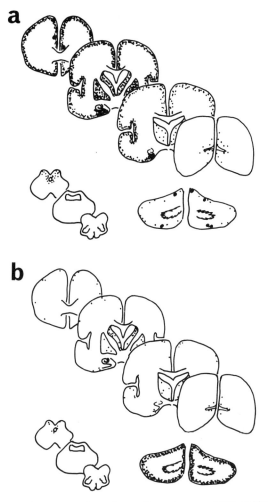

Fig. 7 Diagrammatic representations of spongiform change and PrP-positive plaques in the cerebrum, cerebellum and brainstem of 2 different cases of CJD: (**a**) 66-year-old woman dying after an illness of 12 months which commenced with unsteadiness, proceeding to ataxia followed by confusion and dementia before death. Death occurred from bronchopneumonia. (**b**) 70-year-old man who died 3 months after onset of symptoms. Initial complaints were of unsteadiness and blurred vision proceeding to ataxia and dementia. Death occurred suddenly from pulmonary embolism.

neuronal loss in CJD. Whether this correlates locally with quantity of spongiform change, astrocytosis or deposits of PrP^{CJD}, remains to be determined and is under active investigation in our laboratory. Very careful and detailed mapping studies have been carried out in Japanese cases[102] but these relate to the classical neuropathology rather than to PrP immunocytochemical positivity. Quantitative studies of cerebellar pathology in CJD have documented the loss of granule layer cells and astrocytosis in CJD.[49] Mapping of cerebral neuronal loss and gliosis with clinical correlation was first described in detail in classical studies by Masters and Richardson (1978).[4] Detailed topography of PrP[CJD] deposits may correlate more closely with clinical history and a recent study has suggested that the PrP genotype may dictate the pattern of deposits.[103]

Examination of the pituitary gland, including anterior and posterior lobes, and of the spinal cord reveals no apparent abnormality in routinely stained sections apart from some degeneration of the corticospinal tracts in cases with longer than usual symptomatic history.[4] Staining of these structures with antibodies to PrP is currently in progress. Preliminary results suggest that the pituitary itself is negative using the protocols which yield positive results in the brain although the hypothalamus frequently contains PrP positive plaques. It is possible that PrP[CJD] may be present in these structures at a level too low to detect with present immunocytochemical protocols since the iatrogenic transmission of CJD following use of cadaver pituitary glands does indicate the presence of infective agent in the pituitary.[109,110] Staining results in non-CJD organs will require rigorous validation and repetitive experiments. Studies in animals suggests that the spleen may show positive results[34] and our preliminary investigation suggests that human spleen may show some PrP[CJD] immunopositivity.

As part of the surveillance project which monitors any possible impact of the epidemic of bovine spongiform encephalopathy on human CJD, it will be important to determine whether the pattern of pathology of human CJD shows variation in future from the patterns described above. It has been suggested that novel forms of CJD might result if bovine spongiform encephalopathy were successfully transmitted to man by the oral route.[23,104]

Familial and gene mutation cases

While no genetic abnormality has been determined for sporadic cases of CJD, there are now some well established PrP gene mutations and variants which are associated with the familial forms of human spongiform encephalopathy, including CJD and GSS. These are reviewed elsewhere in this Bulletin. For instance there is a clear association between PrP codon 102 mutation and GSS. It might be expected that specific PrP gene abnormalities might lead to various specific clinical and pathological forms of the disease. In some studies it has been possible to correlate a particular pathological subset with a particular gene mutation. Thus in some studies the ataxic form of GSS seems to correlate with the codon 102 mutation[105] but other workers have not found such clear cut association between genotype and phenotype.[106] There may be better correlation between genotype and PrP deposit but these studies are in their infancy. In fact individual CJD and GSS families are characterised by rather wide clinical and pathological variation despite having the same genetic abnormality,[106] as discussed above. Other, as yet unknown, influences must operate on the expression of the abnormal gene. Collinge et al described a GSS family with inserts in the PrP open reading frame in whom one young member had a history of an illness lasting more than 10 years, with clear cut dementia before the age of 30, but whose brain showed no evidence of spongiform change and very little other abnormality.[23] It is this sort of case which has led to speculation that 'prion diseases' may be numerically more important as causative in dementia than the presence of spongiform encephalopathy would lead us to believe.[5,70] This view has been disputed recently in a study in which large numbers of demented cases were checked for transmissibility and for abnormalities of PrP genetic make-up.[71] No cases of prion abnormality were disclosed in this study. However another example of PrP gene abnormality in which spongiform change may be rather limited is the codon 178 mutation, associated with fatal insomnia, in which thalamic abnormalities predominate.[24,72] Whether PrP immunostaining can become a reliable marker for such atypical cases remains to be seen.[5] The diagnostic difficulties in this challenging area of neuropathology are evident. As long ago as 1978 Masters and Richardson[4] noted that spongiform change may well be absent from cases with long clinical duration and that this did not preclude the diagnosis of CJD. However these cases were characterised by severe gliosis and neuronal loss which are not features of the current controversial cases of atypical dementia. It will also be important to determine whether these atypical cases are transmissible.

In comparing cases of CJD with GSS, it is clear that the pattern of plaque formation is more complex in GSS, particularly in the cerebellum. Compound, multifocal PrP plaques are typical of GSS and although immunocytochemical techniques are not quantitative, it is difficult to escape the impression that the cerebellum carries a larger load of PrP deposits in GSS cases than in CJD. This may be associated with the longer clinical duration of GSS cases. Our preliminary studies of cases of atypical dementia with PrP gene mutations, which lack spongiform change, suggest that PrP immunopositivity can be demonstrated in such cases, usually in glial cells, if a careful regime of pretreatments is used to include those methods most likely to enhance PrP staining. These should include hydrolytic autoclaving in cases which seem negative with other methods.

Iatrogenic cases

Iatrogenic cases of spongiform encephalopathy include those which have been brought about by presumed inoculation of contaminated human tissue during neurosurgery[107] or corneal grafting,[108] as well as by injections of pituitary extracts.[17,109,110] It is clear from study of these two groups of patients that the incubation period from the known date, or period, of exposure to the time of onset of symptoms varies considerably.[17] Those patients inoculated 'centrally' in or near the brain develop disease symptoms very much more quickly than those inoculated 'peripherally', as in the treatment of pituitary dwarfism. This latter group have a rather clearly defined clinical picture[110] in which ataxia, dysarthria and a pancerebellar syndrome precede the signs of dementia and myoclonus and abnormal EEG spikes. The iatrogenic cases which followed neurosurgical and corneal procedures more closely resemble classical CJD in symptomatology. One possible conclusion from this comparison is that the agent is entering the brain by different routes and the variable pathological picture is also suggestive of different patterns of spread of the agent. The part played by a genetic predisposition in the host in iatrogenic CJD has still to be clarified. The role of valine-valine homozygosity at codon 129 in this connection is of particular interest.[111] Since it is possible to surmise the point of entry of the agent into the body, these cases may be particularly rewarding to study in detail with regard to the topography and quantitation of pathological changes and particularly of PrP deposition. Examination of one such case showed numerous PrP-positive plaques in the atrophic and spongiform cerebellum, with little spongiform change elsewhere.

DIFFERENTIAL DIAGNOSIS

Patients suffering from spongiform encephalopathy clearly have a progressive neurodegenerative disorder, which will require neuropathological studies for diagnostic confirmation. In order for the neuropathologist to arrive at a diagnosis, the potential overlap with other neurodegenerative diseases on both clinical and pathological grounds must be recognised and criteria for the diagnosis of spongiform encephalopathy should be stated in each individual case. Recent advances in neuropathology, particularly the use of immunocytochemistry to characterise morphological abnormalities in a way hitherto impossible, have assisted identification of spongiform encephalopathy cases. The use of PrP immunocytochemistry for diagnostic purposes is considered above, and these investigations should be carried out along with other diagnostic neuropathological techniques.

The extremely variable macroscopic pathology of human spongiform encephalopathies, and the absence of any specific macroscopic abnormalities necessitates a comprehensive histological survey for diagnosis. Depending on the presence and distribution of cerebral cortical atrophy, the main differential diagnosis on macroscopic grounds would be Alzheimer's disease. Severe involvement of deep grey matter structures, with atrophy and gliosis in these regions may suggest the possibility of Pick's disease or Huntington's disease. The pronounced cerebellar involvement in some cases of sporadic CJD, iatrogenic CJD, kuru and GSS may suggest other primary cerebellar degenerations, particularly if cerebral involvement is minimal and spinal cord involvement is evident.

In most cases of human spongiform encephalopathy the neuropathological features are characteristic and diagnostic. However, a differential diagnosis may be entertained for cases with unusual distributions of pathology, or where other less characteristic histological abnormalities are identified, e.g. cases with neurofibrillary tangles. Spongiform change is not pathognomonic for spongiform encephalopathies in man. Appearances indistinguishable from spongiform change have been described in certain regions of cerebral cortex, particularly at the medial temporal lobe and temporal pole, in Alzheimer's disease and diffuse Lewy body disease[112,113] (Fig. 1). Other disorders which may exhibit focal spongiform-like change are listed in Table 6a. The distribution of the spongiform change in all cases is strictly limited and extensive cortical involvement with spongiform change has not been described for any of these disorders. However, spongiform change in sporadic CJD can be irregular, with an asymmetrical distribution of lesions in the brain. For this reason, extensive histological sampling is required for accurate diagnosis.

Table 6a Other conditions which may exhibit spongiform-like vacuolation

Alzheimer's disease
Diffuse Lewy body disease
Pick's disease
Dementia of frontal lobe type
Metabolic encephalopathies

It is usually an easy matter to distinguish between Alzheimer's disease and human spongiform encephalopathy, particularly with the use of specialised staining techniques including silver stains or immunocytochemistry to identify characteristic abnormalities, eg phosphorylated tau protein in neurofibrillary tangles, A4 protein or A4 protein precursor deposition in the amyloid plaques in Alzheimer's disease.[114] Studies of GSS cases have indicated that the A4 protein precursor may be involved in the pathogenesis of PrP plaques in this disorder, with apparent co-localisation of these proteins within individual plaques.[115] This clearly has the potential to produce diagnostic confusion, but this can be remedied by a more extensive histological review. Other unrelated disorders may produce spongy degeneration in the brain involving the grey or white matter. Such degenerative changes may be mistaken for CJD; examples of disorders producing this difficulty are listed in Table 6b. PrP immunocytochemistry has enabled precise characterisation of amyloid plaques in human spongiform encephalopathies,[91] with additional PrP deposits around areas of confluent spongiform change with occasional intracellular staining[39] (vide supra). The experience in the Edinburgh CJD Surveillance Unit Laboratory indicates that PrP deposition is not a characteristic feature in Alzheimer's disease, diffuse Lewy body disease or any of the other disorders listed in Table 6a. However, PrP immunocytochemistry may not be able to resolve all diagnostic problems, particularly in cases with poor tissue fixation and preservation.

Table 6b Other conditions which may be mistaken for spongiform change

Status spongiosus
Cerebral oedema
Tissue retraction artefact
White matter rarefaction and gliosis
Neuronal storage disorders
Spongy degeneration of the white matter

Cases of human spongiform encephalopathy with amyloid plaque formation may therefore be recognised by identification of immunocytochemically positive PrP deposits. This approach should help to clarify the diagnostic confusion in some cases between human spongiform encephalopathy and Alzheimer's disease, even in cases with neurofibrillary tangle formation. In cases with extensive neuronal loss, reactive gliosis and status spongiosis the differentiation from Pick's disease on histological grounds may be uncertain. CJD cases with prominent ballooned cortical neurones may also resemble Pick's disease; ballooned neurones have been identified in a wide range of neurodegenerative disorders[116] and are not a reliable diagnostic feature. As before, PrP immunocytochemistry should help to resolve this diagnostic difficulty and a full survey of the fixed brain usually reveals areas with characteristic spongiform change at sites remote from the cerebral cortex, eg the basal ganglia or thalamus. Similarly, a distinction between GSS, kuru and sporadic CJD, and other primary cerebellar degenerative disorders is usually possible through the identification of amyloid plaques, PrP deposition and spongiform change both in the cerebellum and elsewhere in the CNS. In GSS cases with neurofibrillary tangles, differentiation from Alzheimer's disease may not be straightforward on conventional stains, but immunocytochemical investigations should be able to demonstrate PrP in amyloid plaques.

No extensive ultrastructural survey on sporadic CJD has been performed, partly because of the difficulties in the handling of contaminated material in the stages of tissue fixation, processing and cutting for electromicroscopy, but the identification of tubulovesicular structures[64] may facilitate the use of electromicroscopy as a diagnostic investigation. Another use of electronmicroscopy for diagnostic purposes is the study of touch preparations.[117] However, since this technique involves the use of unfixed brain tissue, it is unlikely to come into wide diagnostic application.

SUMMARY AND CONCLUSIONS

The current surge of interest in human spongiform encephalopathies has resulted from the recent enormous strides in molecular pathology of the PrP gene. There is also concern that bovine spongiform encephalopathy may pose a threat to human health. The establishment of reliable methods of PrP immunostaining, allied to gene mutation studies and quantitation of PrP in brain tissue should advance our understanding of this group of neurodegenerative diseases. This will be true not only of classical CJD and spongiform encephalopathies but also in a range of atypical cases with and without PrP gene abnormalities.

Since it is now becoming apparent that the topographical map of PrP immunostaining in CJD does not always co-localise with the map of classical neuropathology, it will be of interest to relate the pattern of PrP deposition to clinical signs and symptoms. When this is done for all CJD cases, including not only sporadic but also familial and iatrogenic cases, it may be possible to deduce the pattern of spread of the agent within the brain, and possibly to uncover the initiation of the disease process.

Review of nomenclature of this group of diseases has rightly been prompted by the remarkable progress in genetic pathology which has focused attention on an extremely interesting group of diseases characterised by dementia and abnormalities of the PrP gene but not by spongiform change. It has been proposed that the term prion dementia should replace spongiform encephalopathy as the generic term for these diseases. This has some appeal in that all spongiform encephalopathy cases do seem to show PrP accumulation in the brain. However, it has yet to be shown that sporadic CJD is regularly associated with PrP gene abnormalities or that atypical 'prion dementias' are transmissible. It is therefore premature to compress all these cases into one disease grouping. In addition, further study is clearly needed of the various histopathological sequelae of PrP perturbation, in order to understand more clearly these fascinating diseases.

ACKNOWLEDGEMENTS

We thank Mr P Hayward for thorough investigation of pretreatment schedules, and Mrs L McCardle and Miss C Barrie for skilled technical assistance. We are indebted to Dr RG Will for clinical information and to Dr S DeArmond, Dr A Taraboulos, Dr SL Yang and Mrs JC Canlas for helpful discussion, and to Ms A Honeyman for typing the manuscript. This study would not have been possible without the provision of cases, and of PrP antibodies, from our many collaborators. The support of the Department of Health, SHHD, AFRC and MRC is gratefully acknowledged.

REFERENCES

1 Creutzfeldt HG. Uber eine eigenartige herdformige Erkrankung des Zentral nervensystems. Z Gesam Neurol Psychitr 1920; 57: 1-18.
2 Jakob A. Uber eigenartige Erkrankung des Zentral nervensystems mit bemerkenswertem anatomischen Befunde. Z Gesam Neurol Psychiatr 1921; 64: 47-228.
3 Masters CL, Gajdusek DC. The spectrum of Creutzfeldt-Jakob disease and the virus-induced spongiform encephalopathies. In: Smith WT, Cavanagh JB, eds. Recent Advances in Neuropathology vol. 2 Edinburgh: Churchill Livingstone, 1982: pp 139-164.
4 Masters CL, Richardson EP. Subacute spongiform encephalopathy (Creutzfeldt-Jakob disease). The nature and progression of spongiform change. Brain 1978; 101: 333-334.
5 Lantos PL. From slow virus to prion: a review of transmissible spongiform encephalopathies. Histopathology 1992; 20: 1-11.
6 Bastian FO, ed. Creutzfeldt-Jakob Disease and Other Transmissible Human Spongiform Encephalopathies. St Louis: Mosby Year Book, 1991.
7 Manuelidis EE. Creutzfeldt-Jakob disease. J Neuropathol Exp Neurol 1985; 44: 1-17.
8 Gerstmann J, Straussler E, Schienker J. Uber eine eigenartige hereditar-familiare Erkrankung des Zentral nervensystems. Z Neurol 1936; 154: 736-762.
9 Boellaard JW, Schlote W. Subakute spongiforme encephalopathy mit multiformer plaquebildung. Acta Neuropathol 1980; 49: 205-212.
10 Hsiao K, Prusiner SB. Inherited human prion diseases. Neurology 1990; 40: 1820-1827.
11 Baker HF, Ridley RM. The genetics and transmissibility of human spongiform encephalopathy. Neurodegen 1992; 1: 3-16.
12 Gajdusek DC, Zigas V. Degenerative disease of the central nervous system in New Guinea. The endemic occurrence of 'kuru' in the native population. N Engl J Med 1957; 257: 974-978.
13 Tomlinson BE. Creutzfeldt-Jakob disease. In: Adams JH, Duchen LW, eds. Greenfield's Neuropathology 5th edn. London: Edward Arnold, 1992: pp 1366-1375.
14 Gajdusek DC, Gibbs CJ, Alpers MP. Experimental transmission of a kuru-like syndrome in chimpanzees. Nature 1966; 209: 794-796.

15 Gibbs CJ, Gajdusek DC, Asher DM et al. Creutzfeldt-Jakob disease (subacute spongiform encephalopathy) : Transmission to the chimpanzee. Science 1968; 161: 388-389.

16 Masters CL, Gajdusek DC, Gibbs CJ. Creutzfeldt-Jakob disease: virus isolations from the Gerstmann-Straussler syndrome. Brain 1981; 104: 559-588.

17 Brown P, Preece MA, Will RG. 'Friendly fire' in medicine: Hormones, homografts, and Creutzfeldt-Jakob disease. Lancet 1992; 340: 24-27.

18 Will RG. An overview of Creutzfeldt-Jakob disease associated with the use of human pituitary growth hormone. Dev Biol Stand 1991; 75: 85-86.

19 Prusiner SB. Molecular biology of prion diseases. Science 1991; 252: 1515-1522.

20 Carlson GA, Hsiao K, Oesch B, Westaway D, Prusiner SB. Genetics of prion infections. Trends Genet 1991; 7: 61-65.

21 Pablos-Mendez A, Netto EM, Defendini R. Infectious prions or cytotoxic metabolites? Lancet 1993; 341: 159-161.

22 Doerr-Schott J, Kitamoto T, Tateishi J, Boellaard JW, Heldt N, Lichte C. Technical communication. Immunogold light and electron microscopic detection of amyloid plaques in transmissible spongiform encephalopathies. Neuropathol Appl Neurobiol 1990; 16: 85-89.

23 Collinge J, Owen F, Poulter M, et al. Prion dementia without characteristic pathology. Lancet 1990; 336: 7-9.

24 Mendori R, Tritschler JH, LeBlanc A, et al. Fatal familial insomnia, a prion disease with a mutation at codon 178 of the prion protein gene. N Engl J Med 1992; 7: 444-449.

25 Petersen RB, Tabaton M, Medori R, et al. Familial thalamic dementia and fatal familial insomnia are prion diseases with the same mutation. Neurobiol Aging 1992; 13: S93.

26 Nieto A, Goldfarb LG, Brown P, et al. Codon 178 mutation in ethnically diverse Creutzfeldt-Jakob disease families. Lancet 1991; 337: 622-623.

27 Goldfarb LG, Brown P, Goldgaber D, et al. Identical mutation in unrelated patients with Creutzfeldt-Jakob disease. Lancet 1990; 336: 174-175.

28 Goldfarb LG, Mitrova E, Brown P, Toh BH, Gajdusek DC. Mutations in codon 200 of scrapie amyloid protein gene in two clusters of Creutzfeldt-Jakob disease in Slovakia. Lancet 1990; 336: 514-515.

29 Will RG. The spongiform encephalopathies. J Neurol Neurosurg Psychiatry 1991; 54: 761-763.

30 Will RG, Matthews WB. Evidence for case-to-case transmission of Creutzfeldt-Jakob disease. J Neurol Neurosurg Psychiatry 1982; 45: 235-238.

31 Gajdusek DC, Gibbs CJ, Asher DM, et al. Precautions in medical care of, and in handling materials from, patients with transmissible virus dementia (Creutzfeldt-Jakob disease). N Engl J Med 1977; 297: 1253-1258.

32 Rohwer RG. Scrapie infectious agent is virus-like in size and susceptibility to inactivation. Nature 1984; 308: 658-662.

33 Committee on Health Care Issues, ANA. Precautions in handling tissues, fluids, and other contaminated materials from patients with documented or suspected Creutzfeldt-Jakob disease. Ann Neurol 1986; 19: 75-77.

34 Kitamoto T, Muramoto T, Mohri S, Doh-Ura K, Tateishi J. Abnormal isoform of prion protein accumulates in follicular dendritic cells in mice with Creutzfeldt-Jakob disease. J Virol 1991; 65: 6292-6295.

35 Kimberlin RH, Walker CA, Millson GC, et al. Disinfection studies with two strains of mouse-passaged scrapie agent. J Neurol Sci 1983; 59: 355-369.

36 Prusiner SB, McKinley MP, Bolton DC, et al. Prions: methods for assay, purification and characterisation. Methods in Virology VIII. New York : Academic Press, 1984: pp 293-345.

37 Advisory Committee on Dangerous Pathogens. Categorisation of pathogens according to hazard and categories of containment, 2 ed. London: HMSO, 1990.

38 Brown P, Liberski PP, Wolff A, Gajdusek DC. Resistance of scrapie infectivity to steam autoclaving after formaldehyde fixation and limited survival after ashing at 360°C: Practical and theoretical implications. J Inf Dis 1990; 161: 467-472.

39 Brown P, Gajdusek DC. Survival of scrapie virus after 3 years' interment. Lancet 1991; 337: 269-270.

40 Esmonde TFG, Will RG, Slattery JM, Knight R, Harries-Jones R, DeSilva R, Matthews WB. Creutzfeldt-Jakob disease and blood transfusion. Lancet 1993; 341: 205-207.

41 Department of Health: Dr JS Metters. Neuro and ophthalmic surgery procedures in patients with, or suspected to have, or at risk of developing CJD or GSS. Letter PL(92)CO/4 to Consultants and Health Managers 7/12/92.

42 Taylor DM. Inactivation of the unconventional agents of scrapie, bovine spongiform encephalopathy and Cruetzfeldt-Jakob disease. J Hosp Inf 1991; 18: 141-146.

43 Brown P, Wolff A, Gajdusek DC. A simple and effective method for inactivating virus infectivity in formalin-fixed tissue samples from patients with Creutzfeldt-Jakob disease. Neurology 1990; 40: 887-890.

44 Taylor DM, McConnell I. Autoclaving does not decontaminate formol-fixed scrapie tissues. Lancet 1988; (i): 1463.

45 Bell JE, Ironside JW. How to tackle a possible Creutzfeldt-Jakob disease necropsy. J Clin Pathol 1993; 46: 193-197.

46 Kitamoto T, Ogomori K, Tateishi J, Prusiner SB. Methods in laboratory investigation: formic acid pretreatment enhances immunostaining of cerebral and systemic amyloids. Lab Invest 1987; 57: 230-236.

47 Tintner R, Brown P, Hedley-Whyte ET, Rappaport EB, Piccardo CP, Gajdusek DC. Neuropathologic verification of Creutzfeldt-Jakob disease in the exhumed American recipient of human pituitary growth hormone. Neurology 1986; 36: 932-936.

48 Weller RO, Steart PV, Powell-Jackson JD. Pathology of Creutzfeldt-Jakob disease associated with pituitary-derived human growth hormone administration. Neuropathol Appl Neurobiol 1986; 12: 117-129.

49 Lafarga M, Berciano MT, Suarez I, Viadero CF, Andres MA, Berciano J. Cytology and organisation of reactive astroglia in human cerebellar cortex with severe loss of granule cells: a study on the ataxic form of Creutzfeldt-Jakob disease. Neurosci 1991; 40: 337-352.

50 Jones HR, Hedley-Whyte ET, Freiberg SR, Baker RA. Ataxic Creutzfeldt-Jakob disease: diagnostic techniques and neuropathologic observations in early disease. Neurology 1985; 35: 254-257.

51 Kim JH, Manuelidis EE. Neuronal alterations in experimental Creutzfeldt-Jakob disease: a Golgi study. J Neurol Sci 1989; 89: 92-101.

52 Nakazato Y, Hirato J,Ishida Y, Hoshi S, Hasegawa M, Fukuda T. Swollen cortical neurons in Creutzfeldt-Jakob disease contain a phosphorylated neurofilament epitope. J Neuropathol Exp Neurol 1990; 49: 197-205.

53 Kato S, Hiran A, Umahara T, Llena JF, Herz F, Ohama E. Ultrastructural and immunohistological studies of ballooned cortical neurons in Creutzfeldt-Jakob disease: expression of αB-crystallin, ubiquitin and stress-response protein 27. Acta Neuropathol 1992; 84: 443-448.

54 Suenaga T, Hirano A, Llena JF, Ksiezak-Reding H, Yen SH, Dickson DW. Ubiquitin immunoreactivity in kuru plaques in Creutzfeldt-Jakob disease. Ann Neurol 1990; 28: 174-177.

55 Ironside JW, McCardle L, Hayward PAR, Bell JE. Ubiquitin immunocytochemistry in human spongiform encephalopathies. Neuropathol Appl Neurobiol 1993; 19: 134-140.

56 Lowe J, McDermott H, Kenward N, et al. Ubiquitin conjugate immunoreactivity in the brains of scrape mice. J Pathol 1990; 162: 61-66.

57 Laslo L, Lowe J, Self T, et al. Lysosomes as key organelles in the pathogenesis of prion encephalopathies. J Pathol 1992; 66: 333-341.

58 Wells GAH, Wilesmith JW, McGill IS. Bovine spongiform encephalopathy. Brain Pathol 1992; 1: 69-78.

59 Kawata A, Masakazu S, Oda M, Hayashi H, Tanabe H. Creutzfeldt-Jakob disease with congophilic kuru plaques: CT and pathological findings of the cerebral white matter. J Neurol Neurosurg Psychiatry 1992; 55: 849-851.

60 Ironside JW, Barrie C, McCardle L, Bell JE. Microglial reactions in human spongiform encephalopathies (Abstract). Neuropathol Appl Neurobiol 1993; 19: 203

61 Hulette CM, Downey BT, Burger PC. Macrophage markers in diagnostic neuropathology. Am J Surg Pathol 1992; 15: 493-499.

62 Humphrey-Smith I, Chastel C. Creutzfeldt-Jakob disease, spiroplasmas, and crystalline artifacts. Lancet 1988; 2: 1199.

63 Lewin PK, Edwards V. Mitochondrial inclusions in neurons of Creutzfeldt-Jakob-like disease. Lancet 1991; 337: 236-237.

64 Liberski PP, Budka H, Sluga E, Barcikowska, Kwiecinski H. Tubulovesicular structures in Creutzfeldt-Jakob disease. Acta Neuropathol 1992; 84: 238-243.

65 Powers JM, Liu Y, Hair LS, Kascsack RJ, Lewis LD, Levy LA. Concomitant Creutzfeldt and Alzheimer diseases. Acta Neuropathol 1991; 83: 95-98.

66 Collinge J, Harding AE, Owens F, et al. Diagnosis of Gerstmann-Sträussler syndrome in familial dementia with prion protein gene analysis. Lancet 1989; 2: 15-17.

67 Collinge J, Brown J, Hardy J, et al. Inherited prion disease with 144 base pair gene insertion. 2. Clinical and pathological features. Brain 1992; 115: 687-710.

68 Miyazono M, Kitamoto T, Doh-ura K, Iwaki T, Tateishi J. Creutzfeldt-Jakob disease with codon 129 polymorphism (valine): a comparative study of patients with codon 102 point mutation or without mutations. Acta Neuropathol 1992; 83: 349-354.

69 Tateishi J, Kitamoto T, Doh-ura K, Boellaard JW, Peiffer J. Creutzfeldt-Jakob disease with amyloid angiopathy: diagnosis by immunological analysis and transmission experiments. Acta Neuropathol 1992; 83: 559-563.

70 Anonymous. Prion disease – spongiform encephalopathies unveiled. Lancet 1990; 336: 21-22.

71 Brown P, Kaur P, Sulima MP, Goldfarb LG, Gibbs CJ, Gajdusek DC. Real and imagined clinicopathological limits of 'prion dementia'. Lancet 1993; 341: 127-130.

72 Manetto V, Medori R, Cortelli P, et al. Fatal familial insomnia: clinical and pathological study of five new cases. Neurology 1992; 42: 312-319.

73 Billette de Villemeur T, Deslys JP, Dormont D, Jardin L, Robain O. Iatrogenic Creutzfeldt-Jakob disease in a 13-year-old growth hormone recipient. Neuropathol Appl Neurobiol 1993 (In press).

74 Bugiani O, Ciaccone G, Verga L, et al. βPP participates in PrP-amyloid plaques of Gerstmann-Straussler-Scheinker disease, Indiana kindred. J Neuropathol Exp Neurol 1993; 52: 66-70.

75 Anano N, Yagishita S, Yokoi S, et al. Gerstmann-Straussler syndrome – a variant type: amyloid plaques and Alzheimer's neurofibrillary tangles in cerebral cortex. Acta Neuropathol 1992; 84: 15-23.

76 Hart J, Gordon B. Early-onset dementia and extrapyramidal disease: clinicopathological variant of Gerstmann-Straussler-Scheinker or Alzheimer's disease. J Neurol Neurosurg Psychiatry 1990; 53: 932-939.

77 de Courten-Myers G, Mandybur TI. Atypical Gerstmann-Straussler syndrome or familial spinocerebellar ataxia and Alzheimer's disease? Neurology 1987; 37: 269-275.

78 Weissmann C. A 'unified theory' of prion propagation. Nature 1991; 352: 679-683.

79 Prusiner SB, DeArmond SJ. Molecular biology and pathology of scrapie and the prion diseases of humans. Brain Pathol 1991; 1: 297-309.

80 Bockman JM, Kingsbury DI, McKinley MP, Bendheim PE, Prusiner SB. Creutzfeldt-Jakob disease prion proteins in human brains. N Engl J Med 1985; 312: 73-78.

81 Taylor DM. Letter to the editor: spongiform encephalopathies. Neuropathol Appl Neurobiol 1991; 17: 345-346.

82 Iggo R, Gatter K, Bartek J, Lane D, Harris AL. Increased expression of mutant forms of p53 oncogene in primary lung cancer. Lancet 1990; 335: 675-679.

83 DeArmond SJ, Mobley WC, Dermott DL, Barry RA, Beckstead JH, Prusiner SB. Changes in the localisation of brain prion proteins during scrapie infection. Neurology 1987; 37: 1271-1280.

84 Doi-Yi R, Kitamoto T, Tateishi J. Immunoreactivity of cerebral amyloidosis is enhanced by protein denaturation treatments. Acta Neuropathol 1991; 82: 260-265.

85 Safar J, Ceroni M, Piccardo P, Gajdusek DC, Gibbs CJ. Scrapie-associated precursor proteins: antigenic relationship between species and immunocytochemical localization in normal, scrapie and Creutzfeldt-Jakob disease brains. Neurology 1990; 40: 513-517.

86 Costa PP, Jacobsson B, Collins VP, Biberfeld P. Unmasking antigen determinants in amyloid. J Histochem Cytochem 1986; 34: 1683-1685.

87 Piccardo P, Safar J, Ceroni M, Gajdusek DC, Gibbs CJ. Immunohistochemical localization of prion protein in spongiform encephalopathies and normal brain tissue. Neurology 1990; 40: 518-522.

88 Kitamoto T, Tateishi J. Immunohistochemical confirmation of Creutzfeldt-Jakob disease with a long clinical course with amyloid plaque core antibodies. Am J Pathol 1988; 131: 435-443.

89 Guiroy DC, Yanagihara R, Gajdusek DC. Localisation of amyloidogenic proteins and sulfated glycosaminoglycans in nontransmissible and transmissible cerebral amyloidoses. Acta Neuropathol 1991; 82: 87-92.

90 Bugiani O, Giaccone G, et al. βPP participates in PrP-amyloid plaques of Gerstmann-Sträussler-Scheinker disease, Indiana kindred. J Neuropathol Exp Neurol 1993; 52: 64-70

91 Lantos PL, McGill IS, Janota I, et al. Prion protein immunocytochemistry helps to establish the true incidence of prion diseases. Neurosci Lett 1992; 147: 67-71.

92 Hashimoto K, Mannen T, Nobuyuki N. Immunohistochemical study of kuru plaques using antibodies against synthetic prion protein peptides. Acta Neuropathol 1992; 83: 613-67

93 Kitamoto T, Shin R, Doh-ura K, et al. Abnormal isoform of prion proteins accumulates in the synaptic structures of the CNS in patients with Creutzfeldt-Jakob disease. Am J Pathol 1992; 140: 1285-1294.

94 McBride PA, Bruce ME, Fraser H. Immunostaining of cerebral amyloid plaques with antisera raised to scrapie associated fibrils (SAF). Neuropathol Appl Neurobiol 1988; 14: 325-336.

95 Clinton J, Lantos PL, Rossor M, Mullan M, Roberts GW. Immunocytochemical confirmation of prion protein. Lancet 1991; 336: 515.

96 Diringer H, Rahn HC, Bode L. Antibodies to protein of scrapie-associated fibrils. Lancet 1984; ii: 345.

97 Serban D, Taraboulos A, DeArmond SJ, Prusiner SB. Rapid detection of Creutzfeldt-Jakob disease and scrapie prion proteins. J Neuropathol Exp Neurol 1990; 49: 290.

98 Jeffrey M, Wilesmith JW. Idiopathic brainstem neuronal chromatolysis and hippocampal sclerosis: a novel encephalopathy in clinically suspect cases of bovine spongiform encephalopathy. Vet Rec 1992; 131: 359-362.

99 Diedrich JF, Bendheim PE, Kim YS, Carp RI, Haase AT. Scrapie-associated prion protein accumulates in astrocytes during scrapie infection. Proc Nat Acad Sci USA 1991; 88: 375-379.

100 Peiffer J, Doerr-Schott J, Tateishi J. Immunohistochemistry with anti-prion protein 27-30 gives reactions with fungi. Acta Neuropathol 1992; 84: 346-347.

101 Will RG, Matthews WB. A retrospective study of Creutzfeldt-Jakob disease in England and Wales 1970-79 I: Clinical features. J Neurol Neurosurg Psychiatry 1984; 47: 134-140.

102 Mizutani T, Shiraki H, eds. Clinicopathological aspects of Creutzfeldt-Jakob disease. Amsterdam: Elsevier, and Nishimura Niigata 1985.

103 Kitamoto T, Doh-ura K, Muramoto T, Miyazono M, Tateishi J. The primary structure of the prion protein influences the distribution of abnormal prion protein in the CNS. Am J Pathol 1992; 141: 271-277.

104 Collee JG. Foodborne illness: Bovine spongiform encephalopathy. Lancet 1990; 336: 1300-1303.
105 Hsiao KK, Doh-ura K, Kitamoto T, Tateishi J, Prusiner SB. A prion protein amino acid substitution in ataxic Gerstmann-Straussler syndrome. Ann Neurol 1989; 26: 137.
106 Brown P, Goldfarb LG, Brown WT, et al. Clinical and molecular genetic study of a large German kindred with Gerstmann-Straussler-Scheinker syndrome. Neurology 1991; 41: 375-379.
107 Bernouilli C, Siegfried J, Baumgartner G et al. Danger of accidental person to person transmission of Creutzfeldt-Jakob disease by surgery. Lancet 1977; i: 438-439.
108 Duffy P, Wolf J, Collins G, De Voc AG, Streeten B, Cowen D. Possible person to person transmission of Creutzfeld-Jakob disease. N Engl J Med 1974; 290: 692-693.
109 Brown P, Gajdusek DC, Gibbs CJ, Asher DM. Potential epidemic of Creutzfeldt-Jakob disease from human growth hormone therapy. N Engl J Med 1985; 313: 728-731.
110 Gibbs CJ, Joy A, Heffner R, et al. Clinical and pathological features and laboratory confirmation of Creutzfeld-Jakob disease in a recipient of pituitary-derived human growth hormone. N Eng J Med 1985; 313: 734-738.
111 Collinge J, Palmer MS, Dryden AJ. Genetic predisposition to iatrogenic Creutzfeldt-Jakob disease. Lancet 1991; 337: 1441-1442.
112 Hansen LA, Masliah E, Terry RD, Mirra SS. A neuropathological subset of Alzheimer's disease with concomitant Lewy body disease and spongiform change. Acta Neuropathol 1989; 78: 194-201.
113 Burkhardt CR, Filley CM, Kleinschmidt-DeMasters BK, de la Monte S, Norenberg MD, Schneck SA. Diffuse Lewy body disease and progressive dementia. Neurology 1988; 38: 1520-1528.
114 Probst A, Langui D, Ulrich J. Alzheimer's disease. A description of the structural lesions. Brain Pathol 1991; 1: 229-239.
115 Miyazono M, Kitamoto T, Iwaki T, Tateishi J. Colocalization of prion protein and β protein in the same amyloid plaques in patients with Gerstmann-Stäussler syndrome. Acta Neuropathol 1992; 83: 333-339.
116 Lowe J, Errington DR, Lennox G, et al. Ballooned neurons in several neurodegenerative diseases and stroke contain αB crystallin. Neuropathol Appl Neurobiol 1992; 18: 341-350.
117 Narang HK, Perry RH. Diagnosis of Creutzfeldt-Jakob disease by electron microscopy. Lancet 1990; 335: 663-664.

British Medical Bulletin (1993) Vol. 49, No. 4, 778–791
©The British Council 1993

Scrapie pathogenesis

J R Scott
AFRC and MRC Neuropathogenesis Unit, Institute for Animal Health, Edinburgh, UK

There is no specific marker for scrapie infectivity, and therefore no means other than prolonged bioassay for estimating levels of infection in tissues. Our knowledge of replication dynamics depends on precise rodent models which have enabled us to determine how the disease spreads and in which cells it replicates. We know, firstly, that infection replicates in the lymphoreticular system, and can identify a candidate cell; secondly, the factors which control the length of the disease process, and how difficult it is to influence this; thirdly, that clinical disease depends on access to the nervous system, and that once neuroinvasion has occurred, the spread of infectivity in both PNS and CNS is along neuroanatomical pathways at a similar rate to slow axonal transport in uninfected mice. Infecting the visual pathways of the CNS through the retina has shown that spongiform pathology occurs as a consequence of replication, and that the *Sinc* gene, which has a major effect on incubation period length in mice, acts by controlling the initiation, but not the rate, of replication. The localisation of PrP, a host protein of unknown function which accumulates in an abnormal form in diseased animals provides an important pointer to pathogenetic mechanisms.

DEFINING PATHOGENESIS

Information about how scrapie spreads and replicates is difficult to gather, largely because the agent is as yet uncharacterised. This means that there is no specific marker for infectivity and that the dynamics of replication can only be estimated by using prolonged bioassays; the mechanism of replication is not known. However, experimental studies using scrapie in rodents have given us many precise models which have generated our current knowledge. The time-course of the disease in laboratory mice can range from 120 days up to mouse life-span depending on the model selected, and it is strictly determined by 4 factors: the site and dose of infection, the strain of scrapie and the genotype of the mouse.

The site of infection determines whether the disease progresses through a phase of replication in the lymphoreticular system, or gains direct access to the nervous system; peripheral and central routes of infection, and the opportunities they offer for interference in the disease process are examined in detail later. One of the enigmas of this disease is that no immune response has been identified.[1]

The precise dose-dependence of the incubation period enables us, as with conventional viruses, to calculate the amount of infectivity in a given tissue in one of two ways. Serial 10-fold dilutions of a tissue homogenate can be injected into groups of recipient mice, and the level of infectivity in the tissue estimated from the ID_{50} (infectious dose, i.e. amount needed to infect 50% of the mice in a group). Mice are killed when clinical disease becomes apparent; the time between infection and killing is defined as the incubation period. The mean incubation periods of these mice provide us with a dose-response (D/R) curve; Figure 1 compares an intracerebral (i.c.) with an intraperitoneal (i.p.) route of infection. Comparison of D/R curves generated by different routes of infection can indicate differences in the mechanism of pathogenesis.

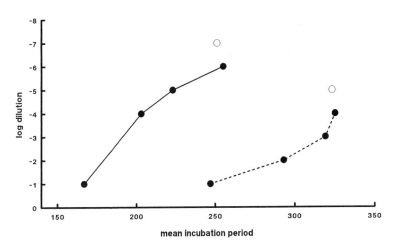

Fig. 1 Dose-response curves for C57BL mice infected intracerebrally (solid line) or intraperitoneally (broken line) with ME7 scrapie. Open symbols show groups in which there were survivors.

Alternatively, infectivity can be estimated by comparing the mean incubation period of a single group of mice which received the same dilution of tissue homogenate with an appropriate D/R curve. Using both methods, the results are expressed as the number of i.c. ID_{50} infectious units either in the infectious dose or per g of tissue. Assays of visual system tissues by both methods give very similar results.[2] However, the importance of using an appropriate D/R curve, i.e. one derived from the tissue being assayed, has been highlighted by Robinson et al.[3] who detected a difference between brain and spleen dilution kinetics using the 263K strain of scrapie in hamsters. This model has the shortest known scrapie incubation period of around 70 days following high-dose intracerebral infection, and produces very high infectivity titres in CNS[4] (around 10^{10} i.c. ID_{50} infectious units per g). A modified incubation period assay has been developed for this model.[5]

The third factor which has an influence on the incubation period length is scrapie strain. Over 15 strains have been isolated in inbred mice from naturally occurring cases in sheep and goats, on the basis of their incubation periods and pattern of vacuolar lesion distribution (see Bruce, this issue).

Mouse genotype is the fourth factor: timing of clinical disease is controlled largely by the *Sinc* gene, although its mode of action is not known. Inbred mice carry either the s7 or p7 allele of this gene, and mouse lines congenic for *Sinc* have been produced in this laboratory.[6] Restriction fragment length polymorphism and DNA sequencing analysis have shown linked differences in the PrP gene.[7] The PrP protein for which it codes is a host protein which becomes more resistant to proteases as a consequence of infection with scrapie or any of the spongiform encephalopathies. The normal metabolic turnover of PrP appears to be compromised by the disease process, and it aggregates to form deposits in a scrapie strain-specific manner. This has provided a valuable early indicator of pathological change (see Fraser and Jeffrey, this issue). Evidence from transgenic mouse studies suggests that PrP is the *Sinc* gene product;[8] however, the congruency of the *Sinc* and PrP genes remains uncertain.[7] In practice, when mice of the 3 *Sinc* genotypes (the s7 and p7 alleles and their F_1 cross) are infected with the same strain of scrapie, the result is three distinctive, reproducible incubation period groups.[9] The order in which the three genotypes produce disease depends on the strain of scrapie.[6]

Once these 4 parameters have been selected, the disease progresses asymptomatically, with uncanny precision, until the terminal stage is reached. The range of individual incubation periods for any group of mice receiving the same treatment is between 1% and 2% of the mean. Although we have no detailed explanation for either the length or precision of scrapie models, studies of pathogenesis have revealed some of the constraints on the spread and replication of infectivity.

PERIPHERAL PATHOGENESIS

Peripheral routes of infection have been used to establish the sequence of events preceding infection of the CNS. The involvement of the lymphoreticular system (LRS) in pathogenesis was established in the 1960s by Eklund et al,[10] who showed that following subcutaneous infection of mice, infection is initially detected in the spleen, and subsequently in lymph nodes, thymus and salivary glands, before spreading to the spinal cord and brain. Many other studies, notably by Kimberlin and Walker[11] have substantiated these results, and the importance of the spleen as a site of replication has been demonstrated by the prolongation of incubation period following intraperitoneal infection of splenectomised[12,13] or genetically asplenic mice.[14] However, the absence of the spleen does not affect all peripheral routes and not all strains of scrapie produce this effect (see review by Fraser et al[15]) Following subcutaneous injection of mink with transmissible mink encephalopathy, for example, peripheral replication is confined to the lymph nodes draining the site of infection, and replication only occurs in the remainder of the LRS after infection has been detected in CNS.[16] Cervical lymph nodes are the primary site of peripheral replication following intraocular infection (J Scott, unpublished observation). Similarly, replication is initiated almost immediately in Peyer's patches following oral (intragastric) infection with 139A scrapie; spleen titres increase subsequently, but the incubation period is unaffected by splenectomy.[17] The disease-specific form of PrP has been detected in spleen early in the incubation period using immunoblotting techniques, indicating a close relationship between this protein and replication.[18,19]

The extent to which replication in the LRS determines incubation period was demonstrated by Kimberlin and Walker,[20] who compared 6 scrapie models infected by the intraperitoneal route. They concluded that once scrapie spread to the PNS, within days to weeks of infection, pathogenesis was decreed by neural replication, and that the length of the incubation period could be predicted from the timing of the initial detection of infectivity in the brain. However, the potential for neuroinvasion varies with the strain of scrapie, and peripheral infection with a long incubation period model can produce chronic infection of the LRS for long periods of time before CNS involvement.[21] This has implications for the natural transmission of scrapie if sheep can harbour infection in the LRS which does not develop into clinical disease within the ovine life span.[22]

In general, the extent of peripheral pathogenesis appears to be determined by the availability of replication sites within a tissue, and the potential for neuroinvasion. For example, immediately following intravenous infection, relatively high levels of infectivity can be recovered from liver compared with spleen.[23] But no detectable replication takes place in liver, from which scrapie is presumably degraded or expelled, although the spleen titres rise steadily. Although peripheral routes have different efficiencies of infection with 139A scrapie, the D/R curves are all similar (but unlike the intracerebral one), suggesting a common pathogenetic mechanism.[24] This mechanism can be modified at the time of infection by a range of treatments: mitogens such as phytohaemaglutinin,[25] methanol extract of BCG[26] and vaccinia virus[27] increase the effective titre and shorten the incubation period, while some immunosuppressants,[28,29] and polyanions such as HPA-23[30,31] and dextran sulphate[31,32] have the opposite effect. None of these treatments influence the disease following intracerebral infection. When mice homozygous for the SCID (severe combined immunodeficiency) gene are infected with Creutzfeldt-Jakob disease (CJD), the peripheral component of pathogenesis is eliminated,[33] suggesting that the sites of lymphoreticular replication are absent in these mice. The intracerebral incubation period remains unaffected. This result has recently been repeated using ME7 scrapie in this laboratory (H Fraser, personal communication).

The role of haematogenous spread in the dissemination of infection within the visceral tissues is not clear. With the 139A strain of scrapie, there is a transient viremia at the time of peripheral infection which could well be important in establishing infection throughout the lymphoreticular system,[23] and a persistent viremia can be detected in mice injected with the Fu strain of CJD.[34] Intravenous infection is the most efficient peripheral route producing shorter incubation periods than intraperitoneal or subcutaneous infection.[24] However, there is no evidence for direct infection of the CNS by a haematogenous route. Some tissues, including the capillary endothelial cells in the CNS, appear to be capable of holding detectable amounts of infectivity, but do not appear to sustain replication.[35]

Where are the sites of replication in the lymphoreticular system? Extensive studies involving irradiation of mice before and after infection had no effect on pathogenesis, indicating that replication must take place in a population of cells which are non-dividing, long-lived cells.[36] The previous suggestion of follicular dendritic cells, a radiation resistant cell population found in the spleen and lymph nodes[37,38] has recently been substantiated by the immunolabelling of these cells with antisera to PrP.[33,39] Follicular dendritic cells are not found in the thymus or in some other non-neural tissues where replication is known to occur; but these tissues contain unidentified, PrP-positive cells.[39] The precise role of the follicular dendritic cell in peripheral pathogenesis remains to be clarified.

In general, lymphoreticular tissues have a meagre innervation; however evidence from various peripheral routes indicates that infection of the PNS determines the route to the CNS. A series of studies by Kimberlin and Walker (*see* review[40]) have demonstrated that following intraperitoneal infection with 139A scrapie, infectivity spreads from spleen and visceral lymph nodes to the thoracic spinal cord, probably through the sympathetic innervation. As previously mentioned, Peyer's patches are the initial site of replication following intragastric infection, from where infectivity spreads to thoracic cord, either via the lymphoid innervation, or directly through nerve endings in the gut.[17] Mild scarification of the skin preceding topical application of infection has been shown in this laboratory to be as effective as intraperitoneal injection in establishing infection (DM Taylor, I McConnell, unpublished observation), probably by facilitating direct infection of nerve endings. It is impossible with many peripheral routes to determine whether CNS infection is directly through neural routes, or if there is a prerequisite for lymphoreticular involvement. SCID mice will be invaluable for future studies in this area.

CENTRAL PATHOGENESIS

Access of infection to replication sites in the CNS appears to be either through the PNS or by direct injection of the CNS. Kimberlin and Walker[41] have shown that the period during which infectivity can be detected in the CNS is shorter when infection is via the PNS, suggesting that this route targets the spread of disease more quickly to vital CNS areas, which they termed clinical target areas. They then substantiated this observation by demonstrating that direct infection of the spinal cord is the only route which will give shorter than intracerebral incubation periods.[42] These findings suggest that the spread of infection within the CNS is restricted to neural pathways, and many subsequent studies have confirmed this. Infection of 5 precise brain areas with 3 strains of scrapie using stereotaxic techniques results in significant changes in incubation period length,[43] and sagittal bisection prior to unilateral infection of the cerebellum prolongs the incubation period and delays the development of vacuolar lesions on the contralateral side.[44] The most fruitful route of infection, however, is via the eye, enabling us to exploit one of the best understood neuroanatomical systems in the CNS. Using this route, Fraser demonstrated that both pathology[45] and

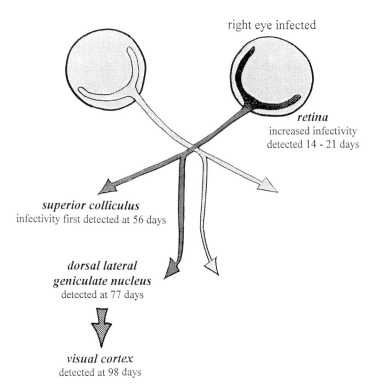

right eye infected

retina
increased infectivity
detected 14 - 21 days

superior colliculus
infectivity first detected at 56 days

dorsal lateral
geniculate nucleus
detected at 77 days

visual cortex
detected at 98 days

Fig. 2 The sequence of detection of infectivity in the neuroanatomical projections of the murine retina determined by tissue assays taken from C57BL mice infected with ME7 scrapie by an intraocular route.

infectivity[46] can be targeted to the neuroanatomical projections of the murine retina (indicated in Fig. 2), and similar findings have been obtained using hamster scrapie models.[47,48] Sequential assays of the visual system projections were made, using a standard murine model of ME7 scrapie in *Sinc* s7 mice, which has an incubation period of around 240 days following intraocular (i.o.) infection.[2] The ME7 titre increased in the retina between 14 and 21 days (above the background level of residual injected inoculum), and was first detected in the superior colliculus (SC) at 56 days, the dorsal lateral geniculate nucleus (dLGN) at 77 days and the optic nerves and visual cortex at 98 days. The level of infectivity in these areas tended to rise rapidly up to between 100 and

140 days; subsequently, a plateau titre of around $10^{4,5}$ i.c. ID_{50} units per injected dose was maintained in retina, SC and optic nerve. Infection in the dLGN and visual cortex continued to rise gradually, which was probably an artefact stemming from the relatively crude dissection of these tissues. The titre in optic nerve was over a log lower than in other tissues; this and the relatively late detection of infectivity in optic nerve suggests that replication does not take place in the axons but in the cell bodies or neurite terminals.[2,48]

This progression of infection is entirely consistent with the antero-grade spread of infection through neuroanatomical pathways; however the time periods involved are much longer than for conventional viruses in the same system; for example, herpes simplex virus (type 2) can be detected in the SC and dLGN from 3 days after intraocular infection.[49] We know from assays of retina following i.c. infection with ME7 and 79A strains that infection can be detected at 60 but not at 20 days, indicating that retrograde spread of infection can also occur.[2] Further evidence for neural spread of infection has come from mice treated as neonates with monosodium glutamate, which results in a degeneration of the retinal ganglion cells, the axons of which form the optic nerve. There was a marked reduction in the severity of the retinopathy which is a primary lesion with the 79A strain following i.c. infection of these mice, and the i.o. incubation period was prolonged.[50]

What can the i.o. route tell us about the rate of spread of infection? When the infected eye was removed at intervals from 12 h to 28 days post-infection, it was found that at least a 14 day period was required to establish infection in the superior colliculus.[51] Mice enucleated before 14 days developed scrapie after a much prolonged incubation period typical of a peripheral infection, and also lacked the asymmetrical lesions which indicate direct infection via the optic nerve. A period of 14 days represents an overall transport rate of slightly over 1 mm per day; this suggests an association with the slow axonal transport rate, which is between 0.5 and 2 mm per day in the normal murine optic nerve, where it is concerned with the translocation of cytoskeletal elements such as tubulin and the MAP proteins.[52] This estimate is in accord with previous studies in CNS[53] and PNS.[54] The molecular and cellular mechanisms involved in the uptake and transport of infectivity in vivo are unknown; some clues from cell culture and immunolocalisation of PrP protein are discussed in the final section.

The pattern of the pathognomonic spongiform lesions of scrapie (see Fraser and Jeffrey, this issue) is definitive for each scrapie strain. Following i.o. infection with ME7 scrapie, these lesions appear about halfway through the incubation period in the same regions, and in the same sequence as infectivity. Lesions develop initially in the contralateral projection to the infected eye, either in SC or dLGN depending on the strain of scrapie, and become more widespread in both contra and ipsilateral sides of the brain during the second half of the incubation period.[45] The relationship between replication in the CNS and subsequent vacuolar pathology is difficult to clarify in the absence of a marker for replication sites. The close correlation demonstrated by i.o. infection suggests that vacuolation occurs as an eventual consequence of replication, in neurones where a high titre has been maintained for several weeks. If replication in clinical target areas in the brain induces clinical disease, then the lengthy delay between replication and its pathological sequelae could resolve the problem of clinical cases with little or no vacuolation which have been reported for scrapie and other spongiform encephalopathies.[55]

The limitations on pathogenesis of controlled neurone-to-neurone spread through neuroanatomical pathways is consistent with the protracted but predictable incubation periods of the spongiform encephalopathies, and the intraocular route has enabled us to identify some of these limitations in a simple neuronal relay. By using a PrP preparation to concentrate the infectious dose, we have shown that the prolongation of the i.o. incubation period, which is 30% to 60% longer than with an i.c. route in all mouse models, is an intrinsic effect of pathogenesis, and not solely due to restrictions on the dose which can be given by the i.o. route.[56] The *Sinc* gene is known from assays of whole brain homogenates to influence replication dynamics by delaying the initiation of replication in p7 mice.[57] When sequential infectivity levels in the visual projections of s7 and p7 mice infected with ME7 were compared, the results show that at each stage in the neuronal relay, replication was delayed by 60 to 100 days in the p7 mice, although the rate remained constant (Fig. 2).[2] If this delay in replication occurs at each junction in the route to the clinical target areas, then we can begin to visualise how the *Sinc*-mediated prolongation of incubation period would retain its precision.

Opportunities for interfering with central pathogenesis require more detailed knowledge of the mechanisms of replication and of infectivity transfer between cells. Treatment of hamsters with the antibiotic amphotericin B prolongs the i.c. incubation period of 263K scrapie,[58] although its mode of action is not known. It is suggested that it either modifies a scrapie receptor on target cells, delays replication, or interferes with the deposition of abnormal PrP.[59] One other way of prolonging pathogenesis in the CNS is by 'blocking' replication of a scrapie strain with a short incubation period by previous infection with a longer incubation period strain.[60] This finding suggests that there are a finite number of replication sites;[61] this idea is substantiated by the plateaux in infectivity levels in CNS which occur in the visual system,[2] and in several other scrapie models with the exception of the rapid 263K hamster model, where the rate of replication increases until death.[48]

CONCLUSION

Despite the difficulties of studying an unidentified agent, we know a great deal about the way in which pathogenesis is controlled both by the disease and its victims. The candidate cells for replication – the follicular dendritic cells in the LRS and the neurones in the CNS – share several features including being non-dividing and relatively radiation resistant, having a large surface area, and supporting a variety of complex functions. The immunolocalisation of infection-specific PrP on and in these cells[39,62] at the light microscope level supports the contention that this protein is closely related to replication. The function of this protein in the normal animal is unknown, although much is known of the structure of the gene and its polymorphisms (see Goldmann, this issue); the cellular and subcellular sites of accumulation of the abnormal protein are therefore regarded as important indications of its role in replication. However, the present evidence is conflicting: early accumulation of PrP in astrocytes following infection with 22L scrapie has given rise to the speculation that these cells are the site of replication.[63] In vitro studies using mouse neuroblastoma cells infected with a Chandler-derived scrapie strain have indicated that the conversion of normal PrP to infection-specific PrP is associated with the plasma membrane or an endocytotic pathway[64] (see also Caughey and Race, this issue). However, similar investigations using a novel hamster brain cell line infected with 263K scrapie found infection-specific PrP confined to the cytoplasm, and particularly to the Golgi complex.[65] At an ultrastructural level, PrP in brain sections has been localised in lysosomes in mice infected with ME7 scrapie,[66] and alternatively to plasmalemma in mice infected with 87V scrapie.[67] The latter observation makes it tempting to speculate that following axonal transport of infectivity in association with cytoskeletal elements,[51] replication and the related conversion to infection-specific PrP occurs at the plasmalemma, since interactions of the plasma membrane and the cytoskeleton are known to be implicated in many cellular processes including specific recognition of cell surface molecules.[68] These conflicting observations may in part be due to the variety of models available as we have described here; different investigators tend to have their own preferred scrapie model.

The controversial question of whether infectious PrP molecules or prions are the sole progenitor of disease remains to be proven, even to the prion protagonists – 'whether prions are composed entirely of PrP^{sc} molecules or contain a second component needs to be resolved'.[69] Many transgenic mouse lines have recently been produced (see Prusiner, this issue) which demonstrate that the properties of infection-specific PrP depend on both the PrP transgene and the source of infection,[70] in the same way that infection of inbred mouse strains with different strains of scrapie produces the variety of scrapie models described earlier. It is interesting that mice lacking the PrP gene develop normally;[71] their long term response to infection is not yet known (see Weissmann, this issue). The mutation in the human PrP gene associated with Gerstmann-Straussler-Scheinker syndrome, an inherited disorder with similarities to CJD, has also been inserted into mice which subsequently developed spontaneous spongiform degeneration;[72] however PrP levels remained near normal, and the results of the attempted transmission from these mice have yet to be reported.

In many ways, the pathogenesis of scrapie still remains an enigma. Current theories on the nature of the infectious moiety and its means of replication[73,74] can draw on a vast range of experimental results dating back to the first sheep transmission in 1936,[75] many of which remain valid today. The future lies in examining at a cellular and molecular level the scrapie models with which we are most familiar and can precisely control the pathogenesis.

REFERENCES

1 Brown P. The phantasmagoric immunology of transmissible spongiform encephalopathy. In: Waksman BH, ed. Immunologic mechanisms in neurologic and psychiatric disease. New York: Raven Press, 1990: pp. 305-315.

2 Scott JR, Davies D, Fraser H. Scrapie in the central nervous system: neuroanatomical spread of infection and *Sinc* control of pathogenesis. J Gen Virol 1992; 73: 1637.

3 Robinson MM, Cheevers WP, Burger D et al. Organ-specific modification of the dose-response relationship of scrapie infectivity. J Infect Dis 1990; 161: 783.

4 Kimberlin RH, Walker CA. Characteristics of a short incubation period model of scrapie in the golden hamster. J Gen Virol 1977; 34: 295.

5 Prusiner SB, Cochran SP, Groth DF et al. Measurement of the scrapie agent using an incubation period time interval assay. Ann Neurol 1982; 11: 353.

6 Bruce ME, McConnell I, Fraser H et al. The disease characteristics of scrapie in *Sinc* congenic mouse lines: implications for the nature of the agent and the host control of pathogenesis. J Gen Virol 1991; 72: 595.

7 Hunter N, Dann JC, Bennett AD et al. Are *Sinc* and the PrP gene congruent? Evidence from PrP gene analysis in *Sinc* congenic mice. J Gen Virol 1992; 73: 2751.

8 Scott M, Foster D, Mirenda C et al. Transgenic mice expressing hamster prion protein produce species-specific scrapie infectivity and amyloid plaques. Cell 1989; 59:847.

9 Dickinson AG, Meikle VMH, Fraser H. Identification of a gene which controls the incubation period of some strains of scrapie in mice. J Comp Pathol 1968; 78: 293.

10 Eklund CM, Kennedy RC, Hadlow WJ. Pathogenesis of scrapie virus infection in the mouse. J Infect Dis 1967; 117: 15.

11 Kimberlin RH, Walker CA. Pathogenesis of experimental scrapie. In: Bock G, Marsh J, eds. Novel infectious agents and the central nervous system (Ciba Foundation Symposium 135). Chichester: Wiley, 1988: p 37.

SCRAPIE PATHOGENESIS   789

12 Fraser H, Dickinson AG. Pathogenesis of scrapie in the mouse: the role of the spleen. Nature 1970; 226: 462-463.
13 Kimberlin RH, Walker CA. The role of the spleen in the neuroinvasion of scrapie in mice. Virus Res 1989; 12: 201-212.
14 Dickinson AG, Fraser H. Scrapie: effect of Dh gene on incubation period of extraneurally injected agent. Heredity 1972; 29: 91.
15 Fraser H, Bruce ME, Davies D et al. The lymphoreticular system in the pathogenesis of scrapie. In: Prusiner SB, Collinge J, Powell J, Anderton B, eds. Prion diseases of humans and animals. New York: Ellis Horwood, 1992.
16 Hadlow WJ, Race RE, Kennedy RC. Temporal distribution of transmissible mink encephalopathy virus in mink inoculated subcutaneously. J Virol 1987; 61: 3235-3240.
17 Kimberlin RH, Walker CA. Pathogenesis of scrapie in mice after intragastric infection. Virus Res 1989; 12: 213-220.
18 Doi S, Shinagawa M, Sato G et al. Western blot detection of scrapie-associated fibril protein in tissues outside the central nervous system from preclinical scrapie-infected mice. J Gen Virol 1988; 69: 955-960.
19 Race RE, Ernst D. Detection of proteinase K-resistant prion protein and infectivity in mouse spleen by 2 weeks after scrapie agent inoculation. J Gen Virol 1992; 73: 3319-3323.
20 Kimberlin RH, Walker CA. Incubation periods in six models of intraperitoneally injected scrapie depend mainly on the dynamics of agent replication within the nervous system and not the lymphoreticular system. J Gen Virol 1988; 69: 2953-2960.
21 Bruce ME. Agent replication dynamics in a long incubation period model of mouse scrapie. J Gen Virol 1985; 66: 2517-2522.
22 Foster JD, Dickinson AG. The unusual properties of CH 1641, a sheep passaged isolate of scrapie. Vet Rec 1988; 123: 5-8.
23 Millson GC, Kimberlin RH, Manning EJ et al. Early distribution of radioactive liposomes and scrapie infectivity in mouse tissues following administration by different routes. Vet Microbiol 1979; 4: 89-99.
24 Kimberlin RH and Walker CA. Pathogenesis of mouse scrapie: effect of route of inoculation on infectivity titres and dose-response curves. J Comp Pathol 1978; 88: 39-47.
25 Dickinson AG, Fraser H, McConnell I et al. Mitogenic stimulation of the host enhances susceptibility to scrapie. Nature 1978; 272: 54-55.
26 Kimberlin RH, Cunnington PG. Reduction of scrapie incubation time in mice and hamsters by a single injection of methanol extraction residue of BCG. FEBS Microbiol Lett 19 ; 3: 169-172.
27 Marsh RF. Effect of vaccinia-activated macrophages on scrapie infection in hamsters. Adv Exp Med Biol 1980; 134: 359-363.
28 Outram GW, Dickinson AG, Fraser H. Reduced susceptibility to scrapie in mice after steroid administration. Nature 1974; 249: 855-856.
29 Outram GW, Dickinson AG, Fraser H. Slow encephalopathies, inflammatory responses and arachis oil. Lancet 1975; i: 198.
30 Kimberlin RH, Walker CA. The antiviral compound HPA-23 can prevent scrapie when administered at the time of infection. Arch Virol 1983; 78: 9-18.
31 Kimberlin RH, Walker CA. Suppression of scrapie infection in mice by heteropolyan-ion 23, dextran sulphate and some other polyanions. Antimicrob Agents Chemother 1986; 30: 409-413.
32 Farquhar CF, Dickinson AG. Prolongation of scrapie incubation period by an injection of dextran sulphate 500 within a month before or after infection. J Gen Virol 1986; 67: 463-473.
33 Kitamoto T, Muramoto T, Mohri S. Abnormal isoform of prion protein accumulates in follicular dendritic cells in mice with Creutzfeldt-Jakob disease. J Virol 1991; 65: 6292-6295.
34 Kuroda Y, Gibbs C, Amyx HL et al. Creutzfeldt-Jakob disease in mice: persistent viremia and preferential replication of virus in low density lymphocytes. Inf and Immun 1983; 41: 154-161.

35 Diringer H. Sustained viremia in experimental hamster scrapie. Arch Virol 1984; 82: 105-109.
36 Fraser H, Davies D, McConnell I et al. Are radiation-resistant, post-mitotic, long-lived (RRPMLL) cells involved in scrapie replication? In: Court LA, Dormont D, Brown P, Kingsbury DT, eds. Unconventional virus diseases of the central nervous system. Fontenay-aux-Roses: Commissariat a l'Energie Atomique: pp. 563-574.
37 Clarke MC, Kimberlin RH. Multiplication of scrapie agent in mouse spleen. Res Vet Sci 1984; 9: 215-225.
38 Fraser H, Farquhar CF. Ionising radiation has no effect on scrapie incubation period in mice. Vet Microbiol 1987; 13: 32-41.
39 McBride PA, Eikelenboom P, Kraal G et al. PrP protein is associated with follicular dendritic cells of spleens and lymph nodes in uninfected and scrapie-infected mice. J Pathol 1992; 168: 413-418.
40 Kimberlin RH, Walker CA. Pathogenesis of experimental scrapie. In: Bock G, Marsh J, eds. Novel infectious agents and the central nervous system. Ciba Foundation Symposium 135, Chichester: Wiley, 1988.
41 Kimberlin RH, Walker CA. Invasion of the CNS by scrapie agent and its spread to different parts of the brain. In: Court LA, ed. Virus non-conventionnels et affections du systeme nerveux central. Paris: Masson, 1983, pp. 15-33.
42 Kimberlin RH, Cole S, Walker CA. Pathogenesis of scrapie is faster when infection is intraspinal instead of intracerebral. Microb Pathogen 1987; 2: 405-415.
43 Kim YS, Carp RI, Callahan SM et al. Incubation periods and survival times for mice injected stereotaxically with three scrapie strains in different brain regions. J Gen Virol 1987; 68: 695-702.
44 Kim YS, Carp RI, Callahan SM. Pathogenesis and pathology of scrapie after stereotactic injection of strain 22L in intact and bisected cerebella. J Neuropath Exp Neurol 1990; 49: 114-121.
45 Fraser H. Neuronal spread of scrapie agent and targeting of lesions within the retinotectal pathway. Nature 1982; 295: 149-150.
46 Fraser H, Dickinson AG. Targeting of scrapie lesions and spread of agent via the retino-tectal projection. Brain Res 1985; 346: 32-41.
47 Buyukmihci N, Goering-Harmon F, Marsh RF. Neural pathogenesis of experimental scrapie after intraocular infection of hamsters. Exp Neurol 1983; 81: 396-406.
48 Kimberlin RH, Walker CA. Pathogenesis of scrapie (strain 263K) in hamsters infected intracerebrally, intraperitoneally or intraocularly. J Gen Virol 1986; 67: 255-263.
49 Kristensson K, Ghetti B, Wisniewski HM. Study on the propagation of herpes simplex virus (type 2) into the brain after intraocular injection. Brain Res 1974; 69: 189-201.
50 Foster JD, Scott JR, Fraser H. The use of monosodium glutamate in identifying neuronal populations in mice infected with scrapie. Neuropathol Appl Neurobiol 1990; 16: 423.
51 Scott JR, Fraser H. Enucleation after intraocular scrapie injection delays the spread of infection. Brain Res 1989; 504: 301.
52 Grafstein B, Forman DS. Intracellular transport in neurons. Physiol Rev 1980; 60: 1167-1283.
53 Kimberlin RH, Walker CA. Pathogenesis of mouse scrapie: patterns of agent replication in different parts of the CNS following intraperitoneal infection. J R Soc Med 1982; 75: 618-624.
54 Kimberlin RH, Hall SM, Walker CA. Pathogenesis of mouse scrapie; evidence for direct neural spread of infection to the CNS after infection of the sciatic nerve. J Neurol Sci 1983; 61: 315-325.
55 Taylor DM. Spongiform encephalopathies. Neuropath Appl Neurobiol 1991; 17: 345-346.
56 Scott JR, Reekie LJD, Hope J. Evidence for intrinsic control of scrapie pathogenesis in the murine visual system. Neurosci Lett 1991; 133: 141.
57 Dickinson AG, Meikle VMH, Fraser H. Genetical control of the concentration of ME7 scrapie agent in the brain of mice. J Comp Path 1969; 79: 15-22.

58 Pocchiari M, Scmittinger S, Masullo C. Amphoteracin B delays the incubation period of scrapie in intracerebrally inoculated hamsters. J Gen Virol 1987; 68: 219.
59 Xi YG, Ingrosso L, Ladogano A et al. Amphoteracin B treatment dissociates in vivo replication of the scrapie agent from PrP accumulation. Nature 1992; 356:598.
60 Dickinson AG, Fraser H, Meikle VM et al. Competition between different scrapie strains in mice. Nature 1972; 237: 244-245.
61 Dickinson AG, Outram GW. The scrapie replication-site hypothesis and its implications for pathogenesis. In: Prusiner SB, Hadlow WJ, eds. Slow transmissible diseases of the nervous system, vol. 2. New York: Academic Press, 1979; pp. 13-31.
62 Bruce ME, McBride PA, Farquhar CF. Precise targeting of the sialoglycoprotein, PrP, and vacuolar degeneration in mouse scrapie. Neurosci Lett 1989; 102: 1-6.
63 Diedrich JF, Bendheim PE, Kim YS et al. Scrapie-associated prion protein accumulates in astrocytes during scrapie infection. Proc Natl Acad Sci 1991; 88: 375.
64 Caughey B, Raymond GJ, Ernst D. N-terminal truncation of the scrapie-associated form of PrP by lysosomal protease(s): implications regarding the site of conversion of PrP to the protease resistant state. J Virol 1991; 65: 6597-6603.
65 Taraboulos A, Serban D, Prusiner SB. Scrapie prion proteins accumulate in the cytoplasm of persistently infected cultured cells. J Cell Biol 1990; 110: 2117-2132.
66 Lowe J, Fergusson J, Kenward N et al. Immunoreactivity to ubiquitin-protein conjugates is present early in the disease process in the brains of scrapie-infected mice. J Pathol 1992; 168: 169-177.
67 Jeffrey M, Goodsir CM, Bruce ME et al. Infection specific prion protein (PrP) accumulates on neuronal plasmalemma in scrapie infected mice. Neurosci Lett 1992; 147: 106.
68 Carraway CAC. Association of cytoskeletal proteins with membranes. In: Carraway KL, Carraway CAC, eds. The cytoskeleton. Oxford: IRL Press, 1992: pp. 123-150.
69 Prusiner SB. Prion biology. In: Prusiner SB, Collinge J, Powell J, Anderton B, eds. Prion diseases of humans and animals. New York: Ellis Horwood, 1992: pp. 533-567.
70 Prusiner SB, Scott M, Foster D et al. Transgenetic studies implicate interactions between homologous PrP isoforms in scrapie prion replication. Cell 1990; 63: 673.
71 Bueler H, Fischer M, Lang Y et al. Normal development and behaviour of mice lacking the neuronal cell-surface PrP protein. Nature 1992; 356: 577.
72 Hsaio K, Scott M, Foster D. Spontaneous neurodegeneration in transgenic mice with mutant prion protein. Science 1990; 250: 1587.
73 Weissman C. A 'unified theory' of prion propagation. Nature 1991; 352: 679-683.
74 Alper T. The infectivity of spongiform encephalopathies: does a modified membrane hypothesis account for lack of immune response? FEMS Microbiol Immunol 1992; 89: 235-242.
75 Cuille J, Chelle PL. La maladie dite tremblante du mouton est-elle inoculable? C R Acad Sci (Paris), 1936; 203: 1552-1554.

British Medical Bulletin (1993) Vol. 49, No. 4, pp. 792–809
©The British Council 1993

Diversity in the neuropathology of scrapie-like diseases in animals

H Fraser
AFRC & MRC Neuropathogenesis Unit, Institute for Animal Health, Edinburgh

The main diagnostic histology in the spongiform encephalopathies consists of a degenerative and usually symmetrical vacuolation of neurons and a spongiform lesion in the neuropil. Sometimes there can be asymmetry. This pathology is usually confined to grey matter, but an additional white matter vacuolation is sometimes typical. The degeneration can progress to neuronal necrosis, with reactive glial changes. Photoreceptor loss in the retina occurs in some experimental models. Cerebral amyloidosis is conspicuous in many types of scrapie-like pathology in animals, but is sometimes not recognised or may be absent. Abnormal immunolabelling with anti-PrP is always associated with both the degenerative and amyloid lesion and precedes the occurrence of the degeneration in experimental scrapie models. All aspects of the pathology are closely controlled by host genetic factors and by the strain of the infecting, causal agent.

The histopathology associated with scrapie-like diseases is confined to the central nervous system (CNS),[1] despite the occurrence and amplification of the infectious causal agent in non-nervous tissues such as in the lymphoid system. Thus, the progressive debility and loss of condition in the terminal disease is not associated with specific peripheral pathology, although the spleen can be atrophic in some experimentally infected rodents. In the naturally-occurring and induced scrapie-like diseases the CNS usually appears grossly normal, although an increase in the amount of cerebrospinal fluid is apparent at brain removal. This review is confined to microscopic changes recognised in the CNS, and is based on experimentally-induced pathology in rodents, but with some reference to scrapie-like diseases which occur spontaneously in several mammals. In all these the histopathology shares common, specific features. It is entirely degenerative and non-inflammatory, and therefore appears to lack any immunopathological pathogenesis. It is usually confined to grey matter where the typical lesion consists of vacuolation of neurons and spongiform degeneration of the neuropil. Some types of experimental scrapie, particularly some models in mice, include vacuolation in white matter. Although this is only seen in one or two models of scrapie, the most widely studied experimental form of murine scrapie shows this severe white matter vacuolar pathology. Amyloidosis in the form of plaques and associated with small blood vessels occurs in some models of scrapie. There is thus considerable diversity in the range and distribution of the degenerative and amyloid lesions. The biological basis of this diversity has been identified mainly in terms of genetic differences in the infected host and variation in the strain of the causal agent.[2-4]

NATURALLY-OCCURRING SCRAPIE-LIKE DISEASES

The neuropathology in haematoxylin or methylene blue and eosin stained sections from sheep and goats with scrapie, from bovine spongiform encephalopathy, and other ruminants such as mule deer, nyala, kudu, and from the scrapie-like disease reported in cats, is essentially similar[1,5] (Fig. 1). The most prominent and consistent degenerative pathology in sheep and the small reported number of goats affected with natural scrapie is the occurrence of single and multiple cytoplasmic vacuolation in neurons in spinal cord, medulla oblongata, pons and mid-brain, accompanied by other evidence of degeneration such as chromatolysis, cell shrinkage, neuron necrosis and neuronophagia, and Wallerian degeneration. Vacuoles often contain eosinophilic, floccular material. The commonly affected sites are the raphe, reticular formation, mesencephalic tegmentum, and the facial, lateral cuneate, dorsal vagal, ambiguus, superior olivary nuclei, and occasionally the red nucleus and cerebellum. The cerebrum is usually unaffected, and this probably accounts for the normal gross appearance of the brain, in contrast to the homologous disease in man, Creutzfeldt-Jakob disease (CJD), where cortical atrophy is sometimes striking. In all species this pathology is accompanied by astrocytic hypertrophy and sometimes hyperplasia, demonstrable with Cajal's stain and by anti-GFAP immunolabelling. In many cases a spongy vacuolation in the neuropil occurs in the brain stem and cranial neuraxis, septum, and hypothalamus.[6] A low incidence of vacuolated neurons occurs in apparently healthy sheep. Some scrapie affected sheep have cerebrovascular amyloid lesions, and these occur mainly in the forebrain basal ganglia.[7] In mule deer affected with chronic wasting disease (CWD) and mink with transmissible mink encephalopathy (TME), in domestic cats and a puma, forebrain and cerebral cortical spongiform lesions are prominent and extensive.[8-11] Field cases of scrapie in goats show severe vacuolar lesions throughout the neuraxis, and amyloid plaques,[12] which also occur in CWD.[13] Disease specific immunostaining with anti-PrP of the amyloid is reported in the goat and other species but the significance of PrP immunostaining in the neuroparenchyma is less clear as staining of normal nervous tissue is known to occur. The 'scrapie-specific' isoform of the PrP protein, and scrapie-associated fibrils (SAF) have been identified in BSE, in cats, kudu and other cases.[14,15]

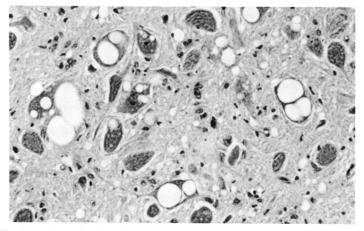

Fig. 1 Dorsal vagal nucleus from a nyala showing neuronal and neuropil vacuolation. Haematoxylin and eosin stain, magnification x 250.

A neurological disease in adult cows associated with chromatolysis of brain stem neurons and hippocampal sclerosis has emerged in the course of BSE diagnosis; there is no reason to suspect a scrapie-like cause.[16] Although the cause of a spongiform encephalopathy identified in ostriches has not been identified, the neuropathology described in these birds is suggestive of a scrapie-like process.[17] A similar uncertainty surrounds the occurrence of a slowly progressive disease in captive white tigers at Bristol Zoo. Spongiform neuropathology occurred, together with gliosis, but with hepatic pathology in some cases, and the survival of a small number of newborn mice injected intracerebrally with brain tissue from one affected tiger was shorter than that of sham-injected mice.[18]

EXPERIMENTAL SCRAPIE

Mice, hamsters, rats, gerbils, sheep, goats and several primate species have been used in experimental transmission studies. Work in mice and hamsters has contributed considerably both to understanding the basic neurobiology, pathogenesis and biochemistry of scrapie and its homologues and to their epidemiology.

The identification of scrapie strain variation has been established almost entirely with work in mice, in particular using strains carrying different alleles of the Sinc gene (*see* Bruce, this issue). There are major differences in lesion targeting between strains of scrapie, as well as between mouse strains, and it is this precise involvement of individual groups of neurons that provides strong evidence that the neuron is the primary candidate for the amplification of the infection and the consequent primary pathology. The very obvious neuronal pathology seen in the natural disease provides additional support for this conclusion, and this is strongly reinforced by a great deal of work in rodents. For instance, the quantitative loss of dendritic spines in Golgi preparations in hamsters suggests a primary neuron lesion,[19] and a loss of neurons has been found in vestibular nuclei in BSE.[20] Wallerian and nerve fibre degeneration occurs in sheep and mice which can be expected to arise both from neuron loss and local encephalopathy.[21] Neuroanatomical and neurochemical diversity provides the most parsimonious argument in advocating the neuron as the basis of differential lesion targeting. An alternative is that glia contribute to regional targeting, for instance in view of some evidence for regional heterogeneity in astrocytes.[22] This would imply a stricter association of these region specific glial properties with particular neuronal groups than is the case.

Lesion distribution differences in mice have been reviewed extensively elsewhere.[2,3,23] For example, depending on scrapie strain, the hippocampus can be unaffected, or develop vacuolar neuronal pathology with or without neuronal necrosis, which can progress to severe 'hippocampal sclerosis'. Or the degeneration can be confined very precisely to the CA2 sector of hippocampus.[2,24,25] The cerebellum is a major focus with the 22L scrapie strain, with which there is white matter vacuolation in some mouse strains but only cortical vacuolation in the molecular and granular layers in others.[2,26] Two strategies of directing the infection and neuropathogenesis directly into very restricted CNS sites have been developed, using intraocular or stereotactic injections,[27,28] which have shown that neurons can be permissive or non-permissive and that groups of neurons differ in the sequence of neuropathogenesis between strains of scrapie [29] (*see* Scott, this issue). Bioassay of discrete areas of the visual system following direct retinal exposure with two strains clearly demonstrates that the Sinc gene controls the initiation of neuronal infection and that spread of infection is restricted to neuroanatomical pathways.[30] Intracerebral injection or stereotaxic exposure of the cerebellum of mice to the 22L strain suggests axonal spread in and selective vulnerability of cerebellum to infection, and that lesion targeting is genetically controlled by Sinc or other host genes.[2,26,31,32] There are also differences in agent replication and degenerative pathology in the retina; the photoreceptor cells being selectively vulnerable to 79A scrapie which produces a severe retinopathy in all mouse strains.[30,33]

LESION PROFILES; QUANTIFICATION OF DEGENERATIVE PATHOLOGY

In view of the lack of in vitro assays of scrapie or strategy of strain discrimination using laboratory culture, the differences in disease manifestation or phenotype in mice has become pivotally important for strain identity, and therefore indirectly for epidemiology. Together with differences in incubation period in mice carrying different alleles of Sinc, the major and subtle differences in neuropathology are a major criterion of agent identity.[34] Therefore an objective means of representing quantitatively the intensity and localisation of the vacuolar and spongiform lesions in the grey and white matter has been established, called the 'lesion profile'.[2] The intensity of spongy change and vacuolation is scored in twelve brain regions on coded sections.[35] Each scrapie strain has its own characteristic and highly repeatable lesion profile.[36,37] Also a distinctive shape of lesion profile, for a scrapie strain, is found with particular mouse genotypes and route of injection; peripheral infection giving much less severe brain lesions and lower profiles than intracerebral infection. In experimental mixed scrapie agent infections, lesion profiles have identified the strain responsible for disease.[38,39] It has recently been shown that lesion profiles in mice infected with 'natural' scrapie and with BSE can provide important information about the identity, origin and epidemiology of the disease in individual animals.[40] The severity of cerebral amyloid and distribution of amyloid plaques also differ between scrapie and mouse strains.[4,41]

SYMMETRICAL AND ASYMMETRICAL LESIONS

Typically the distribution of spongiform degeneration shows strict symmetry but focal asymmetrical lesions occur frequently with some scrapie strains as well as at primary transmission to mice from field cases of scrapie and BSE[2, 40,42] (Fig. 2). The strains with which asymmetry is conspicuous, such as 87A, also produce severe cerebral amyloid. It has also been observed that focal asymmetry occurs with wild-type scrapie strains that are the precursors of mutant strains – the best studied example is the mutation of 87A to ME7,[34,43] although some could produce asymmetrical lesions but not 'viable' mutants. With 87A the asymmetrical lesions are seen in locations where degeneration is usually absent, such as thalamus, cerebral cortex, superior colliculus, dentate gyrus, and is sometimes associated with the needle scar of intracerebral injection. The probability is that asymmetrical focal lesions are sites of the local generation of the mutant strain.[2,42] Asymmetrical lesions can also be produced in retinal projection areas, as a result of monocular infection with several other scrapie strains.[27,29]

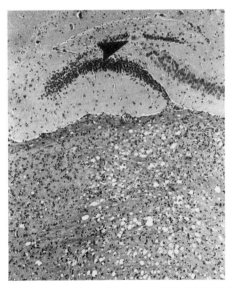

Fig. 2 Vacuolation in thalamus and amyloid plaque (arrow) in dentate gyrus granule cell layer in 87A-scrapie in a mouse. Haematoxylin and eosin stain, magnification x 50.

AMYLOID PLAQUES

Cerebral amyloidosis, in the form of discrete plaques and as small blood vessel-associated amyloid is a prominent lesion with infection with some scrapie strains in mice as well as in sheep and goat affected with natural scrapie, in CWD, and rarely in BSE.[1,12,13,44] There is no conspicuous cerebral amyloidosis with other mouse scrapie strains, in TME or in spongiform encephalopathy in cats, or in scrapie in hamsters, although very small periventricular PrP-staining deposits in hamsters and mice with these strains are designated 'amyloid'. Scrapie-associated amyloid immunolabels with anti-PrP wherever this has been attempted.[1,12,13,45] In mice the occurrence of plaque amyloid is under Sinc-independent host gene control.[46] Amyloid occurrence is not influenced by age in mice, and plaques are absent in very old normal mice.[47] However plaques, probably not containing PrP, have been identified in old rats, dogs, and monkeys.[48–50] In infection with 87A or 87V mouse scrapie, following intracerebral injection, large concentrations of plaque amyloid are situated in the periventricular areas associated with the lateral ventricles and in the corpus callosum. In addition, with any injection route, plaques occur prominently in forebrain regions where spongiform degeneration is inapparent with these strains. The cerebral cortex, hippocampus and dentate gyrus, thalamus and midbrain are the areas most affected, but plaques also occur in the cerebellum, brain stem and spinal cord[4,41,51] (Fig. 2). The pathogenesis of plaque formation, and the reason that plaques are absent or rare in some scrapie models, is not known. There is evidence of neuroanatomical relationships between brain areas undergoing degeneration and areas of amyloidosis. One suggestion ('network hypothesis') is that loss of innervation resulting from degeneration of afferent neurons causes a failure of removal of a plaque precursor (PrP) produced by normal neurons in the vicinity of plaques,[3] while plaques in a periventricular location following intracerebral infection are probably associated with a migration pathway of glial cells following their reaction to the initial injection procedure.

NEUROANATOMICAL PROJECTION PATHWAYS IN SCRAPIE PATHOLOGY AND NEUROPATHOGENESIS

In mice, the intraocular route of infection produces discrete spongiform pathology in the projections which are innervated from the retina.[27,30] Monocular injection of Sinc s7 mice with a high dose of the ME7 scrapie strain, for example, produces the first lesions after 110–120 days in the contralateral superior colliculus (sc). This is halfway through the incubation period of about 240 days. Lesions in the dorsal lateral geniculate nucleus (dlgn) appear about 20 days later. The sc is also affected before the dlgn with the 22L scrapie strain, but lesions in the dlgn precede those in the sc with the 87V, 22A, 22C and 79A strains. Scrapie strains show a consistent preference between one or the other of these two areas, independently of the host's Sinc genotype. As the dlgn and sc receive their retinal innervation from branches of the same ganglion cell axons, the most parsimonious basis for these differences must lie in the target neurons in sc and dlgn. With ME7 infection spongiform lesions start to appear in the visual cortex of the cerebrum from about 190 days. The timing is in direct proportion to the incubation period which varies with the strain of scrapie and the Sinc genotype of the host (*see* Bruce, this issue). Thus the first contralateral lesions in the central retinal target nuclei occur at around 260 days in Sinc p7 mice (VMs) and even later at about 400 days in the sc of Sinc s7 mice (C57BLs).[29] As the sc may not be a permissive site for the 87A strain, the probability exists that the lesions here are due to the ME7 strain being generated as a mutant locally (*see* above 'symmetrical and asymmetrical lesions'). Biological assays of infectivity of precise locations in the visual system show that agent replication precedes the spongiform degeneration in the same locations, and that both events are directly controlled by Sinc,[30] (*see* Scott, this issue). A retinopathy, consisting of photoreceptor loss, occurs with the 79A scrapie strain, but not with ME7 in these mice,[52] and retinal agent titre is over tenfold higher in the former.[30] This, and the occurrence of retinopathy in mice maintained in the dark,[33] suggests that this is a direct consequence of replication of the infectious agent in retina.

PATHOLOGY REVEALED BY IMMUNOLABELLING THE PrP PROTEIN

A precise definition of scrapie and any related diseases must depend on an identification of unique molecular events, which can be distinguished from non-specific and reactive change which are absent in other diseases. There are now convincing reasons for thinking that the primary pathology is closely involved with PrP which is the normal host-coded glycoprotein of neuronal membranes and which assumes altered properties only in the scrapie-like diseases (*see* Goldman, this issue). An alteration of this normally soluble protein into insoluble protease-resistant forms, which can also be identified ultrastructurally as fibrils (scrapie-associated fibrils or SAF) in enriched fractions of affected and infected tissues is a highly specific diagnostic indicator of these diseases. In routine paraffin sections antisera raised to PrP contain antibodies which bind to small amyloid plaque-like structures in periventricular areas of formol-fixed brain of hamsters intracerebrally infected with 263K scrapie.[52] Much stronger immunolabelling of plaques is found in formol-fixed mouse brain affected with the strains scrapie (87A, 87V, 111A) which produce cerebral amyloidosis in conventional histology, and in other models with less conspicuous plaques (ME7 scrapie in Sinc p7 mice and 22A scrapie in Sinc s7 mice). Cerebral and perivascular amyloid in routine sections of sheep and goat scrapie also bind the antibody and pretreatment with formic acid intensifies the immunolabelling,[45] as is the case in Creutzfeldt-Jakob disease.[53] Much more informative PrP-immunostaining is obtained with mild perfusion or immersion fixation with periodate-lysine paraformaldehyde (PLP), when widespread staining of the protein occurs in the neuropil and neurons in those areas where vacuolation and glial reactions occur.[25, 54] Long before other morphological evidence of degeneration can be seen, the PrP-related neuropathology is targeted very precisely to those anatomically-defined areas which become affected in the terminal lesions. In models with restricted terminal lesions, abnormal PrP is restricted to these same sites, and in models with widespread pathology, such as ME7 scrapie, PrP-staining becomes diffuse in areas of spongy degeneration throughout the brain. Thus in the ME7 model the hippocampal staining, although not restricted to any sector, is concentrated in areas of the termination of the granule cell axons in all sectors. In contrast, in the 87V model PrP-staining is confined to, or intense in, the substantia nigra, the ventral pallidum, the ventral thalamic nuclei, the CA2 region of the hippocampus, the dorsal raphe and other discrete areas, and a very striking localisation of abnormal PrP staining is found on the neuronal perikarya and neuritic processes of some neurons. In the 87V model, staining of amyloid plaques is found much more widely than in routine sections, in the same areas as the neuroparenchymal staining but in other areas such as the cerebral cortex, hippocampus (outside CA2), and basal ganglia where diffuse staining and vacuolation are largely absent. Also PLP-fixation reveals PrP in neurons of mice which are not scrapie-infected.[25]

A method of regional mapping of the abnormal PrP-associated pathology in scrapie-infected hamsters, in transgenic mice expressing the hamster PrP gene, and in human CJD brain has been developed.[55] Cryostat sections are mounted on nitrocellulose membranes, protease-digested and immunolabelled with anti-PrP. The resulting 'histoblots', reveal different patterns of staining with two hamster scrapie strains. Also the soluble PrP in normal brains can be mapped if proteolysis is omitted. Immunolabelling of white matter tracts led to the suggestion that infection spreads along neuroanatomical pathways.[55] Histoblots also revealed localisation of β/A4-amyloid protein and abnormal PrP in Alzheimer's and Creutzfeldt-Jakob diseases. Although they lack the resolution of histological sections in which immunolabelling of individual cells is obtained, histoblots provide an elegant method for the topographical localisation of abnormal PrP and for demonstrating overall differences in distribution between strains and models of scrapie.

The very precise and reproducible targeting differences in abnormal PrP-localisation, with different strains and models of scrapie, provide clear evidence that the primary lesion and replication of infection is in the neuron itself. It is clear that neuronal PrP plays a central role in these events, not least because of its closeness or identity with the Sinc gene. However the basis of the differences in lesion targeting is not known and there must remain other unknown molecular abnormalities, with interactions with PrP, which dictate these differences (Fig. 3).

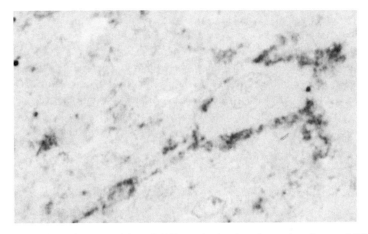

Fig. 3 Anti-PrP immunostaining of 87V-scrapie showing abnormal perineuronal PrP accumulation in lateral hypothalamus in the mouse. Immunostaining is visible on both sides of two neurites arising from the perikaryon, magnification x 1200.

REACTIVE AND SECONDARY PATHOLOGY

It is widely assumed that the primary molecular lesion in scrapie is neuronal, although the possibility that it also occurs in other cells in the CNS cannot be formally excluded. Precise, regional differences in lesion targeting, sometimes to very well defined nuclei or neuronal subgroups, point to a primary neuronal basis. Astrocytic hypertrophy and hyperplasia has been recognised in the neuropathology of these diseases and has been assumed to be a reactive change.[2] However the abnormal isoform of the PrP protein has been detected in astrocytes in mouse scrapie brain which has given rise to the suggestion that these cells have a primary role in pathogenesis,[56] but up-regulation of genes encoding, and translation into glial fibrillary protein, apolipoprotein, cathepsin D, αβ-crystallin, β2microglobulin and transferrin in scrapie and other neurodegenerative diseases[57] suggests that these are secondary. Abnormal immunoreactivity to ubiquitin-protein conjugates, associated with 'lysosome-related' bodies, are a comparatively early change in mouse scrapie, suggesting an intimate role for this pathway in the primary pathology of scrapie and other neurodegenerative disorders.[58,59] Other ultrastructural studies have failed to confirm an association between lysosomes and abnormal PrP immunolabelling but have shown an association with the plasmalemma of neurites, and this finding supports the view that the neuron is the primary site for scrapie neuropathogenesis.[60]

Amyloid plaques form from the deposition of the neuronal membrane PrP protein, including its proteinase-resistant form. The pathogenesis of this deposition is not known, although a contribution from microglial cells and of a haematogenous component has been suggested.[61] Several reports indicate a defect in blood-brain barrier permeability, but this has not been confirmed in murine scrapie.[62] Also, in contrast to AD in which it is suggested that plaque formation involves chronic inflammatory mediators, scrapie plaques do not contain complement factors or an association with microglial cells expressing class II MHC molecules.[63]

ULTRASTRUCTURE OF SCRAPIE NEUROPATHOLOGY

A scaling and sampling dilemma in any ultrastructural analysis of the neuropathology of scrapie arises from variation in the type and distribution of lesions between different models, and the long incubation periods. This diversity may explain some differences in interpretation of ultrastructure by different workers. For example and as described above, some strains of scrapie produce vacuolation largely confined to grey matter while others also produce severe white matter vacuolation and there are wide differences in targeting to particular groups of nerve cells; it is inconceivable therefore that such variation will not impose differences in ultrastructure and its interpretation. The changes which have been identified ultrastructurally include vacuolation of neuropil, amyloid plaques, neuronal autophagy, tubulovesicular bodies and dystrophic neurites. Immuno-electron microscopical techniques have allowed the identification of PrP in amyloid plaques, and have been developed to localise PrP in the neuroparenchyma. Scrapie associated fibrils (SAF or prion rods) are identified ultrastructurally in negatively-stained detergent extracts of infected brains.

Vacuolation has been identified predominantly in dendrites, axon terminals and neuronal perikarya and often contain membranous and granular intravacuolar debris.[60,64,65] However there is no consensus view on the sub-cellular origin or morphogenesis of vacuolation. Some studies have described vacuoles within processes limited by single membranes, while others have described double membrane bound vacuoles. These vacuoles have been interpreted as arising respectively in the smooth endoplasmic reticulum and in mitochondria. Some other vacuoles which lack any identifiable boundary other than the plasmalemma of the neurite, appear to arise from the dispersion of the cytoskeleton.[64,65] Large vacuoles in neurites impinge on adjacent vacuolated neurites and may appear to coalesce with adjacent vacuoles. Double, single membrane and unbounded vacuoles have been identified in an ME7 scrapie model.[66] In studies with other models and in CJD, intramyelinic vacuolation and vacuolation of the inner tongue of oligodendroglial cytoplasm is prominent. An important finding is a small number of vacuoles, indistinguishable from some in scrapie, in normal brain. But in scrapie these increase in frequency early in the incubation period.[66] Another important finding is the sudden increase in vacuole number, just as vacuolation becomes evident by light microscopy, and without any evidence of an obvious precursor of vacuolation. This suggests that vacuolation is a non-specific index of a crisis in neuronal homeostasis associated with the replication of the infective agent and correlated loss of particular functions.

Scrapie associated cerebral amyloid takes different forms.[51] Ultrastructurally, 'classical' plaques are composed of radiating bundles of closely packed filaments, with microglia, hypertrophic astrocytic processes, and dystrophic neurites, at the plaque periphery.[51,67] Diffuse plaques are found adjacent to the ependyma and pia and are composed of irregular and individual amyloid filaments in the extracellular space.[54] The bundles of filaments in classical plaques and single filaments immunostain for PrP.[52,60,68] It has been suggested that cerebral amyloid in scrapie is produced by microglia, but infection-specific accumulations of PrP occur as diffuse and granular accumulations in the neuropil, and immunoelectron microscopy has shown that PrP is located at the neuronal and neuritic plasmalemma both in the vicinity of plaques, at distances from them and in areas of degenerative pathology where both plaques and reactive microglia are remote or inconspicuous[60] (Fig. 4). This suggests that the primary lesion associated with a PrP abnormality is neuronal, that amyloid plaques occur as a consequence of neuronal dysfunction, and that any glial associations are secondary. Amyloid filaments are probably assembled from subunits of presumably normal host PrP located on the neuronal membrane.[60] However wide differences in the morphology of abnormal PrP, in the form of plaques remote from spongy degeneration or only demonstrable by immunolabelling in areas where degeneration occurs, remain to be explained.

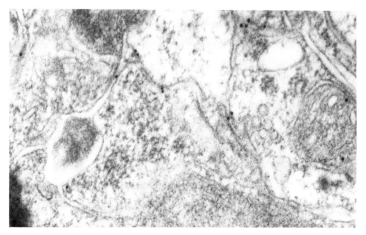

Fig. 4 Subcellular localisation of PrP on the neuronal plasmalemma in immunogold-stained lateral hypothalamus in 87V-scrapie in mouse. Magnification x 42 000.

In early reports a variety of particulate and tubulovesicular structures approximately 23–45nm diameter were reported.[69] In one report similar structures were described in spleen of scrapie infected mice.[70] Tubulovesicular bodies have been reported in axon terminals and neurites and in negatively stained 'touch preparations' of brain. Although their origin remains undetermined, they appear to become more frequent as the incubation period progresses.[71]

Dystrophic neurites, characterised by clusters of pleomorphic membrane bound dense bodies, have been identified throughout the neuropil of terminally diseased animals with scrapie and humans with CJD. These dystrophic neuronal structures are detected in hamsters as early as 2 weeks after experimental infection and appear to increase in frequency thereafter.[72] In murine scrapie these dystrophic structures immunolabel for ubiquitin and other lysosome markers[58] and are concentrated in the close vicinity of amyloid plaques, although they are equally prominent in plaque-forming and non-plaque scrapie models. Another lysosome-related pathological process which has been identified in ultrastructural studies is an autodigestion of neuronal cytoplasm (neuronal autophagy) which has been described in CJD, BSE and scrapie.[65,73]

COMPARISON OF SCRAPIE AND ALZHEIMER'S DISEASE NEUROPATHOLOGY

One of the most striking parallels between scrapie and Alzheimer's disease (AD) is the common occurrence of argyrophilic amyloid plaques which share the same basic structure of an amyloid core surrounded by degenerating neurites containing abnormal tau protein, reactive microglia and astrocytic processes.[44,51,67,74,75] Although the major constituent proteins of the amyloid cores are different (PrP in scrapie, β/A4 in AD), it seems highly probable that parallel mechanisms are involved in the generation of the plaques in both diseases. The availability of more sensitive immunolabelling techniques has revealed extensive abnormal and diffuse accumulations of PrP in scrapie[25] and widespread non-congophilic and diffuse β/A4 in AD.[76] There are several forms of abnormal PrP staining in scrapie, some suggestive of a primary pathology associated with neurons and their processes. An intriguing pattern of PrP deposition in the molecular layer of the cerebellum of ME7-scrapie affected mice is suggestive of a neuronal association, and is strikingly similar to the streaky pattern of abnormal β/A4 staining seen in the cerebellum in AD.[75,77] These β/A4 accumulations in AD differ from classical AD plaques both because they lack the typical and congophilic amyloid core structure and share with scrapie plaques an absence of acute phase proteins, alpha 1-antichymotrypsin, complement C3 and P-component, which are present in AD plaques in the forebrain. There are close similarities in the neuronal association of the β/A4 in AD and Down's syndrome, and the neuritic and perineuronal localisation of abnormal PrP in some scrapie models, in which PrP can be traced as 'tramlines' on both sides of neurites for some distance from cell bodies.[75] However both in scrapie and AD, these respective forms of amyloid protein can sometimes be deposited in clear association with small blood vessels, suggesting common mechanisms involved in amyloid processing in both diseases.

CONCLUSION

The biggest obstacle in understanding the pathogenesis and epidemiology of the scrapie-related diseases is the unknown chemical identity of the infectious agent. With this knowledge and of the biochemistry involved in amplification of the infection, the molecular pathology in the CNS and the molecular pathogenesis of the disease in the whole animal can be approached. The basis of the 'slowness' of these events and action of different allelic combinations of the Sinc gene, the restriction of the pathology only to neurons, without dysfunction associated with replication of the infection elsewhere, can then be addressed. Other questions concern the molecular basis for differences in permissiveness of different groups of neurons between models. The widespread expression of PrP throughout nerve cells suggests that a basis of targeting must involve some other intercedent and primary initiating events, in those permissive neurons which are restricted for a particular host genotype, scrapie strain interaction, and that PrP changes are a consequence of such initiating, and cell restricted steps. Clearly PrP-null mice must contribute to answering these questions. Only an understanding of the chemical basis of these events can lead to their control in individuals and populations.

ACKNOWLEDGEMENTS

I am pleased to acknowledge the generous help of Dr Martin Jeffrey, of the Lasswade Laboratory, both in the preparation of this chapter and with assistance in the section on ultrastructure.

REFERENCES

1 Wells GAH, McGill IS. Recently described scrapie-like encephalopathies of animals: case definitions. Res Vet Sci 1992; 53: 1-10.
2 Fraser H. Neuropathology of scrapie: the precision of the lesions and their diversity. In: Prusiner SB, Hadlow WJ, eds. Slow Transmissible Diseases of the Nervous System, Vol.1 New York: Academic Press, 1979: pp 387-406.
3 Fraser H, McBride PA, Scott JR, Bruce ME. Infectious degeneration of the nervous system. In: Triger DR, ed. Advanced Medicine 22. London: Bailliere Tindall. 1986: pp 371-384.
4 Fraser H, Bruce ME. Experimental control of cerebral amyloid in scrapie in mice. In: Behan PO, Meulen V ter, Clifford Rose R, eds. Immunology of Nervous System Infections. Amsterdam: Elsevier, 1983: pp 381-390.
5 Jeffrey M, Wells GAH. Spongiform encephalopathy in a nyala (Tragelaphus angasi). Vet Pathol 1988; 5: 398-399.
6 Zlotnik I. The histopathology of the brain stem of sheep affected with natural scrapie. J Comp Pathol 1958; 68: 148-165.
7 Gilmour JS, Bruce ME, MacKellar A. Cerebrovascular amyloidosis in scrapie-affected sheep. Neuropathol Appl Neurobiol 1986; 11: 173-183.
8 Williams ES, Young S. Chronic wasting disease of captive mule deer: a spongiform encephalopathy. J Wildlife Dis 1980; 16: 89-98.
9 Burger D, Hartsough GR. Transmissible mink encephalopathy. In: Gajdusek DC, Gibbs CK, Alpers M, eds. Slow, latent, and temporate virus infections, NINDB Monograph No. 2, 1965: pp 297-305.
10 Wyatt JM, Pearson GR, Smerdon T, Gruffydd-Jones TJ, Wells GAH. Naturally-occurring scrapie-like spongiform encephalopathy in five domestic cats. Vet Rec 1991; 129: 233-236.
11 Willoughby K, Kelly DF, Lyon DG, Wells GAH. Spongiform encephalopathy in a captive puma (Felis concolor). Vet Rec 1992; 131: 431-434.
12 Wood JLN, Done SH. Natural scrapie in goats: neuropathology. Vet Rec 1992; 131: 93-96.
13 Guiroy DC, Williams ES, Yanagihara R, Gajdusek DC. Topographic distribution of scrapie amyloid-immunoreactive plaques in chronic wasting disease in captive mule deer (Odocoileus hemionus hemionus). Acta Neuropath 1991; 81: 475-478.

14 Hope J, Reekie LJD, Hunter N, et al. Fibrils from brains of cows with new cattle disease contain scrapie-associated protein. Nature 1988; 336: 390-392

15 Pearson GR, Wyatt JM, Gruffydd-Jones TJ, et al. Feline spongiform encephalopathy: fibril and PrP studies. Vet Rec 1992; 131: 307-310.

16 Jeffrey M, Wilesmith JW. Idiopathic brainstem neuronal chromatolysis and hippocampal sclerosis: a novel encephalopathy in clinical suspect cases of bovine spongiform encephalopathy. Vet Rec 1992; 131: 359-362.

17 Schoon HA, Brunckhorst D, Pohlenz J. A contribution to the neuropathology of the red-necked ostrich (Struthio camelus) – a spongiform encephalopathy. Verh Ber Erkrg Zootiere 1991; 33: 309-314.

18 Kelly DF, Pearson H, Wright AI, Greenham LW. Morbidity in captive white tigers. In: Montali RJ, Migaki G, eds. The Comparative Pathology of Zoo Animals. Washington DC, Smithsonian Institute Press. 1980: pp 183-188.

19 Hogan RN, Baringer JR, Prusiner SB. Scrapie infection diminishes spines and increases varicosities of dendrites in hamsters: a quantitative Golgi study. J Neuropathol 1987; 46: 461-473.

20 Jeffrey M, Halliday WG, Goodsir CM. A morphometric and immunohistochemical study of the vestibular nuclear complex in bovine spongiform encephalopathy. Acta Neuropathol 1992; 84: 651-657.

21 Fraser H. The occurrence of nerve fibre degeneration in brains of mice inoculated with scrapie. Res Vet Sci 1969; 10: 338-341.

22 Schoussboe A, Drejer J, Divac I. Regional heterogeneity in astroglial cells. Implications of neuron-glia interactions. Trends Neurosci 1980; 3: XIII-XIV.

23 Fraser H. Scrapie: a transmissible degenerative CNS disease. In: Behan PO, Clifford Rose F, eds. Progress in Neurological Research with particular reference to motor neuron disease. Tunbridge Wells: Pitman Medical, 1979: pp 194-210.

24 Scott JR, Fraser H. Degenerative hippocampal pathology in mice infected with scrapie. Acta Neuropathol 1984; 65: 62-68.

25 Bruce ME, McBride PA, Farquhar CF. Precise targeting of the pathology of the sialoglycoprotein, PrP, and vacuolar degeneration in mouse scrapie. Neurosci Lett 1989; 102: 1-6.

26 Fraser H. The pathogenesis and pathology of scrapie. In: Tyrrell DAJ, ed. Aspects of slow and persistent virus infections. The Hague: Martinus Nijhoff, 1979: pp 30-58.

27 Fraser H. Neuronal spread of scrapie agent and targeting of lesions within the retino-tectal pathway. Nature 1982; 295: 149-150.

28 Kim YS, Carp RI, Callahan SM, Wisniewski HM. Incubation periods and survival times for mice injected stereotaxically with three scrapie strains in different brain regions. J Gen Virol 1987; 68: 695-702.

29 Fraser H, Dickinson AG. Targeting of scrapie lesions and spread of agent via the retino-tectal projection. Brain Res 1985; 346: 32-41.

30 Scott JR, Davies D, Fraser H. Scrapie in the central nervous system: neuroanatomical spread of infection and Sinc control of pathogenesis. J Gen Virol 1992; 73: 1637-1644.

31 Kim YS, Carp RI, Callahan BS, Natelli M, Wisniewski HM. Vacuolization, incubation period and survival time analysis in three mouse genotypes injected stereotaxically in three brain regions with the 22L scrapie strain. J Neuropathol 1990; 49: 106-113.

32 Kim YS, Carp RI, Callahan BS, Wisniewski HM. Pathogenesis and pathology of scrapie after stereotactic injection of strain 22L in intact and bisected cerebella. J Neuropathol 1990; 49: 114-121.

33 Foster JD, Davies D, Fraser H. Primary retinopathy in scrapie in mice deprived of light. Neurosci Lett 1986; 72: 111-114.

34 Bruce ME, Fraser H. Scrapie strain variation and its implications. In: Cheseboro BW, ed. Current Topics in Microbiology and Immunology, vol 172. Transmissible spongiform encephalopathies, scrapie, BSE and related disorders Berlin: Springer Verlag, 1991: pp 126-138.

35 Fraser H, Dickinson AG. The sequential development of the brain lesions of scrapie in three strains of mice. J Comp Pathol 1968; 78: 301-311.

36 Fraser H, Dickinson AG. Scrapie in mice: agent strain differences in the distribution and intensity of grey matter vacuolation. J Comp Pathol 1973; 83: 29-40.

37 Kim YS, Carp RI, Callahan S, Wisniewski HM. Incubation periods and histopathological changes in mice injected stereotaxically in different brain areas with the 87V scrapie strain. Acta Neuropathol 1990; 80: 388-392.

38 Dickinson AG, Fraser H, Meikle VM, Outram GW. Competition between different scrapie strains in mice. Nature 1972; 237: 244-245.

39 Dickinson AG, Fraser H, McConnell I, Outram GW, Sales DI, Taylor DM. Extraneural competition between different scrapie strains leading to loss of infectivity. Nature 1975; 253: 556.

40 Fraser H, Bruce ME, Chree A, McConnell I, Wells GAH. Transmission of bovine spongiform encephalopathy and scrapie to mice. J Gen Virol 1992; 73: 1891-1897.

41 Bruce ME, Dickinson AG, Fraser H. Cerebral amyloidosis in scrapie in the mouse: effect of agent strain and mouse genotype. Neuropathol Appl Neurobiol 1976; 2: 471-478.

42 Bruce ME, Fraser H. Focal and asymmetrical vacuolar lesions in the brains of mice infected with scrapie. Acta Neuropathol 1982; 58: 133-140.

43 Bruce ME, Dickinson AG. Biological evidence that scrapie agent has an independent genome. J Gen Virol 1987; 68: 79-89.

44 Fraser H, Bruce ME. Argyrophilic plaques in mice inoculated with scrapie from particular sources. Lancet 1973; i: 617-618.

45 McBride PA, Bruce ME, Fraser H. Immunostaining of cerebral amyloid plaques with antisera raised to scrapie-associated fibrils (SAF). Neuropathol Appl Neurobiol 1988; 14: 325-336.

46 Bruce ME, Dickinson AG. Genetic control of amyloid plaque production and incubation period in scrapie-infected mice. J Neuropathol 1985; 44: 285-294.

47 Bruce ME, Fraser H. Effect of age on cerebral amyloid plaques in murine scrapie. Neuropathol Appl Neurobiol 1982; 8: 471-478.

48 Wisniewski HM, Johnson AB, Raine CS, Kay WJ, Terry RD. Senile plaques and cerebral amyloidosis in aged dogs: a histochemical and ultrastructural study. Lab Invest 1970; 23: 287-296.

49 Wisniewski HM, Ghetti B, Terry RD. Neuritic (senile) plaques and filamentous changes in aged rhesus monkeys. J Neuropathol 1973; 32: 566-584.

50 Vaughan DW, Peters A. Structure of neuritic plaques in the cerebral cortex of old rats. J Neuropathol 1981; 40: 472-478.

51 Bruce ME, Fraser H. Amyloid plaques in the brains of mice with scrapie: morphological variation and staining properties. Neuropathol Appl Neurobiol 1975; 1: 189-202.

52 DeArmond SJ, McKinley MP, Barry RA, Braunfeld MB, McColloch JR, Prusiner SB. Identification of prion amyloid filaments in scrapie-infected brain. Cell 1985; 41: 221-235.

53 Kitamoto T, Ogomori K, Tateishi J, Prusiner SB. Formic acid pretreatment enhances immunostaining of cerebral and systemic amyloids. Lab Invest 1987; 57: 230-336.

54 DeArmond SJ, Mobley WC, DeMott DL, Barry RA, Beckstead JH, Prusiner SB. Changes in the localisation of brain prion proteins during scrapie infection. Neurology 1987; 37: 1271-1280.

55 Taraboulos A, Jendroska K, Serban D, Shu-Lian Yang, DeArmond SJ, Prusiner SB. Regional mapping of prion proteins in brain. Proc Natl Acad Sci USA 1992; 89: 7620-7624.

56 Diedrich JF, Bendheim PE, Kim YS, Carp RI, Haase AT. Scrapie-associated prion protein accumulates in astrocytes during scrapie infection. Proc Natl Acad Sci, USA 1991; 88: 375-379.

57 Diedrich JF, Minnigan H, Carp RI, Whitaker JN, Race R, Frey W, Haase AT. Neuropathological changes in scrapie and Alzheimer's disease are associated with increased expression of apolipoprotein E and cathepsin D in astrocytes. J Virol 1991; 65: 4759-4768.

58 Lowe J, Fergusson J, Kenward, N, et al. Immunoreactivity to ubiquitin-protein conjugates is present early in the disease process in the brains of scrapie-infected mice. J Pathol 1992; 168: 169-177.
59 Mayer RJ, Landon M, Laszlo L, Lennox G, Lowe J. Protein processing in lysosomes: the new therapeutic target in neurodegenerative disease. Lancet 1992; 340: 156-159.
60 Jeffrey M, Goodsir CM, Bruce ME, McBride PA, Scott JR, Halliday WG. Infection specific prion protein (PrP) accumulates on the neuronal plasmalemma in scrapie infected mice. Neurosci Lett 1992; 147: 106-109.
61 Moretz RC, Wisniewski HM, Lossinsky AS. Pathogenesis of neuritic and amyloid plaques in scrapie. Ultrastructural study of early changes in the cortical neuropil. In: Samuel D, ed. Aging of the brain. Raven Press, 1983: pp 61-79.
62 Eikelenboom P, Scott JR, McBride PA, Rozemuller JM, Bruce ME, Fraser H. No evidence for involvement of plasma proteins or blood-borne cells in amyloid formation in scrapie-affected mice. An immunohistoperoxidase study. Virchows Archiv B 1987; 53: 251-256.
63 Eikelenboom P, Rozemuller JM, Kraal G, Stam FC, McBride PA, Bruce, ME, Fraser H. Cerebral amyloid plaques in Alzheimer's disease but not in scrapie-affected mice are closely associated with a local inflammatory process. Virchows Archiv B Cell Biol 1991; 60: 329-336.
64 Lampert PW, Hooks J, Gibbs CJ, Gajdusek DC. Altered plasma membranes in experimental scrapie. Acta Neuropathol 1971; 19: 81-93.
65 Jeffrey M, Scott JR, Williams A, Fraser H. Ultrastructural features of spongiform encephalopathy transmitted to mice from three species of bovidae. Acta Neuropathol 1992; 84: 559-569.
66 Jeffrey M, Scott JR, Fraser H. Scrapie inoculation of mice: light and electron microscopy of the superior colliculus. Acta Neuropathol 1991; 81: 562-571.
67 Wisniewski HM, Bruce M, Fraser H. Infectious etiology of neuritic (senile) plaques in mice. Science 1975; 190: 1108-1110.
68 Wiley CA, Burrola PG, Buchmeir MJ, et al. Immunogold localisation of prion filaments in scrapie infected hamster brain. Lab Invest 1987; 57: 646-656.
69 David Ferreira JF, David Ferreira KL, Gibbs CJ, Morris JA. Scrapie in mice: ultrastructural observations in the cerebral cortex. Proc Soc Exp Biol Med 1968; 127: 313-320.
70 Siakotis AN, Raveed D, Longa G. The discovery of a particle unique to brain and spleen subcellular fractions from scrapie infected mice. J Gen Virol 1979; 43: 417-422.
71 Narang H HK, Asher DM, Gajdusek DC. Tubulofilaments in negatively stained scrapie-infected brains: relationships to scrapie associated filaments. Proc Nat Acad Sci USA 1987; 84: 7730-7734.
72 Liberski PP, Yanagihara R, Gibbs CJ, Gajdusek DC. Scrapie as a model for neuroaxonal dystrophy: ultrastructural studies. Exp Neurol 1989; 106: 133-141.
73 Boellard JW, Kao M, Schlote W, Diringer H. Neuronal autophagy in experimental scrapie. Acta Neuropathol 1991; 81: 225-228.
74 Brion JP, Fraser H, Flament-Durand J, Dickinson AG. Amyloid scrapie plaques in mice, and Alzheimer senile plaques, share common antigens with tau, a microtubule-associated protein. Neurosci Lett 1987; 78: 113-118.
75 Bruce ME, McBride PA, Jeffrey M, Rozemuller JM, Eikelenboom P. PrP in scrapie and β/A4 in Alzheimer's disease show similar patterns of deposition in the brain. In: Corain B, Iqbal K, Nicolini M, Winblad B, Wisniewski H, Zatta P, eds. Alzheimer's disease: Advances in clinical and basic research. Chicester: Wiley, 1993: pp 481-487.
76 Rozemuller JM, Eikelenboom P, Stam FC, Beyreuther K, Masters C. A4 protein in Alzheimer's disease: primary and secondary events in extracellular amyloid deposition. J Neuropathol 1989; 48: 647- 663.
77 Yamaguchi H, Harai S, Morimatsu M, Shoji M, Nakazato Y. Diffuse type of senile plaques in the cerebellum of Alzheimer-type dementia demonstrated by β protein immunostain. Acta Neuropathol 1989; 77 314-319.

British Medical Bulletin (1993) Vol. 49, No.4, pp 810–821
©The British Council 1993

Inactivation of SE agents

D M Taylor
AFRC & MRC Neuropathogenesis Unit, Institute for Animal Health, Edinburgh, UK

The transmissible agents of the spongiform
encephalopathies are relatively resistant to inactivation,
and accidental transmission has occurred in animals
and man. Rigorous chemical or physical procedures
are required to achieve decontamination, and their
effectiveness can only be determined by bioassay in
animals. The best-defined model is scrapie in mice or
hamsters, and this has been used in many of the studies
to establish practical inactivation procedures. Although
a number of techniques had been considered to be
effective, more recent observations suggest that some of
these may not always be completely reliable. Research
continues on scrapie inactivation, and work is in progress
to extend this knowledge to the BSE agent.

As discussed in other chapters of this issue there are uncertainties concerning the aetiology of the spongiform encephalopathies (SE) and the
nature of their causal agents. Although experimental studies have not
yet revealed the molecular identity of SE agents it is evident that an
abnormal, protease-resistant form of the host PrP protein is implicated
in the pathological process; the 'prion' hypothesis argues that this is
per se the transmissible causal factor. The 'virino' theory proposes that
normal PrP protein is a putative attachment/replication site for an informational molecule which adopts this host protein as its protective coat
in a novel but quasi-viral fashion, and suggests that this 'hermit-crab'
type of association between the informational molecule and normal
PrP protein induces the conformational modification of the latter to its
pathological, protease-resistant form. The attractiveness of the 'virino'
theory is that it provides an explanation for the variety of agent-specific,
host-independent characteristics of cloned strains of scrapie agent, and
explains the absence of any immunological response in the host. The
most obvious candidate informational molecule is a nucleic acid but
none has been detected. However, such a molecule could be extremely
small since there is no requirement for it to possess any protein-coding

information. The 'prion' model can account equally for the failure of any immune reaction but is less able to accommodate the existence of 14 or more strains of scrapie agent, each with its own distinctive biological characteristics, unless it can be demonstrated that at least an equivalent number of different post-translational modifications of normal PrP protein can occur spontaneously within the host; all such modifications would have to result in the production of protease-resistant PrP protein.

STABILITY OF SE AGENTS

Theoretical aspects

It has been recognised for many years that the unconventional transmissible agents of SE are relatively resistant to chemical and physical inactivation but the reasons are not understood.

One argument used to support the 'prion' hypothesis is that procedures which degrade proteins result in greater inactivation of infectivity compared with treatments known to denature nucleic acids. However, the protein-denaturing techniques used have had to be more rigorous than those which would achieve inactivation of conventional microorganisms and may simply indicate that a nucleic acid enveloped by the hardy PrP protein may be relatively impervious to the effects of nucleic acid denaturants. This uncertainty is confounded by the known hydrophobicity of PrP protein and the neuronal cell-membrane domains with which it is predominantly associated, and consequently the protective aggregation which occurs in tissue homogenates used for experimental purposes.[1,2] Because of such constraints there are problems in interpreting the data from inactivation experiments as far as the nature of SE agents is concerned. This is epitomised by the disparate views which have been expressed on the interpretation of data derived from experiments where scrapie agent was irradiated; on the one hand it was suggested that the transmissible agent is not dependent upon a nucleic acid[3] but an alternative interpretation was that the agent could be an unusual but conventional virus.[2] Such studies have stimulated considerable thought and discussion but have not revealed the molecular nature of SE agents. This is not surprising since the molecular changes which occur during inactivation even of conventional microorganisms are generally not clearly defined.

Practical considerations

A further reason for conducting inactivation studies is to establish decontamination standards for SE agents whereby those involved in animal and human health-care might be guided with regard to their own safety and that of their patients; this concern extends obviously to others such as research workers who may also be subjected to occupational exposure.

The first indication of the unusual stability of SE agents was signalled by the occurrence of scrapie in several hundred of 14 000 sheep which received the same batch of louping-ill vaccine. Preparation of the vaccine involved prolonged exposure of sheep CNS tissue infected with louping-ill virus to formalin. From the outcome of the vaccination programme it was construed that the formalin treatment had inactivated the louping-ill virus as anticipated, but failed to inactivate scrapie agent which had been present unsuspectedly in the donor sheep tissue.[4] This early incident provided the first clue that scrapie agent might be different from conventional viruses, and stimulated further and continuing interest in the theoretical and practical aspects of inactivation of SE agents.

It is now known that scrapie agent is relatively resistant to a variety of other practical procedures which are effective against conventional microorganisms; these include exposure to gravity-displacement autoclaving,[5] hot air,[6] gamma and UV irradiation,[3] ethylene oxide[7] and peracetic acid.[1] It has also been demonstrated that after treatment with formalin the agent is resistant to an autoclaving regime which would otherwise be effective.[8] These and other inactivation data have been discussed in recent reviews.[9–13]

Studies involving the agents of Creutzfeldt-Jakob disease (CJD), kuru and transmissible mink encephalopathy (TME) have confirmed that inactivation resistance is a general property of SE agents but most of the work has involved scrapie agent as the acknowledged model for the group.

Environmental contamination

The known capacity for SE agents to survive environmental rigours such as desiccation, thermal extremes and UV exposure are considered to explain the emergence of scrapie in a previously-unaffected flock of sheep when introduced to pastures which had been grazed by affected sheep 3 years earlier.[14]

Although known to be transmissible accidentally and experimentally it has been suggested that CJD, and Gerstmann-Straussler-Scheinker syndrome (GSS), cannot normally be infectious because of their very low incidence in the human population; therefore it has been postulated that these diseases arise because of mutations in the PrP gene which result in the direct synthesis of a protease-resistant form of PrP protein (prion) which is pathogenic in its own right. However, what is not ruled out is the existence of a transmissible agent which is either: (a) ubiquitous in the environment; or (b) commonly present in the human population as a silent infection, e.g. of the lymphoreticular system, which does not progress to produce neurological disease within a normal lifespan. Given these possibilities, a small group of individuals compromised by virtue of inherited or somatic PrP gene abnormalities, or by traumatic events which permit access of the transmissible agent to critical replication sites, might develop neurological disease. Such hypotheses are not entirely speculative but are based upon experimental studies in mice. In one model, animals challenged with scrapie agent by the intraperitoneal route fail to succumb to disease within their normal lifespan but, by serial passage of brain tissue, can be shown to have had a neurological infection which would have been fatal if they were capable of greater longevity. In another model, scrapie infectivity injected by the intraperitoneal route is detectable only within the lymphoreticular system throughout the natural lifespan of the recipient mice; this suggests that these animals would not have developed neurological disease regardless of how long they lived, even though intracerebral passage of their spleen tissue produced typical disease in other mice. Support for the 'pathogenic gene' concept was considered by some to have been provided by the spontaneous development of a scrapie-like disease in mice with an induced mutation of the PrP gene; in humans the same mutation is associated with SE. However, the disease was confined to mice with high copy numbers of the transgene and there was little evidence of the presence of disease-specific PrP protein; animals with low copy numbers were unaffected.[15] It is considered that meaningful conclusions cannot be drawn from this study.

Accidental transmission

The louping-ill episode (vide supra) represents the earliest known example of accidental SE transmission but there have since been other instances where transmission has occurred as a known or suspected consequence of inactivation resistance. Bovine spongiform encephalopathy (BSE) may be viewed in this light since it is considered to represent transmission of scrapie from sheep to bovines via scrapie-contaminated meat and bone meal which had been a constituent of commercial cattle diets. Epidemiological evidence suggests that more recent manufacturing procedures in the UK may have permitted greater survival of scrapie infectivity than earlier methods, and that this was sufficient to establish an effective oral challenge.[16]

Iatrogenic transmission associated with neurosurgery is suspected but unproven for some cases of CJD[17] but in others there is a known association between surgical intervention, the subsequent development of CJD, and the failure to have used appropriate decontamination standards for instrument sterilisation.[18,19] There are also individuals who have developed CJD following surgical implantation of commercially-processed cadaveric human dura mater; it has been recognised that CJD agent would not have been inactivated by the original manufacturing methods which now include exposure to 1M sodium hydroxide.[20]

The therapeutic use of growth hormone and gonadotrophin derived from cadaveric human pituitary glands has also been associated with the occurrence of CJD in some recipients. Because of the prolonged nature of growth hormone therapy these patients had typically received multiple doses from various batches.[21] A validation study of the production method used most recently in the UK until the product ban in 1985 concluded that the procedure was capable of removing an infectivity challenge many times greater than that which could be encountered in practice but that infectivity which was retained, e.g. by gel filtration or chromatography columns would probably remain viable and could be a source of cross-contamination if handled inappropriately.[22] In another study designed to test the effectiveness of a similar process, a slightly lower reduction factor was reported; in contrast to the previous study, residual infectivity was detectable but the starting material had a much higher titre of infectivity.[23] This has been interpreted as evidence that the conclusions drawn from the UK study may be inappropriate[20,21] but the extraction method used in the second study was not exactly the same as that used in the UK. It is re-emphasised that the clearance factor obtained in the UK study was greater than that required to accommodate a worst-case scenario, and that the maximum reduction of infectivity was achieved before the final chromatographic step which is capable of removing a further 5.5 logs of infectivity;[23] it is considered that these factors negate criticism that the number of animals used in the UK study, although typical,[24] was inadequate.[25] Also, a common factor among the UK cases which have occurred so far is that they received treatment between 1974 and 1976 with hormone prepared by procedures which preceded the chromatographic method.[26]

CJD has occurred in a neurosurgeon,[27] a neuropathologist[28] and two histopathology technicians.[29,30] Although none of these cases had any clear link with occupational exposure this could be difficult to demonstrate for a disease with such a long incubation period. Because of the resistance of SE agents to inactivation by formalin, infectivity survives in tissue blocks and sections processed by traditional histopathological methods.

There have therefore been ample opportunities for transmission to have occurred, e.g. through accidents involving microtome blades, but there is no evidence that it has. Also, during the forty year gap between the recognition of CJD as a clinical entity and the first suspicion that it might be transmissible, brain tissue would have been handled without precautions but this does not appear to have resulted in any detectable occupational risk.

THE SCRAPIE MODEL

The sheep disease, scrapie, is known to have existed for at least 250 years, and was shown to be transmissible experimentally to sheep in 1936. Human SE had been described as early as 1920 in the case of CJD but their clinical and neurohistopathological similarities to scrapie, and therefore their potential transmissibility, were not recognised until 1959. The first successful experimental transmission (of kuru) to primates was achieved in 1966, and transmission of CJD to mice was achieved in 1976. By this time the mouse scrapie model had been established for 15 years and had facilitated – e.g. the detection of strain variation in the scrapie agent, and genetic influences of the host on scrapie incubation period. These facts, together with the perceived greater occupational risk of working with human SE agents in rodents, firmly established mouse and (later) hamster scrapie as the model experimental SE. A further advantage of the hamster and mouse models is that because strains of scrapie agent have been cloned and purified by serial passage, they display consistent and predictable characteristics, e.g. in terms of incubation period and topography of brain lesions. Similar strain purification has not been attempted for other SE agents except BSE, as described elsewhere in this issue (see Bruce).

Because SE agents have not been characterised or purified it is necessary to use infected tissue as the substrate for experimental studies, and then determine infectivity titres by bioassay in animals; the most commonly-used tissue used is brain because it has the highest infectivity titre, at least during the terminal stage of disease. Studies on scrapie in mice have demonstrated that there is an inverse relationship between the dose of infectivity administered and the ensuing incubation period. When a dose-response curve has been plotted for any given strain within a specific mouse genotype which has received a standard injection dose by a defined route, the concentration of agent in further samples can be estimated from the incubation period of a single dilution group.[31] The same consistency, and therefore appropriateness of the incubation period assay, has also been demonstrated for scrapie in hamsters.[32,33] Unfortunately, this does not apply to infectivity which has been subjected to chemical or physical treatment because such procedures can modify the dose-response curve. Prolongation of dose-response curves has been observed in mice by endpoint titration following exposure of the 139A strain of scrapie agent to lithium chloride,[32] sodium deoxycholate,[34] sodium dodecyl sulphate[32] or a combination of octyl glucoside and sulphobetaine 3–14;[35] a similar phenomenon was observed with strain ME7 after boiling.[31] The amount of infectivity in such samples would have been underestimated by incubation period assay. There was no alteration of the dose-response curve in hamsters after strain 263K had been boiled, but heating to 121°C resulted in a 1 log underestimate of titre by the incubation period assay.[36]

Because of its short incubation period and its high titre of infectivity in the brain (about two logs higher than in most mouse models), the 263K strain of scrapie in Syrian hamsters has been used preferentially for a variety of research purposes including decontamination studies. When injected intracerebrally with a high concentration of 263K the mean incubation period in hamsters is ~70 days with a small standard error. As with mouse scrapie models, incubation periods and standard errors increase in hamsters as the dose of infectivity is reduced; at limiting dilutions the mean incubation period increases to ~150 days. In contrast, mouse scrapie models have longer incubation periods; for example, when a high concentration of the ME7 strain of scrapie is injected intracerebrally into C57BL mice, the mean incubation period is ~160 days but at limiting dilutions extends to ~280 days.[31] In the experiments with ME7 where prolongation of the dose-response curve occurred due to boiling, the average maximum incubation period increased to ~370 days;[5,31] such animals would need to be observed for up to 14 months to be sure of detecting late cases. Use of the hamster model for inactivation studies is compromised by a number of factors. Despite the maximum mean incubation periods of ~150 days for recipients of untreated 263K infectivity, it has been our experience that exposure of the agent to chemical or physical treatments can result in incubation periods exceeding 400 days (DM Taylor & I McConnell, unpublished observations). Others have found that such animals require observation for up to 18 months[23] or 2 years[37] to ensure that late cases are not missed. Another difficulty is that, unlike mice, specific-pathogen-free (SPF) hamsters are not available; for unidentified reasons it has not yet been possible to produce germfree hamsters which would be the customary route to establish SPF stocks. Consequently, all hamsters harbour proscribed microorganisms thus creating problems for those who wish to house hamsters and SPF mice within a common facility. The microbiological status of hamsters is more than a theoretical problem: it has been proposed that a study claiming to have produced a scrapie-like disease in hamsters injected with leucocytes from relatives or cases of Alzheimer's disease[38] may have been compromised by an unsuspected late-onset wasting disease in the hamsters caused by *Clostridium difficile*, and that the same problem may have confounded the interpretation of important SE transgenic studies.[39] A further complicating factor is that Syrian hamsters, especially females, have a predisposition to systemic amyloidosis which is fatal on average by about 62 weeks of age in multiply-caged animals; individually-housed animals survive on average for 35 weeks more, and crowding stress is thought to be the precipitating factor,[40] but infection may have a role in the aetiology of the amyloidosis as has been observed in conventional but not germfree mice.[41]

Because of the general usefulness of the 263K model, attempts have been made to achieve SPF status for hamsters by chemotherapeutic eradication of proscribed microorganisms; this has been relatively successful[42-44] but *Pasteurella pneumotropica* has still to be eliminated.

Current decontamination standards for SE agents

Data from extensive studies involving CJD and/or scrapie agent[37,45] have been used to establish standards in the UK[46] and USA[47] for the decontamination of CJD and other SE agents, and these have been largely adopted worldwide. Because the aim of these studies was to define practical conditions for decontamination, macerates or homogenates of infected brain were used in contrast to biochemically-purified preparations. Although the latter can contain higher titres of infectivity, they lack the high level of organic matter which is known to be an essential challenge factor in studying decontamination of conventional microorganisms. The UK study involved the use of two strains of scrapie agent, one of which (22A) was known to be relatively thermostable.[6] This showed that porous-load autoclaving at 136°C for periods in excess of 3 minutes, or exposure to sodium hypochlorite solution yielding 14 000 ppm available chlorine for 30 minutes were effective. The standards which have subsequently been recommended in the UK are (a) porous-load autoclaving at 134–138°C for 18 minutes, or (b) exposure to sodium hypochlorite solution providing at least 20 000 ppm of available chlorine for an hour. This concentration of hypochlorite is contra-indicated by some USA data but the apparent anomalies have been discussed.[9] The USA studies demonstrated that inactivation was achieved by gravity-displacement autoclaving at 132°C for an hour or by a one hour exposure to 1M sodium hydroxide. However, the latter data are challenged by pre-existing[48] and later findings which indicate that the hydroxide treatment is not entirely effective;[49-51] results from recent experiments suggest that these anomalies are attributable to the relative insensitivity of the original bioassays (DM Taylor et al, unpublished observations). Also, the effectiveness of the recommended gravity-displacement autoclaving regime has been questioned by other data derived from studies using the same model, i.e. 263K scrapie agent in Syrian hamsters.[52] Reciprocally, there are challenges relating to the UK studies concerning (a) the validity of regarding 22A as the most thermostable known strain of scrapie agent, and (b) the security of the UK autoclaving standard. These questions have arisen because of the survival of some infectivity of strain 263K following gravity-displacement autoclaving at 134°C.[53] However, the gravity-displacement method of autoclaving is known to be less efficient than the porous-load technique, and the titre of infectivity in brain of the 263K model in hamsters is about two logs higher than for the mouse models. Therefore, even if the exposure conditions had been identical for the 22A and 263K strains, it would have been difficult to interpret the outcome in terms of intrinsic strain resistance, given the differences in starting titres. Nevertheless, recent data suggest that the lower end of the temperature-range recommended for porous-load decontamination of SE agents in the UK (134°C) may not be entirely secure in all practical circumstances (DM Taylor et al, unpublished observations), and further studies are in progress.

A major improvement in safety within the neurohistopathology laboratory has been achieved by the demonstration that treatment of formalin-fixed brain tissue with > 90% formic acid results in substantial inactivation of CJD or scrapie infectivity while retaining good tissue morphology.[54]

CONCLUSION

Research activity on SE has been stimulated in recent years by two dominant features. The application of molecular biological techniques has demonstrated that there is a frequent association between the inheritance of aberrant PrP genes and the overt expression of familial CJD or GSS; the development of transgenic animal technology has permitted the insertion of these genes or their analogues into laboratory species. Despite some expectation that the animal and human studies would collectively provide substantial support for the validity of the 'prion' hypothesis this has not yet proved to be the case.

The other major stimulus to SE research has been the emergence of a novel SE, i.e. BSE. Although the disease has been largely confined to the British Isles, the severity of the epidemic has created anxiety worldwide. Apart from obvious concern about endemic cattle infection, there has been the hyperventilated issue of potential transmission to the human population via the food-chain or biopharmaceutical products of bovine origin. Although those knowledgeable in this area consider these putative risks to be minimal, precautionary measures have been introduced. Dietary exposure has been minimised in the UK by excluding tissues containing (theoretically) high infectivity titres as a source of food for humans and animals. The putative risk associated with treatment involving medicinal products of bovine origin has also been minimised by a variety of statutory and voluntary codes which define policy and methods for sourcing raw materials together with relevant inactivation procedures and the conditions required for experimental validation procedures. At present it is assumed reasonably that the inactivation spectrum for BSE agent is much the same as for other SE agents, pending the outcome of current BSE decontamination studies.

In view of the accidental animal-to-animal and human-to-human transmissions which have occurred with the SE, it is clear that stringent standards for decontamination and prevention of cross-contamination need to be maintained.

REFERENCES

1 Taylor DM. Resistance of the ME7 scrapie agent to peracetic acid. Vet Microbiol 1991; 27: 19-24.
2 Rohwer RG. Scrapie infectious agent is virus-like in size and susceptibility to inactivation. Science 1984; 308: 658-662.
3 Alper T, Cramp WA, Haig DA, Clarke MC. Does agent of scrapie replicate without nucleic acid? Science 1967; 214: 764-766.
4 Gordon WS, Brownlee A, Wilson DR. Studies in louping-ill, tick-borne fever and scrapie. Report of the Proceedings of the Third International Congress for Microbiology. Baltimore: Waverley, 1940: pp 362-363.
5 Zlotnik I, Rennie JC. The effect of heat on the scrapie agent in mouse brain. Br J Exp Path 1967; 48: 171-179.
6 Dickinson AG, Taylor DM. Resistance of scrapie agent to decontamination. N Engl J Med 1978; 229: 1413-1414.
7 Dickinson AG. Scrapie in sheep and goats. In: Kimberlin RH, ed. Slow Virus Diseases of Animals and Man. Amsterdam: North-Holland, 1976:pp 209-241.
8 Taylor DM, McConnell I. Autoclaving does not decontaminate formol-fixed scrapie tissues. Lancet 1988; i: 1463-1464.
9 Taylor DM. Inactivation of BSE agent. Develop Biol Standard 1991; 75: 97-102.
10 Taylor DM. Inactivation of the unconventional agents of scrapie, bovine spongiform encephalopathy and Creutzfeldt-Jakob disease. J Hosp Infect 1991; 18(Suppl A): 141-146.
11 Taylor DM. The Kelsey lecture: Inactivation of slow viruses including CJD. J Sterile Services Management 1991; 4-8.
12 Taylor DM. Decontamination of scrapie-like agents. In: Bradley R, Savey M, Marchant B, eds. Sub-acute Spongiform Encephalopathies. Dordrecht: Kluwer Academic, 1991: pp 153-159.
13 Taylor DM. Inactivation of unconventional agents of the transmissible degenerative encephalopathies.In: Russell AD, Hugo WB, Ayliffe GAJ,eds. Principles and Practice of Disinfection, Preservation and Sterilization. Oxford: Blackwell, 1992: pp 171-179.
14 Palsson PA. Rida (scrapie) in Iceland and its epidemiology. In: Prusiner SB, Hadlow WJ, eds. Slow Transmissible Diseases of the Nervous System, vol 1. London: Academic Press,1979: pp 357-366.
15 Hsiao KK, Scott M, Foster D, Groth DF, DeArmond SJ, Prusiner SB et al. Spontaneous neurodegenerative disease in transgenic mice with mutant PrP protein. Science 1990; 250: 1587-1590.
16 Wilesmith JW, Wells GAH, Cranwell MP, Ryan JBM. Bovine spongiform encephalopathy: Epidemiological studies. Vet Record 1988; 123: 638-644.

17 Will RG, Matthews WB. Evidence for case-to-case transmission of Creutzfeldt-Jakob disease. J Neurol Neurosurg Psychiatr 1982; 45: 235-238.
18 Bernoulli C, Siegfried J, Baumgartner G et al. Danger of accidental person-to-person transmission of Creutzfeldt-Jakob disease by surgery. Lancet 1977; i: 478-479.
19 Foncin JF, Gaches J, Cathala F, El Sherif E, Le Beau J. Transmission iatrogene interhumaine possible de maladie de Creutzfeldt-Jakob avec alteinte des grains du cervulet. Rev Neurol 1980; 136: 280.
20 Brown P, Preece MA, Will RG. 'Friendly fire' in medicine: hormones, homografts, and Creutzfeldt-Jakob disease. Lancet 1992; ii: 24-27.
21 Fradkin JE, Schonberger LB, Mills JL et al. Creutzfeldt-Jakob disease in pituitary growth hormone recipients in the United States. J Am Med Assoc 1991; 265: 880-884
22 Taylor DM, Dickinson AG, Fraser H, Robertson PA, Salacinski PR, Lowry PJ. Preparation of growth hormone free from contamination with unconventional slow viruses. Lancet 1985; ii: 260-262.
23 Pocchiari M, Peano S, Conz A et al. Combination ultrafiltration and 6M urea treatment of human growth hormone effectively minimizes risk from potential Creutzfeldt-Jakob disease virus contamination. Horm Res 1991; 35: 161-166.
24 Taylor DM, Dickinson AG. Safety of human growth hormone. Lancet 1985; ii: 837-838.
25 Brown P. Virus sterility for human growth hormone. Lancet 1985; ii: 729-730.
26 Griffin JP. Transmission of Creutzfeldt-Jakob disease by investigative and therapeutic procedures. Adverse Drug React Toxicol Rev 1991; 10: 89-98.
27 Schoene C, Masters CL, Gibbs CJ et al. Transmissible spongiform encephalopathy (Creutzfeldt-Jakob disease). Atypical clinical and pathological findings. Arch Neurol 1981; 38: 473-477.
28 Gorman DG, Benson DF, Vogel DG, Vinters HV. Creutzfeldt-Jakob disease in a pathologist. Neurology 1992; 42: 463.
29 Miller DC. Creutzfeldt-Jakob disease in histopathology technicians. N Engl J Med 1988; 318: 853-854.
30 Sitwell L, Lach B, Atack E, Atack D. Creutzfeldt-Jakob disease in histopathology technicians. N Engl J Med 1988; 318: 854.
31 Dickinson AG, Fraser H. Modification of the pathogenesis of scrapie in mice by treatment of the agent. Nature 1969; 222: 892-893.
32 Kimberlin RH, Walker CA. Characteristics of a short incubation period model of scrapie in the golden hamster. J Gen Virol 1977; 34: 295-304.
33 Kimberlin RH, Walker CA. Pathogenesis of scrapie (strain 263K) in hamsters infected intracerebrally, intraperitoneally or intraocularly. J Gen Virol 1986; 67: 255-263.
34 Lax AJ, Millson GC, Manning EJ. Can scrapie titres be calculated accurately from incubation periods? J Gen Virol 1983; 64: 971-973.
35 Somerville RA, Carp RI. Altered scrapie infectivity estimates by titration and incubation period in the presence of detergents. J Gen Virol 1983; 64: 2045-2050.
36 Prusiner SB, Cochran SP, Groth DF, Downey DE, Bowman KA, Martinez HM. Measurement of the scrapie agent using an incubation time interval assay. Ann Neurol 1982; 11: 353-358.
37 Brown P, Rohwer RG, Gajdusek DC. Newer data on the inactivation of scrapie virus or Creutzfeldt-Jakob disease virus in brain tissue. J Infect Dis 1986; 153: 1145-1148.
38 Manuelidis EE, De Figuiredo JM, Kim JH, Fritch WW, Manuelidis LL. Transmission studies from blood of Alzheimer's disease patients and healthy relatives. Proc Natl Acad Sci USA 1988; 85: 4898-4901.
39 Rohwer RG. Alzheimer's disease transmission: Possible artifact due to intercurrent illness. Neurology 1992; 42: 287-288.
40 Germann P-G, Kohler M, Ernst H, Baumgart H, Mohr U. The relation of amyloidosis to social stress induced by crowding in the Syrian hamster (Mesocricetus auratus). Z Versuchstierkd 1990; 33: 271-275.
41 Taylor DM, Fraser H, Bruce ME. Altered clinical and histological features of male MM mouse pyelonephritis associated with a change in its microbiology. Lab Anim 1988; 22: 35-45.

42 Taylor DM. Eradication of pinworms (Syphacia obvelata) from Syrian hamsters in quarantine. Lab Anim Sci 1992; 42: 413-414.

43 Taylor DM, Farquhar CF, Neal DL. Studies on the eradication of intestinal protozoa of Syrian hamsters in quarantine and their transfaunation to mice. Lab Anim Sci (in press).

44 Taylor DM, Neal DL, Farquhar CF. Elimination of Giardia muris from Syrian hamsters in quarantine. Lab Anim Sci (submitted).

45 Kimberlin RH, Walker CA, Millson GC et al. Disinfection studies with two strains of mouse-passaged scrapie agent. J Neurol Sci 1983; 59: 355-369.

46 DHSS. Management of patients with spongiform encephalopathy (Creutzfeldt-Jakob disease [CJD]) 1984; DHSS Circular: DA(84)16.

47 Rosenberg RR, White CL, Brown P et al. Precautions in handling tissues, fluids, and other contaminated materials from patients with documented or suspected Creutzfeldt-Jakob disease. Ann Neurol 1986; 19: 75-77.

48 Prusiner SB, McKinley MP, Bolton DC et al. Prions: methods for assay, purification, and characterization. In: Maramorosch K, Koprowski H, eds. Methods in Virology vol VII: New York: Academic Press, 1984: pp 293-345.

49 Diringer H, Braig HR. Infectivity of unconventional viruses in dura mater. Lancet 1989; i: 439-440.

50 Tamai Y, Taguchi F, Miura S. Inactivation of the Creutzfeldt-Jakob disease agent. Ann Neurol 1988; 24: 466.

51 Tateishi J, Tashima T, Kitamoto T. Inactivation of the Creutzfeldt-Jakob disease agent. Ann Neurol 1988; 24: 466.

52 Pocchiari M. Validation of methods to remove spongiform encephalopathy agents from biological materials. Dev Biol Standard (in press).

53 Brown P, Liberski PP, Wolff A, Gajdusek DC. Resistance of scrapie infectivity to steam autoclaving after formaldehyde fixation and limited survival after ashing at 360°C: Practical and theoretical implications. J Infect Dis 1990; 161: 467-472.

54 Brown P, Wolff A, Gajdusek DC. A simple and effective method for inactivating virus infectivity in formalin-fixed tissue samples from patients with Creutzfeldt-Jakob disease. Neurology 1990; 40: 887-890.

British Medical Bulletin (1993) Vol. 49, No. 4, 822–838
©The British Council 1993

Scrapie strain variation and mutation

M E Bruce
AFRC & MRC Neuropathogenesis Unit, Institute for Animal Health, Edinburgh, UK

There are many strains of scrapie, distinguishable by their disease characteristics in genetically-defined mice. Numerous distinct strains have been isolated in the same mouse strain, indicating that scrapie agents have an informational molecule, independent of the host. Strain characteristics are stable on serial mouse passage under constant passaging conditions. However, changes in the species or mouse genotype used for passage may lead to changes in properties which are consistent with the selection of variants which replicate faster in the new host, rather than active modification of the agent by the host. The fact that this has been observed with biologically cloned strains is evidence for mutation in the scrapie agent. Transmissions to mice from natural scrapie and BSE suggest that strain variation exists in the field. These findings have important implications when considering the molecular nature of the scrapie agent and the details of agent-host interactions.

It has been known for many years that scrapie-like agents, like conventional microorganisms, exhibit strain variation. This was first observed over 30 years ago in two experimentally passaged scrapie isolates, which produced dramatically different clinical signs in goats, either a 'drowsy' or a 'scratching' syndrome.[1] Since then strain variation has been well documented for experimental scrapie in sheep,[2] mice[3,4] and hamsters,[5,6] CJD in mice[7,8] and transmissible mink encephalopathy in hamsters.[9]

Our current understanding of strain diversity in scrapie is based largely on the long-term studies of Alan Dickinson and coworkers, working at the Neuropathogenesis Unit in Edinburgh, who have concentrated mainly on experimental mouse models.[10,11] About 20 phenotypically distinct strains have been isolated in mice by serially passaging scrapie or BSE from a wide range of sheep, goat and cattle sources. The methods used for strain discrimination have, of necessity, relied on simple measurements of disease characteristics, particularly the incubation period and the severity and distribution of pathological changes in the brain. Scrapie strains have also been found to differ in their clinical manifestations,[12] their ease of transmission to new species[5] and their susceptibility to thermal inactivation.[13,14]

There has been much speculation in recent years about the molecular nature of the scrapie agent. Its unusual physico-chemical properties (*see* Taylor, this issue), together with the failure to identify scrapie-specific nucleic acids in highly infectious brain extracts,[15] have prompted the hypothesis that the agent is a protein devoid of nucleic acid.[16] The candidate protein, PrP, is host coded, accumulates in abnormally protease-resistant forms in infected organs and copurifies with infectivity in extracts from these organs.[17] The alternative view is that there are scrapie-specific nucleic acids which have not yet been detected because of the limitations of currently available techniques. According to the 'virino' hypothesis,[18] these nucleic acids would be closely associated with and protected by host tissue components, which could be abnormal forms of PrP. Another view is that there is still the possibility that the scrapie agent is a virus, despite its unconventional properties.[19]

The existence of many distinct strains of scrapie is crucial to these arguments as it clearly demonstrates that the scrapie agent has an informational molecule which is independent of the host. We review here the characteristics of strains and their behaviour on passage in different host species and genotypes and go on to discuss the implications of these observations for molecular models of the scrapie agent.

INCUBATION PERIODS AND BRAIN PATHOLOGY

The most obvious way in which scrapie strains differ is in their incubation periods between initial infection and clinical disease in genetically defined hosts.[3] If all experimental variables are kept constant, this measurement is remarkably repeatable; a single scrapie strain injected intracerebrally at high dose into a group of inbred mice will generally give standard errors of less than 2% of the mean incubation period. In mice the host *Sinc* (*scrapie incubation*) gene also exerts a major influence on the incubation period and this has been exploited to extend the scope of strain discrimination. Two alleles of *Sinc* have been identified, designated s7 and p7.[20] It is almost certain that the *Sinc* gene encodes PrP and *Sinc*s7 and *Sinc*p7 mice consistently differ in the sequence of the protein, by two amino acids.[21–23]

Each scrapie strain, injected under standard conditions, has a characteristic and highly reproducible pattern of incubation periods in the 3 *Sinc* genotypes of mice (the two homozygotes and the heterozygote F_1 cross) (Fig. 1).[4,11] Scrapie strains differ, not only in their incubation periods within a single *Sinc* genotype, but also in their relative incubation periods in the two homozygotes; for example, the ME7 scrapie strain has a shorter incubation period in *Sinc*[s7] mice than in *Sinc*[p7] mice, but this ranking is reversed for 22A. Another striking difference between strains is in the dominance characteristics shown by the 2 *Sinc* alleles; with ME7 the incubation period in the F_1 heterozygote lies between those of the two parental genotypes, whereas with 22A the incubation period in the heterozygote lies beyond the parental range.

Scrapie strains also show dramatic and reproducible differences in the type, severity and distribution of pathological changes they produce in the brain (*see* also Fraser, this issue). The most prominent change seen in routine histological sections is a vacuolation of the neuropil, which is targeted to different parts of the brain, depending mainly on the strain of scrapie, but also to some extent on *Sinc* and other mouse genes. The distribution of vacuolar degeneration is the basis of a semi-quantitative method of strain discrimination in which the severity of pathology is scored from coded sections in nine grey matter and three white matter brain areas to construct a 'lesion profile'.[24] Each combination of scrapie strain and mouse genotype has a characteristic lesion profile[4,10] which, unlike the incubation period, is not sensitive to the initial infecting dose. Lesion profiles can therefore be used to identify strains in samples with low levels of infectivity and to determine which strain kills the animal when a mixture of strains is injected.

The differences in pathology between scrapie strains can be demonstrated even more clearly in sections immunostained with PrP-specific antisera. There are extensive accumulations of PrP in the brain with all strains of scrapie, mostly in the form of diffuse or granular deposits in the neuropil in areas of vacuolar degeneration and amyloid plaques. As with vacuolation, there are clear and reproducible differences between scrapie strains in the distribution and severity of these changes.[25] As an illustration, Figure 2 shows PrP accumulation in different parts of the hippocampus with 4 strains of scrapie. The most selective strain, 87V, targets pathology precisely to a narrow sector, which correlates exactly with the distribution of the dendritic processes of pyramidal neurons within this sector. Precise targeting to particular identifiable groups of neurons is also seen elsewhere in the brain with 87V and other strains.

These results suggest that a fundamental difference between scrapie strains is their ability to recognize and replicate in different neuronal populations. However, as there is considerable overlap in target-

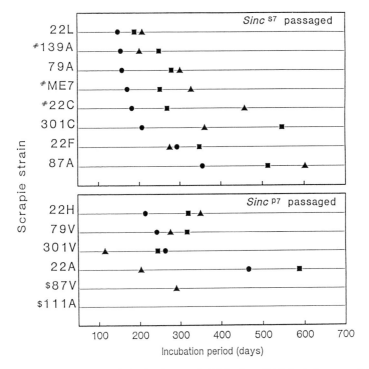

Fig. 1 Incubation periods following intracerebral injection of 1% brain homogenates for 14 scrapie/BSE strains in mice of the three *Sinc* genotypes: C57BL(*Sinc*^s7^)(●), VM(*Sinc*^p7^)(▲) and C57BLxVM(*Sinc*^s7p7^)(■).
‡The properties of 139A, ME7 and 22C are unchanged when they are passaged in *Sinc*^p7^ mice.
$ The incubation periods for C57BL and C57BLxVM mice with 87V and for all three genotypes for 111A are longer than 700 days and some individuals do not develop clinical disease within their lifespan.

ing patterns seen with different strains, it is probable that a uniform group of neurons is capable of supporting the replication of more than one strain. Indeed, it has been demonstrated recently that two distinct scrapie strains can replicate in neuronal cultures containing a single cloned cell type.[26] Further evidence that different strains can use the same replication sites has come from 'blocking' experiments in which the intracerebral injection of a strain with a comparatively long incubation period has been shown to delay or prevent the replication of a shorter incubation period strain injected some time later.[27]

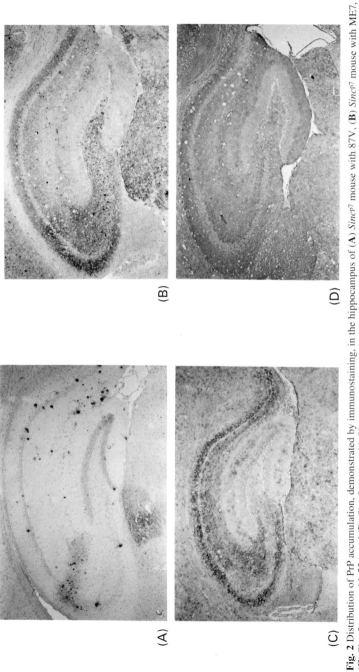

Fig. 2 Distribution of PrP accumulation, demonstrated by immunostaining, in the hippocampus of (**A**) *Sinc*p7 mouse with 87V, (**B**) *Sinc*p7 mouse with ME7, (**C**) *Sinc*p7 mouse with 22A and (**D**) *Sinc*s7 mouse with 79A.

ISOLATION OF STRAINS IN MICE

On transmission of a scrapie-like disease from its natural host to mice the incubation period is usually very long and there may be survivors. On subsequent mouse-to-mouse passage in a single genotype the incubation period shortens and stabilises after a few passages to give a strain with characteristic properties. These properties are stable indefinitely on further mouse-to-mouse passage, as long as the conditions of passage, particularly the mouse genotype, remain constant. In Edinburgh alone, 14 unequivocally distinct strains of scrapie and BSE have been isolated in mice (Fig. 1).[11] A further 5 isolates have unique disease characteristics, indicative of new strains, but are not yet fully stable.

Most primary sources have given rise to two different scrapie strains when passaged in $Sinc^{s7}$ and $Sinc^{p7}$ mice.[10,11] Clearly, these differences are not simply imposed by the host as numerous strains have been isolated in the same mouse genotype and the same strain (e.g. ME7) has occasionally been isolated in both genotypes. On the other hand, this resolution of isolates into two distinct stable strains has always been consistent with the selection of strains which replicate more rapidly in the mouse genotype used for passage.[10] For example, 79A and 79V were isolated from the goat 'drowsy' source, by passage in $Sinc^{s7}$ and $Sinc^{p7}$ mice respectively; 79A is quicker than 79V in $Sinc^{s7}$ mice and 79V is quicker than 79A in $Sinc^{p7}$ mice. Interestingly, for a single scrapie strain the incubation period is not necessarily shorter in the mouse genotype in which it has been isolated.

Once the incubation periods and pathological properties have stabilised, it cannot be assumed that the isolate contains only a single strain, as it is possible that minor variants are passaged together with the major strain in a stable mixture. For many experimental purposes this may not be significant, but it may become important if the isolate is passaged in a new host, as described below. In order to remove minor strains from an isolate it is necessary to biologically clone the strain, by several sequential passages using the minimum infecting dose.[28] This procedure has been shown to lead to a permanent change in the characteristics or behaviour of several isolates.

STABILITY OF MOUSE-PASSAGED STRAINS

The existence of many strains indicates clearly that scrapie-like agents carry some form of information which is independent of the host. As both the hypothetical 'protein-only' and 'virino' structures include a host component, an important question is whether and to what extent this strain-specific information is modified by the host in which the isolate is passaged. To investigate this, several mouse-passaged strains have been serially passaged in new mouse genotypes or species. Scrapie strains have been found to differ dramatically in the stability of their properties on passage in their new hosts (Fig. 3).

The characteristics of some scrapie strains, such as ME7, 22C and 139A, remain constant when the mouse genotype in which they are passaged is changed from $Sinc^{s7}$ to $Sinc^{p7}$. In contrast, some isolates change their properties when passaged in the alternative $Sinc$ genotype. Whenever such changes have occurred they have been consistent with the selection of strains with shorter incubation periods under the new passaging conditions. In the case of an uncloned isolate this could simply be the separation of strains which have been propagated as a mixture since the original transmission to mice. However, there are examples of changes occurring in cloned strains, suggesting the generation and selection of new mutant strains. There is no evidence that the $Sinc$ genotype of the mouse can actively modify the properties of a strain.

Much of the work on strain stability on passage in different $Sinc$ genotypes has involved two strains derived from the SSBP/1 experimental sheep isolate, 22C and 22A; these studies are described in detail in a recent review.[11] Both 22C and 22A are stable when serially passaged in the genotype in which they were isolated, $Sinc^{s7}$ in the case of 22C and $Sinc^{p7}$ in the case of 22A. However, when uncloned 22C is passaged in $Sinc^{p7}$ mice its properties change gradually over several passages to give a new strain, 22H, which is clearly different from 22A. This change in properties is not seen when cloned 22C is passaged in $Sinc^{p7}$ mice, showing that the change from 22C to 22H is not the result of modification by the new host. Rather, this is evidence that 22C and 22H coexisted in the early mouse passages of the isolate and that 22H was removed from the mixture by cloning. These results emphasise the need to use cloned strains in studies seeking host modifications of strain characteristics.

In contrast, 22A is unstable when the $Sinc$ genotype in which it is passaged is changed, even after it has been cloned. On serial passage in $Sinc^{s7}$ mice the incubation period characteristics gradually change, eventually stabilising after several passages to give yet another new strain, 22F. The fact that this has been seen using cloned 22A suggests that 22F has been generated from 22A, either by a host-induced modification or by mutation, in the sense of a change in the scrapie-specific information of the agent. The same change has been seen in 16 separate $Sinc^{s7}$ passage lines, although the number of passages required to regain stability has varied considerably. In some of these lines little or no change has been seen at the first passage in the new genotype, making it unlikely that the phenomenon is due to a modification of the agent by the host. These results are more consistent with the gradual selection of

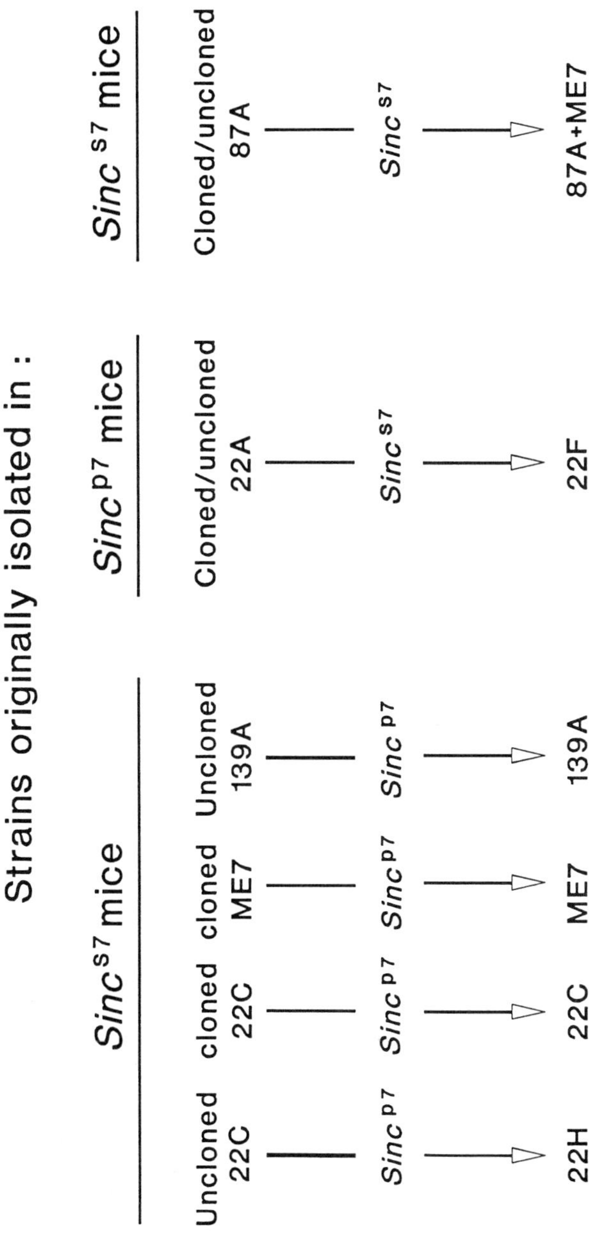

Strains originally isolated in :

Sinc s7 mice				Sinc p7 mice	Sinc s7 mice
Uncloned 22C	cloned 22C	cloned ME7	Uncloned 139A	Cloned/uncloned 22A	Cloned/uncloned 87A
Sinc p7	Sinc p7	Sinc p7	Sinc p7	Sinc s7	Sinc s7
→	→	→	→	→	→
22H	22C	ME7	139A	22F	87A+ME7

Fig. 3 Summary of experiments in which well-characterised scrapie strains were passaged through different Sinc genotypes of mouse.

a mutant strain, 22F, which has a shorter incubation period in the new passaging genotype than the parental strain, 22A.

Other evidence that scrapie strains can mutate has come from studies with 87A, which is unstable even when passaged in the *Sinc* genotype in which it was originally isolated.[29] The characteristics of 87A are stable when it is passaged at low dose in *Sinc*[s7] mice but often change suddenly when it is passaged at higher dose in the same mouse genotype, to give a strain with much shorter incubation periods. This new strain is stable, even when passaged at high dose, and is always identical to ME7. This sudden change in properties is seen even after 87A has been cloned, suggesting that ME7 is a shorter incubation period mutant strain derived from 87A.

The studies described above show that the *Sinc* (or PrP) genotype of mouse used for passage has no consistent effect on the characteristics of scrapie strains, apart from selecting strains which replicate more quickly. Studies showing a change in properties when a 'Chandler'-derived isolate was passaged in a new *Sinc* genotype[30] cannot be taken as evidence of a host modification, as the authors claim, because an uncloned isolate was used; the 'Chandler' isolate has been shown elsewhere to contain a mixture of strains[10] and the results reported by Carlson and coworkers are consistent with the resolution of this mixture on the basis of incubation periods in the two genotypes.

INTERSPECIES TRANSMISSION

As already noted, when scrapie is transmitted from one species to another the incubation period is usually long compared with later passages in the new species, a phenomenon referred to as the 'species barrier'. Even for the same change of passage species, the species barrier is highly variable between scrapie isolates. For example, the 263K strain transmits from hamsters to mice only with difficulty, producing very long incubation periods, whereas the 431K hamster-passaged strain has been transmitted to *Sinc*[s7] mice with a minimal species barrier effect.[5] There is also one natural scrapie-derived strain in mice, 111A, which has been passaged four times in *Sinc*[p7] mice without the usual shortening of the incubation period (*see* Fig. 1).

In a series of experiments in which mouse-passaged scrapie strains were passaged in rats or hamsters and then repassaged in mice (Fig. 4), Kimberlin and coworkers demonstrated that the species barrier has a number of contributing factors.[6,31] They found that cloned 22A and cloned ME7 were completely unchanged after serial passage in hamsters and subsequent reisolation in mice. In contrast, the properties of cloned 139A and cloned 22C were permanently changed by passage in hamsters, giving rise to new strains which were stable on serial passage in mice. Cloned 139A was unchanged by passage through rats. These results are evidence that the species barrier effect can be partly due to the selection of strains in the new host species, other than the major strains present in the original host.

Cloned mouse-passaged strains

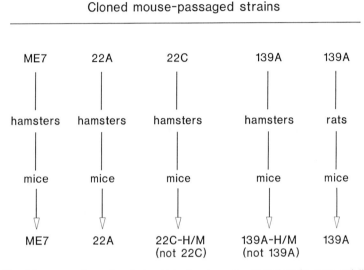

Fig. 4 Summary of experiments in which cloned mouse-passaged strains were serially passaged several times through Syrian hamsters or rats and then repassaged in mice.[6,31]

The fact that a species barrier is seen even when the strain characteristics remain unchanged shows that other factors are involved, but only at the first passage in a new species. These are likely to depend on the association of infectivity with tissue components derived from the 'donor' species. The simplest effect is a reduction in the efficiency of initial infection, possibly as a result of more effective clearance and inactivation by the host of infectivity from the inoculum. There are also differences in pathogenesis between the first and subsequent passages in the new species. When there is no change in passaging species, the incubation period following intraperitoneal infection is longer than that following direct intracerebral infection, usually by about 50%. However, in at least some interspecies passages, the intracerebral and intraperitoneal routes produce similar incubation periods (H Fraser and M Bruce, unpublished results; R H Kimberlin, personal communication).

A possible explanation is that the agent is unable to establish itself directly in the brain when it is associated with foreign tissue, but must be processed in peripheral organs, such as spleen, before it can replicate in the new host.

The assertion that there is the equivalent of a species barrier between mouse strains of different *Sinc* genotypes[30] is misleading. Transmission of scrapie strains between *Sinc* genotypes may sometimes result in the selection of new strains, as described above, but there is no great reduction in the efficiency of infection and there is the usual large difference in incubation periods between intracerebral and intraperitoneal routes.[4,18]

STRAIN VARIATION IN NATURAL SCRAPIE-LIKE DISEASES

Because of the possibility of the selection of minor variants, it is not clear to what extent the mouse-passaged strains isolated from natural cases are representative of field strains. However, transmissions to mice can give some information about the extent of strain variation in the natural diseases.

In the case of transmissions of natural scrapie to mice the incubation periods and pathology in standard panels of mouse strains have varied widely between sources. However, on further passage in mice the majority, but not all, of the isolates from cases occurring in the UK have given varying combinations of the same 3 strains, 87A and ME7 in *Sinc*[s7] mice and 87V in *Sinc*[p7] mice (M Bruce, unpublished observations). Therefore these sources may not be as diverse as they appear on primary transmission to mice. A series of transmissions from Icelandic sheep have given at least 3 strains in mice, which are not yet fully characterised but clearly differ from those isolated from UK cases. In the USA, mouse passages have been set up from 5 natural scrapie sheep; again, the resultant strains have not yet been fully characterised, but differ between sources.[32] It is likely that the variation in transmission results between sources depends on scrapie strain variation in the natural host, but it is also possible that 'donor' effects make some contribution at the first passage in mice, as described in the previous section.

Recent transmissions of BSE from cattle to mice[33] have been much more straightforward. So far, BSE has been transmitted from 6 unrelated cattle sources, collected at different times during the epidemic and from widely separated geographical locations within the UK. The results of these transmissions were remarkably similar to each other and differed from those in all previous and contemporary transmissions of scrapie (Fig. 5). All 6 BSE sources produced a characteristic pattern of incubation periods and pathology in a standard panel of inbred mouse strains and crosses. There were large and consistent differences in incubation period between mouse strains of different *Sinc* genotypes and also, surprisingly, between mouse strains of the same *Sinc* genotype (e.g. C57BL and RIII). This incubation period difference within *Sinc* genotypes was lost at the first mouse-to-mouse passage. Further passages in *Sinc*[s7] and *Sinc*[p7] mice have produced two strains, 301C and 301V, which differ from all strains derived from sheep or goat scrapie (Fig. 1).

The uniformity of transmission results with different sources of BSE suggests that each cow was infected with the same major strain of agent. The consistency of the pathology reported in cattle with BSE[34] also suggests that a single or a limited number of strains is involved. It is generally accepted that BSE originated from rendered scrapie-infected offal, included in high-protein feed supplements. The transmission studies described above suggest that the major strain of agent causing BSE in cattle is different from the strains causing scrapie in sheep. A possible explanation is that the high temperatures involved in rendering and subsequent passage through cattle have selected variant strains from sheep scrapie.

Recently, transmissions to mice have been achieved from other species with novel scrapie-like diseases, which were suspected to be related to the BSE epidemic; the sources were 3 cats, a greater kudu and a nyala. The results of all 5 transmissions were strikingly similar to results from cattle sources, indicating that these species were infected with BSE (H Fraser and G Pearson, personal communication). BSE from cattle has also been transmitted experimentally to sheep, goats and pigs and then from each of these species to mice. Again, the results of these mouse transmissions were similar to direct transmissions of BSE (unpublished observations). These results show, firstly, that the BSE agent is unchanged when passaged through a range of species and, secondly, that the donor species has little influence on the disease characteristics of BSE on transmission to mice.

PrP IN AGENT-HOST INTERACTIONS

There is little doubt that PrP plays a central role in pathogenesis, as it is almost certainly the *Sinc* gene product (*see* Scott, this issue). The biological effects of *Sinc* probably depend on one or both of the two amino acid differences observed between PrPs from *Sinc*[s7] and *Sinc*[p7] mice.[22] As described above, the phenotypic properties of a mouse-passaged strain depend on specific and precise interactions between the scrapie informational molecule and the *Sinc* or PrP genotype of the host. It has been suggested that the incubation periods of mouse-passaged

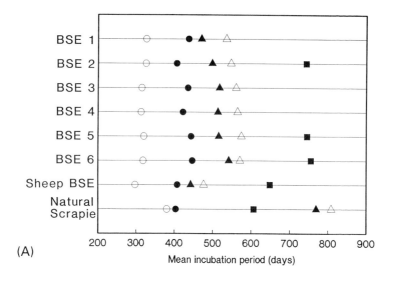

(A)

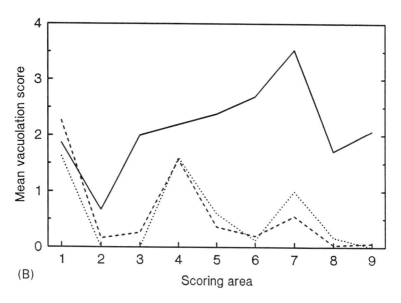

(B)

Fig. 5 (A) Comparison of incubation period characteristics in a panel of mouse strains on primary passage to mice of 6 sources of cattle BSE, one source of experimental BSE in sheep and one contemporary source of natural sheep scrapie. The mouse strains were RIII($Sinc^{s7}$) (○), C57BL($Sinc^{s7}$) (●), VM($Sinc^{p7}$) (▲), IM($Sinc^{p7}$) (△) and C57BLxVM($Sinc^{s7}p^7$) (■). Data are not yet available for BSE 5 and 6 sources in C57BLxVM mice. **(B)** Lesion profiles at the primary passage for RIII mice infected with cattle BSE (— — —), sheep BSE (······) and natural sheep scrapie (————).

strains depend on the compatibility of PrPs between donor and recipient mice[30] but there is no experimental support for this. In fact, many of the observations cited in this review argue that the donor mouse genotype has no direct effect on strain characteristics. At the simplest level, it can be seen from Figure 1 that the incubation period for a single strain is not necessarily shorter in the genotype which matches that of the donor. Also, 3 out of 4 cloned strains tested have been unchanged by passaging in the alternative genotype and the fourth strain has changed only gradually, suggesting a host-permitted selection of a new strain, rather than a host modification.

Mismatching of PrPs in donor and recipient species may, on the other hand, be involved in some way in the species barrier. Transgenic mice carrying multiple copies of the hamster PrP gene have short incubation periods when intracerebrally infected with the Sc237 hamster-passaged scrapie strain (identical to the 263K strain used elsewhere), in contrast with the extremely long incubation periods seen in non-transgenic mice with this strain.[35] Also, there is evidence that the abnormal PrP in these animals is derived from the hamster rather than the mouse protein.[36] This shows that the Sc237 strain interacts preferentially with hamster PrP in the transgenic recipients, as would be expected from its very short incubation period in hamsters and its very long incubation period in non-transgenic mice. However, these results give no information about whether donor PrP type is critical in this interaction or about the effect of the transgene on efficiency of infection and details of pathogenesis.

Other investigations in transgenic mice into various aspects of the agent-host interaction and species barrier have so far been difficult to interpret. Problems in these studies have included the effects of trans-gene copy number and endogenous gene expression on incubation periods and the use of uncloned, poorly characterised scrapie isolates. The insertion of foreign or altered PrP genes into mice lacking their own PrP gene[37] will avoid some of these problems in future.

MOLECULAR MODELS OF SCRAPIE-LIKE AGENTS

The existence of many strains of scrapie is crucial to speculation about the nature of the scrapie agent as any valid model must include a molecule which carries strain-specific information. It is relatively easy to explain strains in terms of an agent-specific nucleic acid, in which case the genetic variation would be analogous to that seen in conventional microorganisms. It is more difficult to envisage how a protein alone could specify strain diversity. According to protein-only models the scrapie pathogen is PrP which has been modified in some specific but as yet unknown way. This abnormal protein is suggested to induce the same modification in host PrP molecules, either by direct interaction or by causing a mistranslation of the gene.[38,39,40]

The characteristics of strains do not depend, to any great extent, on the primary sequence of PrP in the animals in which they are passaged. Therefore, if scrapie-like agents do consist solely of PrP, strain-specific information is likely to reside in post-translational modifications of the protein. The relevant modifications could either be conformational or chemical, for example involving differences in glycosylation. There must be as many specific modifications as there are distinct strains and each must be able to 'replicate' itself accurately over many serial passages, apart from predictably generating other specific modifications. Also, multiple forms of modified PrP must be capable of retaining their separate identities when passaged as mixtures and such mixtures must be resolvable by biological cloning. A crucial question is whether a protein alone can fulfil all these criteria or whether it requires a separate informational molecule, such as a nucleic acid, as proposed in the 'virino' and virus hypotheses.

In order to reconcile the protein-only and 'virino' hypotheses, it has recently been speculated that the agent consists of a modified host protein which confers transmissibility and an inessential nucleic acid which determines strain characteristics.[41] Such a model predicts that strain characteristics and infectivity can be separated by treatments which remove or destroy nucleic acids. At present there is no evidence that this separation is possible and, in fact, the phenotypic properties of several strains have survived exposure to high doses of ionizing or UV radiation (D Taylor and M Bruce, unpublished observations). A simpler explanation is still that the agent contains an essential small nucleic acid which is protected by its close association with host tissue components such as PrP (the 'virino' hypothesis).

Despite much speculation, there is very little direct evidence concerning the molecular basis of strain variation. No specific differences have been found in PrP from the same host species/genotype infected with different scrapie strains.[42] On the other hand, the scrapie nucleic acid, if it exists, remains obstinately elusive.[15] The issue will remain controversial until there is a direct identification of the informational molecule of the agent and the variations in it which lead to phenotypic diversity.

ACKNOWLEDGEMENTS

I would like to thank Aileen Chree and Laurence Doughty for their help in preparing the figures.

REFERENCES

1 Pattison IH, Millson GC. Scrapie produced experimentally in goats with special reference to the clinical syndrome. J Comp Pathol 1961; 71: 101-108.

2 Foster JD, Dickinson AG. The unusual properties of CH1641, a sheep-passaged isolate of scrapie. Vet Rec 1988; 123: 5-8.

3 Dickinson AG, Meikle VMH. Host-genotype and agent effects in scrapie incubation: change in allelic interaction with different strains of agent. Mol Gen Genet 1971; 112: 73-79.

4 Bruce ME, McConnell I, Fraser H, Dickinson AG. The disease characteristics of different strains of scrapie in *Sinc* congenic mouse lines: implications for the nature of the agent and host control of pathogenesis. J Gen Virol 1991; 72: 595-603.

5 Kimberlin RH, Walker CA. Evidence that the transmission of one source of scrapie agent to hamsters involves separation of agent strains from a mixture. J Gen Virol 1978; 39: 487-496.

6 Kimberlin RH, Walker CA, Fraser H. The genomic identity of different strains of mouse scrapie is expressed in hamsters and preserved on reisolation in mice. J Gen Virol 1989; 70: 2017-2025.

7 Mori S, Hamada C, Kumanishi T et al. A Creutzfeldt-Jakob disease agent (Echigo-1 strain) recovered from brain tissue following the "panencephalopathic type" disease. Neurology 1989; 39: 1337-1342.

8 Kitamoto T, Yi R, Mohri S, Tateishi J. Cerebral amyloid in mice with Creutzfeldt-Jakob disease is influenced by the strain of infectious agent. Brain Res 1990; 508: 165-167.

9 Kimberlin RH, Cole S, Walker CA. Transmissible mink encephalopathy (TME) in Chinese hamsters: identification of two strains of TME and comparisons with scrapie. Neuropathol Appl Neurobiol 1986; 12: 197-206.

10 Bruce ME, Fraser H. Scrapie strain variation and its implications. In: Chesebro BW, ed. Transmissible spongiform encephalopathies. Curr Top Microbiol Immunol 1991; 172: 125-138.

11 Bruce ME, Fraser H, McBride PA, Scott JR, Dickinson AG. The basis of strain variation in scrapie. In: Prusiner S, Collinge J, Powell J, Anderton B, eds. Prion diseases of humans and animals. Chichester: Ellis Horwood, 1992: 497-508.

12 Carp RI, Callahan SM, Sersen EA, Moretz RC. Preclinical changes in weight of scrapie-infected mice as a function of scrapie agent-mouse strain combination. Intervirology 1984; 21: 61-69.

13 Dickinson AG, Taylor DM. Resistance of scrapie to decontamination. N Engl J Med 1978; 299: 1413-1414.

14 Kimberlin RH, Walker CA, Millson GC et al. Disinfection studies with two strains of mouse-passaged scrapie agent. J Neurol Sci 1983; 59: 355-369.

15 Riesner D, Kellings K, Meyer N, Mirenda C, Prusiner SB. Nucleic acids and scrapie prions. In: Prusiner S, Collinge J, Powell J, Anderton B, eds. Prion diseases of humans and animals. Chichester: Ellis Horwood, 1992: pp 341-353.

16 Prusiner SB. Novel proteinaceous infectious particles cause scrapie. Science 1982; 216: 136-144.

17 Bolton DC, McKinley MP, Prusiner SB. Properties and characteristics of scrapie PrP 27-30 protein. In: Prusiner SB, McKinley MP, eds. Prions: novel infectious pathogens causing scrapie and Creutzfeldt-Jakob disease. San Diego: Academic Press, 1987: 173-196.

18 Dickinson AG, Outram GW. Genetic aspects of unconventional virus infections: the basis of the virino hypothesis. In: Bock G, Marsh J eds. Ciba Foundation symposium 135: Novel infectious agents and the central nervous system. Chichester: Wiley, 1988: 63-83.

19 Rohwer RG. The scrapie agent: "a virus by any other name". In: Chesebro BW, ed. Transmissible spongiform encephalopathies. Curr Top Microbiol Immunol 1991; 172: 195-232.

20 Dickinson AG, Meikle VMH, Fraser H. Identification of a gene which controls the incubation period of some strains of scrapie in mice. J Comp Pathol 1968; 78: 293-299.

21 Carlson GA, Kingsbury DT, Goodman PA et al. Linkage of prion protein and scrapie incubation time genes. Cell 1986; 46: 503-511.

22 Westaway D, Goodman PA, Mirenda CA, McKinley MP, Carlson, GA, Prusiner SB. Distinct prion proteins in short and long scrapie incubation period mice. Cell 1987; 51: 651-662.

23 Hunter N, Dann JC, Bennett AD, Somerville RA, McConnell I, Hope J. Are *Sinc* and the PrP gene congruent? Evidence from PrP gene analysis in *Sinc* congenic mice. J Gen Virol 1992; 73: 2751-2755.

24 Fraser H, Dickinson AG. The sequential development of the brain lesions of scrapie in three strains of mice. J Comp Pathol 1968; 78: 301-311.

25 Bruce ME, McBride PA, Farquhar CF. Precise targeting of the pathology of the sialoglycoprotein, PrP, and vacuolar degeneration in mouse scrapie. Neurosci Lett 1989; 102: 1-6.

26 Rubenstein R, Deng H, Race RE et al. Demonstration of scrapie strain diversity in infected PC12 cells. J Gen Virol 1992; 73: 3027-3031.

27 Dickinson AG, Fraser H, Meikle VMH, Outram GW . Competition between different scrapie agents in mice. Nature 1972; 237: 244-245.

28 Dickinson AG, Outram GW. Operational limitations in the characterisation of the infective units of scrapie. In: Court LA, Cathala F, eds. Virus nonconventionnels et affections du systeme nerveux central. Paris: Masson, 1983: 3-16.

29 Bruce ME, Dickinson AG. Biological evidence that scrapie agent has an independent genome. J Gen Virol 1987; 68: 79-89.

30 Carlson GA, Westaway D, DeArmond SJ, Peterson-Torchia M, Prusiner SB. Primary structure of prion protein may modify scrapie isolate properties. Proc Natl Acad Sci USA 1989; 86: 7475-7479.

31 Kimberlin RH, Cole S, Walker CA. Temporary and permanent modifications to a single strain of mouse scrapie on transmission to rats and hamsters. J Gen Virol 1987; 68: 1875-1881.

32 Carp RI, Callahan SM. Variation in the characteristics of 10 mouse-passaged scrapie lines derived from five scrapie-positive sheep. J Gen Virol 1991; 72: 293-298.

33 Fraser H, Bruce ME, Chree A, McConnell I, Wells GAH. Transmission of bovine spongiform encephalopathy and scrapie to mice. J Gen Virol 1992; 73: 1891-1897.

34 Wells GAH, Hawkins SAC, Hadlow WJ, Spencer YI. The discovery of bovine spongiform encephalopathy and observations on the vacuolar changes. In: Prusiner S, Collinge J, Powell J, Anderton B, eds. Prion diseases of humans and animals. Chichester: Ellis Horwood, 1992: 256-274.

35 Scott M, Foster D, Mirenda C et al. Transgenic mice expressing hamster prion protein produce species-specific scrapie infectivity and amyloid plaques. Cell 1989; 59: 847-857.

36 Prusiner SB, Scott M, Foster D et al. Transgenic studies implicate interactions between homologous PrP isoforms in scrapie prion replication. Cell 1990; 63: 673-686.

37 Bueler H, Fischer M, Lang Y et al. Normal development and behaviour of mice lacking the neuronal cell-surface PrP protein. Nature 1992; 356: 577-582.

38 Bolton DC, Bendheim PE. A modified host protein model of scrapie. In: Bock G, Marsh J eds. Ciba Foundation symposium 135: Novel infectious agents and the central nervous system. Chichester: Wiley, 1988: 164-181.

39 Prusiner SB. Prion biology. In: Prusiner S, Collinge J, Powell J, Anderton B, eds. Prion diseases of humans and animals. Chichester: Ellis Horwood, 1992: 533-567.

40 Wills PR. Induced frameshifting mechanism of replication for an information-carrying scrapie prion. Microb Pathogen 1989; 6: 235-249.

41 Weissmann C. A 'unified theory' of prion propagation. Nature 1991; 352: 679-683.

42 Somerville RA, Ritchie LA. Differential glycosylation of the protein (PrP) forming scrapie-associated fibrils. J Gen Virol 1990; 71: 833-839.

British Medical Bulletin (1993) Vol. 49, No. 4 pp 839–859
©The British Council 1993

PrP gene and its association with spongiform encephalopathies

W Goldmann
AFRC & MRC Neuropathogenesis Unit, Institute for Animal Health, Edinburgh, UK

The PrP or prion protein plays a key role in the pathogenesis of the transmissible spongiform encephalopathies. This 33-35 kD sialoglycoprotein is the product of a single host gene which is composed of 2 or 3 exons, a single open reading frame and a cytidine/guanidine rich promoter. The structure of the gene and the sequence of the protein are highly conserved in various mammals. Primarily, transcription of the PrP gene is found in neurons of the central and peripheral nervous system but other tissues do express PrP at least at some stages of development. Translation of the PrP mRNA and processing of the initial gene product result in a 210 amino acid protein with asparagine-linked glycosylation of the complex type which attaches itself to the outer leaflet of the plasma membrane lipid bilayer by a C-terminal glycosylinositol phospholipid. The function of this protein is unknown. Development of the transmissible spongiform encephalopathies, and increasing titre of the causative pathogen, are associated with the accumulation in and around cells of pleiomorphic aggregates of PrP which are partially resistant to proteolytic hydrolysis. These abnormal deposits of PrP, and the normal isoform, are transcribed from the same gene and so any disease-linked modification of the protein must be post-transcriptional. No disease-specific, covalent modifications of PrP have yet been found and some simple, conformational change in its secondary, tertiary (or quaternary) structure may underlie its role in these diseases. Polymorphisms in the PrP gene of different species have been associated with disease but none of these changes in primary structure appear to cause protease resistance per se. Preclinical inference of disease susceptibility can already be made using PrP genotype analysis in man and some animals but developing a cure for these diseases, whether by drug or gene therapy, will require a much greater understanding of the molecular and cell biology of this gene and its products. This article presents current views and understanding of the PrP gene.

The spongiform encephalopathies (SEs) are difficult to classify because their characteristics combine the transmissibility, strain variation and mutational features of a viral disease with the molecular genetics and epidemiology (in man) more closely associated with non-infectious, genetic disorders. No virus or viral genome has been identified in infectious fractions and a host membrane protein (PrP) is the only candidate molecule which has been consistently found to be associated with the infectious particle. The pathology of these diseases is associated with aggregation of PrP (as amyloid plaques, scrapie-associated fibrils or amorphous deposits) and disease susceptibility in man and animals is closely linked to mutations in its gene. Therefore, three lines of SE research have converged to focus on the PrP gene and its product: from one side, virologists seeking to characterise the infectious particle and understand the molecular coding of strain phenotype are investigating PrP and its relationship to infectivity, while in independent lines of research geneticists and neuropathologists seeking to describe the host's response have linked polymorphisms in the PrP gene to the incubation period, incidence and brain pathology of these diseases in man and animal.

Normal PrP protein (PrP^C) is converted into a protease-resistant isoform (PrP^{Sc}) and accumulates in the brain and other affected tissues. Ostensibly, this is similar to the amyloidoses seen in other neurodegenerative diseases such as Alzheimer's disease but, in this case, the mechanism and the nature of this conversion is unknown. It is widely believed that both normal and disease specific PrP protein are encoded by the same gene and that the conversion of PrP^C into PrP^{Sc} is introduced post-translationally. Hence the basic unit of the conversion process could be the primary translation product or the polypeptide with its normal modifications. Similarly, variations in the amino acid sequence of the protein within a species affect individual susceptibility and incubation period of the disease. Thorough analysis of the structure and regulation of this gene and the amount, distribution and variety of its products are needed to help understand the mechanisms that link these PrP-related phenotypes with SE agents and disease.

This article presents a current view and understanding of the PrP gene: in its first part, there is a molecular description of the PrP gene and its RNA transcripts, including those DNA and RNA elements which are essential for its regulated expression; the second part will cover the PrP protein itself, its normal and disease-specific isoforms, including the major post-translational modifications and the concluding part describes the potential application of some of this data.

THE PrP GENE

PrP gene is a single gene with only one protein coding exon

The PrP gene (*PRNP* in human, *Prn-p* in mouse and PrP gene in other species) appears to be a single gene in the genomes of rodents, man and ruminants.[1-4] Its chromosomal location has been established for human *PRNP* on chromosome 20 (20pter-12)[3,5,6] and for mouse *Prn-p* on chromosome 2.[5] Only one homologous gene (PrLP) in a non-mammalian organism (chicken) has so far been described.[7] PrP-related DNA hybridisation signals have been detected in organisms such as Drosophila, the nematode Caenorhabditis elegans and even yeast.[2] However, attempts to prove the existence of PrP-like proteins in these organisms have failed. Interestingly, Iwasaki et al. isolated a novel gene from C. elegans using a hamster PrP cDNA probe.[8] The encoded protein was homologous to nuclear ribonucleoproteins but not to mammalian PrP. These results make it more likely that PrP is a late gene in evolutionary terms, confined to mammals and some other vertebrates. Whether that restricts the potential to become affected with SEs to mammals (or vertebrates) remains to be established. The first description of an almost full-length PrP cDNA (hamster)[1] in 1985 was followed by descriptions of partial PrP gene sequences of other rodents,[9-11] man,[3,6,12] ruminants[4,13,14] and a carnivore.[15] In summary, the PrP gene structure can be described as follows (Fig. 1): (I) 'ORF-EXON': A single exon coding for the entire PrP open reading frame (orf) and the entire 3′ untranslated mRNA region; (II) '5prime-EXON(S)': 1 or 2 small exons coding for 5′ leader sequence of PrP mRNA; (III) a PROMOTER with regulatory elements and 1 or 2 introns (combined ≥10 kb) separating the 5prime-EXON(S) and PROMOTER from the ORF-EXON. The following paragraphs will highlight some of these characteristic features of PrP genes.

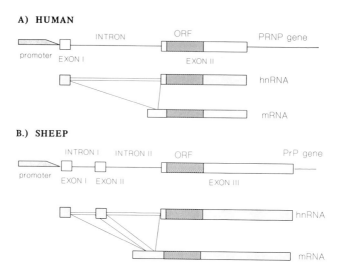

Fig. 1 Schematic diagram of human *PRNP* gene and sheep PrP gene and their transcription products. Illustration of two different types of PrP gene structure represented by (**A**) human *PRNP*[6] and (**B**) sheep PrP gene[7] (and H. Baybutt, personal communication). For details see text. ORF, open reading frame (PrP coding region); hnRNA, primary transcription product; mRNA, messenger RNA; promoter (transcription start site and regulatory region). The 5′ leader sequence of the transcript is encoded either on EXON I only (*PRNP* and hamster,[9] not shown) or EXON I and EXON II together (sheep and mouse,[33] not shown).

The ORF-EXON

The PrP open reading frame (orf) is not interrupted by introns

The boundaries of this exon are given by the intron/exon border and the sequence for the poly(A) addition site (end of the mRNA). The length of the ORF-EXON is about ≥85% of the total mRNA length. Human (2350 basepairs (bp))[3,6,12] and rodent ORF-EXON (about 2000 bp)[1,9,10,16] are of similar size whereas ruminants possess a much larger ORF-EXON (about 4000 bp).[4] These differences reside within the 3′ untranslated region of PrP mRNA, whereas all ORFs are of similar length (about 760 bp).[4] The ORF start codon AUG is 10 bp downstream of the intron/exon border and represents an arrangement precisely conserved in all mammalian PrP genes analyzed. The AUG codon is part of a consensus sequence which facilitates initiation of protein translation and is followed by a signal peptide sequence for membrane transport. The continuous open reading frame of 253 to 257 codons is rather larger than the average for eukaryotic genes. Exons might have evolved as units which can be shuffled to generate new proteins and, quite frequently, encode common protein domains or motifs, e.g. signal peptides, cytoplasmic domains. The PrP ORF-EXON provides little opportunity in evolution for exon shuffling, a fact reflected in the observation that PrP shows little if any homology to other proteins of the mammalian genome[2] (and unpublished observations).

PrP coding region contains short GC-rich repeats

The first half of the PrP coding region contains about 170 bp with a high content (about 80%) of the nucleotides guanidine (G) and cytidine (C). Most of this sequence is organized in 24 bp (or 27bp) repeats.[1] Little DNA sequence variation between repeats within the same ORF or between repeats of PrP genes from different mammals has been observed.[1,3,4,10-15] All repeats encode almost identical glycine-rich octapeptides (or nonapeptides), again with little variation (Table 1B). However variability does exist in the number of copies of these repetitive sequences. The most frequent allele of a species or population usually contains five copies. An exception is found in cattle, where the most common allele has 6 repeat copies and the 5 copy variant represents a minor haplotype of the gene pool.[13,14] Similar polymorphisms in this region of PrP ORF have been described recently for human *Prn-p* (for detail see elsewhere in this issue). Here, variation in the repeat copy number (from 4 to 14 copies) alters the protein considerably, with a maximal increase of the molecular weight of 20%. That the enlargement of this region is detrimental to health is implied by the association of 10 or more copies with familial Creutzfeldt Jakob disease (CJD) and Gerstmann-Sträussler-Scheinker syndrome (GSS).[17] Whether this is due to an increased susceptibility to the SE agents or a result of a disrupted PrP metabolism remains to be investigated.

Control and fidelity of PrP mRNA translation may be mediated through the high G/C rich elements of this region. Several groups have suggested the high G/C content might impose stable folding (i.e. stem-loops) onto the overall secondary structure of PrP mRNA with consequences for its metabolism and translation. One folding model for elements of PrP RNA predicts stemloop structures similar to the TAR-stemloops characteristic of the human immunodeficiency virus.[18] Indeed, preliminary in vitro analysis suggests that this stemloop structure has a positive effect on the translation rate of PrP, with the implication of a novel mechanism for PrP expression control.[19] Interestingly, a TAR RNA-binding protein has recently been isolated from a HeLa cell cDNA library.[20]

Another calculation predicted pseudoknot RNA structures with homology to ribosomal frameshift sites in this region. Structurally-enhanced frame 'slipping and sliding' at these sites has been proposed to lead to aberrant PrP.[21] In turn, this PrP containing an inappropriate peptide segment may be involved in the generation of the protease-resistant forms of PrP such as scrapie-associated fibrils (SAF). If these 'frame-shift' mutants were of low abundance, they may not have been detected during initial sequencing of SAF protein.[22-25] Future investigations will show if these structures can induce such 'slippage' and result in mistranslation of the PrP mRNA. Short (18 bp) repeats (encoding hexapeptides as shown in Table 1A) have also been found in chicken PrLP coding region.[7]

Table 1 Repeated peptide sequences are a feature of mammalian PrP proteins and the chicken PrP-like protein (PrLP)

	Variation of peptide sequences[1]
A. PrLP hexapeptide repeats	RQPSYP; RQPGYP; HNPGYP; QNPGYP
B. Hexapeptide repeats	GGSRYP; GGNRYP
Octapeptide repeats	PQGGGWGQ; PQGGTWGQ; PHGGGWGQ; PHGGSWGQ
Nonapeptide repeats	PQGGGGWGQ; PHGGGGWGQ
Tandem repeat	YYRxxMxxYxNQ; YYRxxVxxYxNQ
Palindromic sequence	RYYxxNxYRYxNxxYYR; RYYxxNxHRYxNxxYYR; RYYxxNxNRYxNxxYYR

[1]Sequence in one letter amino-acid code, x representing nonconsensus positions.

The 3′ untranslated mRNA contains highly conserved areas

Exons are not only protein coding gene segments, but also templates for untranslated regions of mRNA. These mRNA sequences usually carry various regulatory functions, i.e. sequence elements for mRNA processing. They are also responsible for mRNA stability, transport, cellular segregation or translation. It is known from other mRNAs that information for accuracy and efficiency of these processes can be encoded within the 3′ mRNA region.[26,27] The 3′ untranslated region of PrP mRNA is quite long and well conserved between species, although there are some sheep-specific insertions.[4] These insertions are partially homologous to ruminant-specific retroposons,[28] which are usually not part of mRNA. Whether they play a role in PrP expression remains to be established, but repetitive sequences have been shown to be involved in post-transcriptional control of gene expression.[29]

Intriguingly, a polymorphism linked to scrapie in sheep is located within the 3′ untranslated region of ovine PrP mRNA.[30] One of the more-obviously conserved regions of PrP mRNA is a A/T-rich sequence upstream of the poly(A) attachment sites (Fig. 2A), which might function as a signal for mRNA processing, because other consensus sequences for poly(A) addition located further upstream in PrP mRNAs do not appear to be used in the brain. However, smaller transcripts can be detected in RNA extracts of tissues such as heart using PrP probes,[31] and it will be interesting to see if these transcripts are PrP mRNAs with shorter 3' untranslated regions. The use of alternative poly(A) addition sites in gene regulation has recently been shown for, among others, the Alzheimer precursor protein gene.[32]

THE 5PRIME-EXON(S)

The 5' leader sequence of PrP mRNA is variable in length

The length of the PrP mRNA 5' leader sequence is dependent on the transcription start site. Recent results for *Prn-p* suggest that PrP transcription in brain tissue starts at one site only, resulting in a 136 nucleotide long 5' leader (Fig. 2B).[6] In contrast, transcription in mouse (and hamster) brain starts at multiple sites producing variable mRNAs with 5' leader sequences of 119-155 nucleotides (55-85 in hamster brain mRNA).[9,16] A similar size for this region has been estimated for sheep PrP mRNA (150 to 300 nucleotides, deduced from the total mRNA length and the sequenced ORF-EXON)[4] and bovine PrP mRNA (Fig. 2B).[14] The 5' leader sequence of PrP mRNA is encoded by one exon in the human[6] and hamster PrP gene[9] or 2 exons in murine *Prn-p*[33] (J Cameron, personal communication) and ovine PrP (H Baybutt, personal communication, and Fig. 1A).

Elements for PrP translational control may reside in the 5' leader mRNA

The role of the 5' leader sequence in PrP regulation is unknown, but a variety of viral genes and some eukaryotic genes are post-transcriptionally regulated by factors which bind to this region. For example, the ferritin gene expression is regulated via an iron responsive element in its 5' leader sequence.[34] Only future experiments will show if transcriptional control of PrP expression in brain or other tissues is dependent on the 5' sequence of its RNA. It is intriguing that in mouse and sheep PrP (and probably bovine PrP) an additional exon may allow alternative splicing to generate different transcripts coding an identical protein but which may be under different control (Fig. 1). That PrP translation is controlled in normal and scrapie infected brain is implied indirectly by the discrepancy between the distribution of PrP mRNA (measured by *in situ* hybridisation) and PrP protein (measured with immunohistochemistry).[35]

Partitioning of PrP mRNA into translationally active and inactive compartments is another of several possible mechanisms of control of

```
Human      UCCUUAGGCU .UACAAUGUG CACUGAAUCG UUUCAUGUAA GAAUCCAAAG  50
Ovine      UCCUUAGCCU .UACAGUGUG CACUGAAUAG UUUUGUAUAA GAAUCCAGAG
Mouse      CCCUUGGGCU UU.CAGCGUG CACU...CAG UUCCGU..AG GAUUCCAAAG
consensus  uCCUUaGgCU UUaCAguGUG CACUgaauaG UUucgU:uAa GAaUCCAaAG

Human      UGGACACCAU UAACAGGUCU UUGAAAUAUG CAUGUACUUU AUAUUUUCUA 100
Ovine      .......... ....UGAUAU UUGAAAUACG CAUGUGCUU. AUAUUUUUUA
Mouse      CAGACCCC.U .AGCUGGUCU UUGAA.UCUG CAUGUACUUC ACGUUUUCUA
consensus  ::GAC:CC:U :A:CuGgUcU UUGAAaUauG CAUGUACUU: AuaUUUUcUA

Human      UAUUUGUAAC UUUGCAUGUU CUU.GUUUUG UUAUAUAAAA AAAUUGUAAA 150
Ovine      UAUUUGUAAC UUUGCAUGUA CUU.GUUUUG ...UGUUAAA AGUUUAUAAA
Mouse      UAUUUGUAAC UUUGCAUGUA UUUUGUUUUG UCAUAUAAAA AGUUUAUAAA
Consensus  UAUUUGUAAC UUUGCAUGUa cUU:GUUUUG ucaUaUaAAA AguUUaUAAA

Human      UGUUUAAUAU CUGACUGAAA UUAAAC..GA GCGAAGAUGA GCACCA☺
Ovine      UAUUUAAUAU CUGACUAAAA UUAAACA☺
Mouse      UGUUUGCUAU CAGACUGACA UUAAAUAGAA GCUAUGAUG☺
consensus  UgUUUaaUAU CuGACUgAaA UUAAAca::A GC:A:GAUG
```

Fig. 2A Examples for sequence conservation in the 5′ and 3′ untranslated regions of PrP mRNA's. Comparison of the last 200 nucleotides of PrP mRNAs deduced from cDNA and gene sequence. These regions exhibits a sequence conservation comparable to the protein coding regions and might play a role in RNA processing.

```
Human       CGCCGCGGAG CGCCGCCCGU UCCCUUCCCC GCCCCGCGUC CCUCCCCGCC    50

Human       UCGGCCCCGC GCGUCGCCUC CAGUCGCCUG CAGUCGCUGA CAGCCGCGGC   100
Hamster     ACUGCCCCGC CCGCUCCCCC GCGGCG.UCC GAGCAGCAGA CCGAGAAGGC
Bovine      ---------  ---------  --------GC CAGUCGCUGA GAGCCGCAGA
consensus   :::GCCCCGC :CG:::CC:C ::G:CG:UgC cAGucGcugA cagccgcggc

Human       GCCGCGAGCU UCUCCCUCUCC UCACGACCGA GGCAG.....              150
Hamster     ACAUCGA... .UCCACUCG  UCGCGUCGGU GGCAG..... AUAUAUUUC
Bovine      GCUGAGAGCG UCUUCUCUC. UCGCAGAAGC AGGACUUCUG AAUAUAUUUC
Mouse       ---------  ---------  ---------  ---------  AAU.UCCUUC
consensus   gC:gcAgc:  ucUcCuCUC: UCgCg:c:G: ggcAg::::: AAU:U::UUC

Human       .......... .......... .......... ..........              200
Hamster     AAAACUGAAC AGUUUCAACC AGCCGAAGC  A.UCUGUCUU CCCAGAGACA
Bovine      AGAACUGAAC CAUUUCAACC GAGCUGAAGC AUUCUGCCUU CCUAGUGGUA
Mouse       ---------  ---------  ---------  ---------  ..........
consensus   A:AACUGAAC ::UUUCAACC :AGC:GAAGC A:UCUG:CUU CC:AG:G::A

Human       .......... ..........             .AGCAGUCA UU
Hamster     .......... ..........             ..AUCAGCCA UC
Bovine      CAAAUCCAAC UUGAGCUGAA UCACACCAGA .UAUAAGUCA UC
Mouse       CCAGUCCAAU UU.AGGAGAG .CCAAGCAGA CUAUCAGUCA UC
consensus   C:A:UCCAA: UU:AG::GA: :C::A:CAGA :UAUcAgucA C
```

Fig. 2B Examples for sequence conservation in the 5′ and 3′ untranslated regions of PrP mRNA's. Comparison of 5′ untranslated mRNA sequences deduced from gene or cDNA clones. The arrows indicate an inserted sequence in mouse and bovine PrP genes which are probably encoded by a second 5PRIME EXON (EXON II in Fig. 1B). These mRNA regions might be involved in post-transcriptional gene regulation. The consensus sequences (A and B) are shown in shaded areas, with upper case letters indicating identical nucleotides in all sequences, lower case indicating identical nucleotides in the majority of sequences and colons standing for no consensus in this position. Dashed lines represent unsequenced regions, dotted lines are deletions/insertions. Human PRNP,[6,12] hamster PrP gene,[9] bovine PrP gene,[14] ovine PrP gene[4] and mouse Prn-p.[10]

PrP expression. Denman et al. showed the distribution of PrP mRNA between translational active polysomes (70 % of PrP mRNA) and inactive ribonucleoprotein particles (30% of PrP mRNA) and concluded that this sequestration could be responsible in part for the observed imbalance of PrP mRNA and protein concentration.[36] They also suggest this mechanism might account for some selective expression of protein according to cell-type or brain area.

PrP GENE PROMOTER

PrP gene transcription is initiated at a GC-rich sequence region
It is difficult to define the PrP promoter region from its sequence alone. Only experiments using PrP promoter segments in so-called reporter gene constructs tested for expression in vitro or in transgenic animals will tell us what parts of this gene region are essential for constitutive or regulated PrP expression.

PrP promoter regions (transcription start sites) have been described for human *PRNP* (about 70 bp)[6] and hamster PrP gene (about 330 bp).[9] They exhibit some typical characteristics of so-called house-keeping genes. The major feature is the lack of the typical regulatory elements found in most other genes. Especially, sequence elements known to control the precise initiation of the transcription complex are missing in the hamster PrP gene (and probably mouse *Prn-p*), consequently PrP gene expression starts at several nucleotides (multiple start sites) rather than one precise position.[9,16] In contrast human *Prn-p* exhibits a major start site within its promoter, although a consensus sequence for initiation of transcription appears to be missing.[6] Thus the mechanisms involved in the start of PrP gene expression appear to be variable. The second feature is the high content of the nucleotides G and C (83% in human) near the transcription start site in form of repeated elements such as GCCCCGCCC (3 times, hamster) or CCGCCC (4 times, human). Similar elements are found in other house-keeping promoters and have recently been shown to bind proteins in the Alzheimer precursor protein gene.[37] Transcription factor SP1 is one of the DNA binding proteins with specificity for GC-rich elements and a consensus sequence can be detected in the hamster PrP promoter region (nucleotides 285-293).[9] Interestingly, some of the GC-rich elements in human *PRNP* are located downstream of the transcription start site.[6] They are therefore also part of the mRNA and could form secondary structures with the GC-rich region of the ORF.

The importance of the PrP intron(s) (10 kb ~ 14 kb total size)[9,33] has been highlighted in transgenic mice. Here, the lack of any expression in mice transgenic for an intron-less PrP gene may have indicated a more significant role than previously anticipated.[38] Apart from its normal role, intron sequences could be utilised to decrease PrP expression. A first in vitro experiment using PrP pre-mRNA with self-cleaving ribozyme activity in the intron region demonstrated a viable approach of gene expression control, although application in SEs will depend on improved information about the conditions, under which these mechanisms can happen in vivo.[39]

PrP is predominantly, but not exclusively expressed in neuronal cells

The amount of PrP mRNA in brain of an adult mouse is estimated as almost 1.4 ng/μg total RNA. A third of this is found in brainstem. Hippocampus, thalamus and neocortex contain nearly equal amounts of 250 ng/μg each.[40] In situ and northern blot hybridization analysis have revealed that PrP is expressed in most if not all neurons of the adult mouse brain as well as ganglia and nerves of the peripheral nervous system.[41,42] It also showed that it is not exclusively CNS and neurons that contain PrP transcripts: i.e. kidney, heart, lung and spleen all contain transcripts.[1,42,43] In contrast, liver appeared negative.[42] A puzzling result is the localisation of PrP transcripts in axons of cranial nerves (i.e. optic nerve).[42] This may be explained by PrP expression in surrounding glial cells, or by mRNA in transit through axons.[44]

PrP expression can be regulated by other gene products

There is evidence for indirect control of PrP expression, i.e. in embryonal development and cell-specific expression.[42] PrP also appears inducible by other gene products. Mobley et al. reported that nerve growth factor (NGF) injection elevates PrP mRNA expression almost 9 fold and PrP protein levels about 3 times.[40] They concluded that this increase was brain region specific. In another example, mouse chimeras for trisomy 16, unexpectedly exhibited a slight but significant increase of PrP mRNA expression in brain and skin.[45] This kind of control might become important in the course of therapeutic intervention.

PrP PROTEIN

PrP protein acquires distinct biochemical properties in disease

The cellular PrP (PrP^C) is a glycoprotein anchored to the external surface of cells by a glycoinositol phospholipid moiety.[25,47-49] Homogenates of normal brain contain PrP^C of apparent molecular weight (Mr) 33~35 kilodalton (kD) and some minor species of lower Mr.[25,47,48] PrP^C is soluble and digested entirely by proteinase K.[48] In contrast, PrP^{Sc} (the scrapie specific isoform), is insoluble and partially protease resistant in non-denaturing detergents.[1] Preparations of PrP^{Sc}

contain a 33-35 kD sialoglycoprotein,[23,25] which is reduced to 27-30 kD with proteinase K (PrP27-30).[22-25,46-48] The N-terminal sequence of PrP27-30 is heterogeneous with the major fraction starting within the octapeptide repeat region.[22,24] This partial proteinase K resistance is a hallmark of all SEs and widely used for purification of PrP^{Sc} and SE diagnosis. The size and charge heterogeneity observed with electrophoretic separation techniques reflects the considerable extent of post-translational modifications. However, the similarities in size and charge between both isoforms suggest that only a slight structure modification or a conformational change is associated with protease resistance.[23-25] PrP^C has been isolated from normal and SE infected brain. If PrP^C is the precursor molecule of PrP^{Sc}, then its conversion has to be established within the constraints of its primary polypeptide structure as encoded on its gene and its post-translational modifications.

The primary structure (amino acid sequence) creates the basic unit for modifications

Amino acid sequences of PrP have been deduced from genomic and cDNA sequences (see above and Fig. 3), and some have been confirmed partially by protein sequencing.[22-25] PrP proteins exhibit a very high identity ($\geq$85%) between each other (Fig. 3). The overall polypeptide length varies only slightly between 253 (human) and 257 amino acids (mink) and most sequence (and structural) features are conserved. The primary sequence begins with a typical signal peptide of 22 amino acids (sheep, cattle and mink 24 amino acids), which co-translationally guides PrP through the membrane of the endoplasmatic reticulum and is eventually cleaved off to generate the N-terminus Lys-Lys-Arg- found in mature PrP protein. PrP contains 3 different groups of short peptide repeats. In the first 2 groups, hexapeptides and octapeptides (nonapeptides) are repeated in human PrP twice and 5 times, respectively (see Table 1B). They show little sequence variation between various PrPs and might fulfil a major biological or structural function. The third group contains 2 peptides in the form of a tandem repeat (Table 1B). All repeats appear to be unique to PrP proteins, although the Gly-Gly-Gly-Trp core sequence of the octapeptides resemble sequences found in keratin. Recently, Sulkowsi defined an aromatic palindrome motif (amino acids 147 to 163), which coincides in part with the tandem repeats (Table 1B).[50] Palindromic sequences play a key role in DNA as protein binding sites, but a function in protein remains to be established. It is possible that the palindromic symmetry of this region enhances dimerization of PrP or binding of other proteins to PrP. We can not yet assign a function to any of these repeated peptides, but have to recognize them as a characteristic feature of PrP. Whether they are involved in PrP^C to PrP^{Sc} conversion remains to be shown. Finally, there are 2 hydrophobic regions (codons 111 to 134 and 231 to 253) of which the second can be regarded as the signal sequence for attachment of a glycoinositol-phospholipid (GPI) moiety.[49] Other well known peptide motifs are Asn-glycosylation sites in codon 181 (Asn-Ile-Thr) and codon 197 (Asn-Phe-Thr), 2 threonine phosphorylation consensus sequences in positions 183 and 192, and a tyrosine sulphation motif (codon 145) (this site is not present in rodent PrP due to a substitution of Tyr with Trp). A tyrosine phosphorylation site (codon 155) is found in all sequences except human PrP, although its role as a substrate for tyrosine kinases has not been established.

Both PrP isoforms carry post-translational modifications

Cleavage of the N- and C-terminal peptides in normal post-translational modification reduces the number of amino acids to about 210 (Mr=23 kD). The apparent Mr of about 33-35 kD as determined by SDS-PAGE indicates micro-heterogeneity and post-translational modifications (such as carbohydrates) of the mature PrP protein.

Both Asn-glycosylation sites are modified with oligosaccharides, probably of the complex type. Deglycosylation experiments reduce the Mr by about 7 kD.[51] A detailed carbohydrate structure analysis has only been performed for PrP^{Sc}: it revealed that nearly 400 oligosaccharide combinations might exist in PrP^{Sc}.[51] Whether this is also the case for PrP^C remains to be examined. These carbohydrates will contribute to the charge heterogeneity observed for isolated PrP protein. PrP was found to contain an intramolecular disulfide bond, which creates a loop of 36 amino acids containing the two Asn-linked oligosaccharides.[25]

PrP^{Sc} and PrP^C display a structurally heterogeneous GPI moiety (2-2.5 kD), of which 30% contain sialic acid as part of the carbohydrate structure.[9,52,53] Sialic acid as a GPI component is a novel feature which has only been observed in the GPI of PrP.[52] It remains to be established whether the number and position of sialic acids in both structures influence the fate of the cellular or scrapie PrP isoforms. The majority of PrP^{Sc} molecules (hamster brain) have their GPI anchor attached to Scr-231, but about 15% showed a carboxyl terminal Gly-228.[53] This truncated form could be the precursor of secreted PrP protein, which is found in normal and scrapie infected cell cultures and even detected in CSF of normal individuals.[54-56] Further experiments are needed to clarify whether this secreted form corresponds to the Gly(228)-truncated PrP or is simply intact PrP (including GPI) which has been released into the CNS by membrane sloughing. Future experiments will also show whether PrP^C is primarily a membrane protein or a secretory molecule.

```
1        (1)MetAlaAsnLeuGlyCysTrpMetLeuValLeuPheValAlaAlaThrTrpSerAspLeuGlyLeuCysLysLysArg
2                                   Tyr Leu                ThrMet    Thr  Val
3        MetValLysSerHisIle         Ser Ala       Met                Val  Ile
4        MatValLysSerHisIle         Ser Leu                               Phe

1       (26)ProLysProGlyGly---TrpAsnThrGlySerArgTyrProGlyGlnGlySerProGlyGlyAsnArgTyr
2                 ---
3                 Gly
4                 Gly
3+4

1       (50)ProProGlnGlyGlyGlyTrpGlyGlnProHisGlyGlyGlyTrpGlyGlnProHisGlyGlyGlyTrpGlyGlnGlyGlyGlyThrTrpGlyGly
2                                                                                             Ser
3+4              ---Thr

1       (75)GlnProHisGlyGlyGlyTrpGlyGlnProHisGlyGlyGlyTrpGlyGly---TrpGlyGlnGlyGlyGlyThrHisSerGln
2              Ser                                                                           Asn
3                                                                    Gly             ---Ser Ser
4                                                                    Gly                   Asn

1       (99)TrpAsnLysProSerLysProLysThrAsnMetLysHisMetAlaGlyAlaAlaAlaAlaGlyAlaValValGlyGly
2                                          Leu          Val
3+4                                                     Val
5        ProTrpLysProProProLysProLysThrAsnPheLysHisValAlaGlyAlaAlaAlaAlaGlyAlaValValGlyGly

1      (124)GlyLeuGlyGlyTyrMetLeuGlySerAlaMetSerArgProIleIleHisPheGlySerAspTyrGluAspArg
2                                                                   Met            Asn
3+4                                                                 Leu            Asn
5        GlyLeuGlyGlyTyrValAlaMetGlyArgValMetSer

1      (149)TyrTyrArgGluAsnMetHisArgTyrProAsnGlnValTyrTyrArgProMetAspGluTyrSerAsnGlnAsn
2+3                             Tyr                              Lys Gln
4                               Tyr                              Val Gln

1      (174)AsnPheValHisAspCysValAsnIleThrIleLysGlnHisThrValThrThrThrLysGlyGluAsnPhe
2                                                      Val
3+4

1      (199)ThrGluThrAspValLysMetMetGluArgValValGluGlnMetCysIleThrGlnTyrGluArgGluSerGln
2+3                                                Val                           GlnLys
3                                                  Val                           Gln    Glu
4                                                                                Gln    Glu

1      (224)AlaTyrTyr---GlnArgGlySerSer---MetValLeuPheSerSerProProValIleLeuLeuIleSerPhe
2             AspGly Arg          SerThr
3             ---                 ---Val Ile
4                                 ---Ala Ile                Pro
                                                                                        Leu

1      (247)LeuIlePheLeuIleValGlyGly
2+3          Leu
4                                Leu
```

Fig. 3 PrP amino-acid sequence deduced from cDNA sequence of human *PRNP* and differences to other PrP protein sequences. The full human PrP sequence[12] is shown in line in standard three letter amino-acid code. The signal peptide sequence, the putative signal sequence for GPI attachment and the Asn-glycosylation sites are indicated as shaded areas. The N-terminal octapeptide repeats (numbered 1 to 5) are shown in italics. Amino-acid differences of three other PrP sequences are displayed as follows: 2, mouse[10]; 3, sheep[4]; 4, mink.[15] The underlined sequence (5) represents the chicken PrLP[7] region with highest homology to mammalian PrPs.

Another form of PrP^{Sc} modification is the conversion of arginine residues (Arg-3, Arg-15) into citrulline.[57] Its function is unknown. The importance of this modification might become clear when the distribution of citrulline within PrP and the percentage of modified PrP molecules has been investigated. Although PrP has the peptide motifs used for phosphorylation and sulphation (see above) their utilisation has not been proven experimentally. It is probable that some modifications of PrP^C or PrP^{Sc} have not been detected if only a small fraction of total PrP, obscured by the extensive heterogeneity, displays the alteration.

Conformational models of PrP differ depending on the experimental system

Secondary structure predictions of PrP seem to define two distinct regions: A N-terminal part (amino acid 1 to 80) with random coiled structures and a C-terminal part (81-210) with a more common composition of well defined secondary peptide structures, namely beta sheets, alpha-helices and turns[58] (and personal observation). Caughey et al. determined the content of these structures for PrP27-30, resulting in a higher beta-sheet percentage (beta-sheet 47%, alpha-helices 17%, turns 31%) in this isoform than originally predicted from the amino acid sequence.[59] Whether this is an indication for a conformational alteration between PrP^C and PrP^{Sc} or just reflects the inaccuracy of structure predictions has to be established. However, a high beta-sheet content is not unexpected because of the PrP^{Sc} aggregation as amyloid.

In vitro translation experiments and structure predictions have been interpreted as evidence for PrP as an integral membrane protein with two membrane spanning regions.[54,60] In this model both protein termini would be located in the extracytoplasmic compartment. Intriguingly, PrP contains a stop transfer sequence comprised of a 16 amino acid long charged and polar region (codons 96-111) and a 24 residue long hydrophobic sequence (codons 112-136) which can span the membrane once.[61,62] These sequences might direct PrP into the integral membrane topology. However, the discovery of the C-terminal GPI moiety and the enzymatic (GPI-specific phospholipase C) release of PrP^C from cultured cells led to a new model of protein topography in which PrP is attached to the membrane by the GPI anchor.[49]

Allelic variation of PrP primary structure is associated with disease

The C-terminal domain of the PrP protein carries most of the modifications of normal PrP and almost all of the detected single amino acid polymorphisms. Linkage analysis of human and animal SEs have over the last years demonstrated that some clinical and neuropathological features of these disorders are associated with mutations (poly-morphisms) of PrP protein sequence (for details on the molecular ge-netics of CJD and GSS see Gajdusek and Will, this issue). Different PrP genotypes have been associated with onset and incubation period of scrapie in sheep and mice. PrP haplotypes of inbred mice contain two amino acid differences (108 Leu or Phe, 189 Thr or Val).[16] The resulting two PrP protein variants (Fig. 4B) are linked to short and long incubation periods in experimentally challenged animals, although we do not know whether both or only one of these polymorphic sites is linked with the phenotype, as they have always occured together on the same haplotype. Additionally, a correlation between incubation period and primary structure of PrP has been described in PrP-trans-genic mice[38] (see also Prusiner, this issue). PrP polymorphisms are also linked with scrapie in various sheep breeds. Five ovine PrP variants have already been described with polymorphisms in codons 112, 136, 154, 171 (Fig. 4A).[4,63-65] One PrP variant (codon 136:valine) has been linked with susceptibility to disease (with short incubation period) after experimental infection with a specific scrapie isolate.[63] There is also ev-idence that ovine PrP variants are associated with susceptibility to other isolates and natural scrapie[30,64,65] (and unpublished observation). None of these polymorphisms is part of known post-translational modification sites and their influence might therefore be conformational. Neither the murine nor the ovine PrP mutations give clues to the mechanisms that produce the PrP-related phenotype of disease control, but it appears likely that 2 protein 'domains' (or 3 'domains' in human PrP) (see Fig. 4) are involved in modulation of the disease phenotype in scrapie, similar to CJD and fatal familial insomnia in man.[66]

The normal biological function of PrP is still enigmatic

Several proposals for PrP function have been made over the years, most recently the copurification of a chicken PrP-like protein (PrLP) with acetylcholine-receptor inducing activity (ARIA) fuelled specula-tion about an equivalent role for mammalian PrP.[7] This hypothesis has not been experimentally supported with mice lacking a functional PrP gene ($Prn-p^{0/0}$ mice). Their nerve-muscle synapses have normally de-veloped cholinergic receptors.[67] Even more surprisingly, $Prn-p^{0/0}$ mice lack any pathological or behavioural abnormalities up to the age of 7 months, contrary to all expectations based on its significant expression in brain and other tissues as well as during embryonal development.[42] Do other proteins substitute PrP function? Does pathology develop only at a certain age or under stress? Can these $Prn-p^{0/0}$ mice get spongiform encephalopathies? These are key questions which should be answered in the next phase of research on the PrP gene.

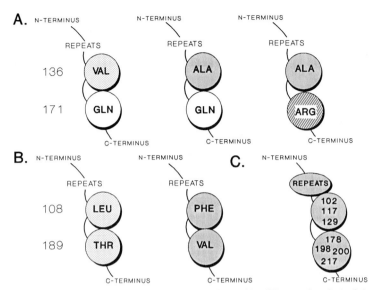

Fig. 4 Disease-associated PrP polymorphisms are located in different 'domains' of the protein. Schematic diagram of PrP variants of sheep (**A**), mouse (**B**) and man (**C**). The distribution of the single amino acid polymorphisms (codon numbers; three letter amino acid code) which appear to be associated with different phenotypes of disease suggest a 'two domain model' for PrP protein of sheep and mouse and a 'three domain model' for human PrP. In this model mutations in different 'domains' are either associated with disease incidence or in the modulation of disease phenotypes such as length of incubation period or neuropathology. (**A**) The presented sheep PrP variants have been reported in disease association. The 136 mutation is associated with onset of some forms of scrapie, whereas modulation of the length of incubation period is linked to mutations in 136 and 171.[63] This association can be reversed with other isolates of scrapie (unpublished results). (**B**) In mouse the two presented variants produce three different genotypes which are linked with different incubation times of scrapie,[16] in contrast to sheep it remains to be established which mutation ('domain') contributes to the various observed phenotype differences in different forms of experimental scrapie. (**C**) Human PrP variants appear to have three different domains (additionally there is disease linkage with the repeat region) with different disease phenotypes depending on which domains (and their mutations) occur together.

CONCLUSION

Spongiform encephalopathies are phenotypically associated with the structure and expression of the host encoded PrP protein. All data so far demonstrate that the same gene encodes PrP^C as well as PrP^{Sc}, which leaves PrP^C as the precursor molecule for a modified PrP^{Sc} isoform. Every PrP polymorphism can therefore be seen as new basic unit for modification and might be linked with a different disease phenotype.[66] Resolving the puzzle of this linkage might ultimately be achieved with a improved understanding of the function and expression of the PrP gene. Of course the agent itself is a decisive participant in the determination of

SE characteristics and further studies into agent properties (*see* Bruce, this issue) and neuropathology (*see* Fraser, this issue) will facilitate our understanding of SEs. The most obvious benefit of PrP gene analysis appears to be the evaluation of disease risk, based on the association of PrP polymorphisms with disease susceptibility. This will lead to preclinical counselling in familial CJD and GSS, much in the same way other inherited disorders such as Huntington's disease are managed. However, in about 80% of all CJD cases there are as yet no apparent PrP mutations, so that a continuation in the search for PrP variants is still essential. In the management of farm animals, such as sheep and cattle, similar risk assessments have also become important. There is already one breeding program to reduce scrapie incidence from a flock of sheep which is now using PrP genotypes as selection method[65] and comparable programs might be used to prevent the spread of bovine spongiform encephalopathy (BSE).

Data from PrP gene analysis could eventually lead to therapeutic intervention, for instance by interference with PrP expression or, even more radical, a total inhibition of PrP production. The preliminary results from *Prn-p$^{0/0}$* mice lacking a functional PrP protein suggest that loss of PrP can be tolerated.[33] Whether this genotype prevents the development of SEs entirely has to be established, but it appears to prolong the incubation period significantly (*see* Weissmann, this issue).

ACKNOWLEDGEMENT

I would like to thank J. Hope and N. Hunter for their invaluable help in preparation of this manuscript and H. Baybutt and J. Cameron for communicating data on gene structure prior to publication.

REFERENCES

1 Oesch B, Westaway D, Wälchli M, et al. A cellular gene encodes scrapie PrP 27-30 protein. Cell 1985; 40: 735-746.
2 Westaway D, Prusiner SB. Conservation of the cellular gene encoding the scrapie prion protein. Nucl Acids Res 1986; 14: 2035-2044.
3 Liao YJ, Lebo RV, Clawson GA Smuckler EA. Human prion protein cDNA: Molecular cloning, chromosomal mapping and biological implications. Science 1986; 233: 364-367.
4 Goldmann W, Hunter N, Foster JD, Salbaum JM, Beyreuther K, Hope J. Two alleles of a neural protein gene linked to scrapie in sheep. Proc Natl Acad Sci USA 1990; 87: 2476-2480.
5 Sparkes RS, Simon M, Cohn VH et al. Assignment of the human and mouse prion protein genes to homologous chromosomes. Proc Natl Acad Sci USA 1986; 83: 7358-7362.
6 Puckett C, Concannon P, Casey C, Hood L. Genomic structure of the human prion protein gene. Am J Hum Genet 1991; 49: 320-329.

7 Harris DA, Falls DL, Johnson FA, Fishbach GD. A prion-like protein from chicken brain copurifies with an acetylcholine receptor-inducing activity. Proc Natl Acad Sci USA 1991; 88: 7664-7668.
8 Iwasaki M, Okumura K, Kondo Y, Tanaka T, Igarashi H. cDNA cloning of a novel heterogeneous nuclear ribonucleoprotein gene homologue in Caenorhabditis elegans using hamster prion protein cDNA as a hybridization probe. Nucl Acids Res 1992; 20: 4001-4007.
9 Basler K, Oesch B, Scott M et al. Scrapie and cellular PrP isoform are encoded by the same chromosomal gene. Cell 1986; 46: 417-428.
10 Locht C, Chesebro B, Race R, Keith JM. Molecular cloning and complete sequence of prion protein cDNA from mouse brain infected with the scrapie agent. Proc Natl Acad Sci USA 1986; 83: 6372-6376.
11 Liao YL, Tokes Z, Lim E et al. Cloning of rat 'prion-related protein' cDNA. Lab Investigation 1987; 57: 370-374.
12 Kretzschmar HA, Stowring LE, Westaway D, Stubblebine WH, Prusiner SB, DeArmond SJ. Molecular cloning of a human prion protein cDNA. DNA 1986; 5: 315-324.
13 Goldmann W, Hunter N, Martin T, Dawson M, Hope J. Different forms of the bovine PrP gene have five or six copies of a short, G-C-rich element within the protein-coding exon. J Gen Virol 1991; 72: 201-204.
14 Yoshimoto J, Iinuma T, Ishiguro N, Horiuchi M, Imamura M, Shinegawa M. Comparative sequence analysis and expression of bovine PrP gene in mouse L-929 cells. Virus Genes 1992; 6: 343-356.
15 Kretzschmar HA, Neuman M, Riethmueller, Prusiner SB. Molecular cloning of a mink prion protein gene. J Gen Virol 1992; 73: 2757-2761.
16 Westaway D, Goodman PA, Mirenda CA, McKinley MP, Carlson GA, Prusiner SB. Distinct prion proteins in short and long scrapie incubation period mice. Cell 1987; 51: 651-662.
17 Goldfarb LG, Brown P, Gajdusek DC. The molecular genetics of human transmissible spongiform encephalopathies. In: Prusiner SB, Collinge J, Powell J, Anderton B, eds. Prion diseases of humans and animals. Chichester: Wiley, 1992: 139-153.
18 Will PR, Hughes AJ. Stem loops in HIV and prion protein mRNAs. J Acquir Immune Defic Syndr 1990; 3: 95-97.
19 Müller WEG, Pfeifer K, Forrest J, et al. Accumulation of transcripts coding for prion protein in human astrocytes during infection with human immunodeficiency virus. Biochim Biophys Acta 1992; 1139: 32-40.
20 Gatignol A, Buckler-White A, Berkhout B, Jeang KT. Characterisation of a human TAR RNA-binding protein that activates the HIV-1 LTR. Science 1991; 251: 1597-1600.
21 Will PR.Potential pseudoknots in the PrP-encoding mRNA. J Theor Biol 1992; 159: 523-527.
22 Prusiner SB, Groth DF, Bolton DC, Kent SB, Hood LE. Purification and structural studies of a major scrapie prion protein. Cell 1984; 38: 127-134.
23 Hope J, Morton LJD, Farquhar CF, Multhaup G, Beyreuther K, Kimberlin H. The major polypeptide of scrapie-associated fibrils (SAF) has the same size, charge distribution and N-terminal protein sequence as predicted for the normal brain protein (PrP). EMBO J 1986; 5: 2591-2597.
24 Hope J, Multaup G, Reekie LJD, Kimberlin RH, Beyreuther K. Molecular pathology of scrapie-associated fibril protein (PrP) in mouse brain affected by the ME7 strain of scrapie. Eur J Biochem 1988; 172: 271-277.
25 Turk E, Teplow DB, Hood LE, Prusiner SB. Purification and properties of the cellular and scrapie hamster prion protein. Eur J Biochem 1988;176:21-30.
26 Jackson RJ, Standart N. Do the poly(A) tail and 3′ untranslated region control mRNA translation? Cell 1990; 62: 15-24.
27 Carter BZ, Malter JS. Biology of disease: Regulation of mRNA stability and its relevance to disease. Lab Invest 1991; 65: 610-621.

28 Goldmann W, Hunter N, Manson J, Hope J. The PrP gene of the sheep, a natural host of scrapie. 8th International Congress of Virology, Berlin, 1990: abstract, p.284

29 Vidal F, Mougneau E, Glaichenhaus N, Vaigot P, Darmon M, Cuzin F. Coordinated posttranscriptional control of gene expression by modular elements including Alu-like repetitive sequences. Proc Natl Acad Sci USA 1993; 90: 208-212.

30 Hunter N, Foster JD, Benson G, Hope J. Restriction fragment length polymorphisms of the scrapie-associated fibril protein (PrP) gene and their association with susceptibility to natural scrapie in British sheep. J Gen Virol 1991; 72: 1287-1292.

31 Robakis NK, Sawh PR, Wolfe GC, Rubenstein R, Carp RI, Innis MA. Isolation of a cDNA clone encoding the leader peptide of prion protein and expression of the homologous gene in various tissues. Proc Natl Acad Sci USA 1986; 83: 6377-6381.

32 Sauvage F de, Kruys V, Marinx O, Huez G, Octave JN. Alternative polyadenylation of the amyloid protein precursor mRNA regulates translation. EMBO J 1992; 11: 3099-3103.

33 Büeler H, Fischer M, Lang Y, et al. Normal development and behaviour of mice lacking the neuronal cell-surface PrP protein. Nature 1992; 356: 577-582.

34 Goosen B, Caughman SW, Harford JB, Klausner RD, Hentze MW. Translational repression by a complex between the iron-responsive element of ferritin mRNA and its specific cytoplasmic binding protein is position-dependent in vivo. EMBO J 1990; 9: 4127-4133.

35 Manson J, McBride P, Hope J. Expression of the PrP gene in the brain of *Sinc* congenic mice and its relationship to the development of scrapie. Neurodegeneration 1992; 1: 45-52.

36 Denman R, Potemska A, Wolfe G, Ramakrishna N, Miller DL. Distribution and activity of alternatively spliced Alzheimer amyloid peptide precursor and scrapie PrP mRNAs on rat brain polysomes. Arch Biochem Biophys 1991; 288: 29-38.

37 Pollwein P, Masters CL, Beyreuther K. The expression of the amyloid precursor protein (APP) is regulated by two GC-elements in the promoter. Nucl Acids Res 1992; 20: 63-68.

38 Scott M, Foster D, Mirenda C, et al. Transgenic mice expressing hamster prion protein produce species-specific scrapie infectivity and amyloid plaques. Cell 1989; 59: 847-857.

39 Denman RB, Purow B, Rubenstein, Miller DL. Hammerhead ribozyme cleavage of hamster prion pre-mRNA in complex cell-free model systems. Biochem Biophys Res Commun 1992; 186: 1171-1177.

40 Mobley WC, Neve RL, Prusiner SB, McKinley MP. Nerve growth factor increases mRNA levels for the prion protein and the β-amyloid protein precursor in developing hamster brain. Proc Natl Acad Sci USA 1988; 85: 9811-9815.

41 Kretzschmar HA, Prusiner SB, Stowring LE, DeArmond SJ. Scrapie prion proteins are synthesized in neurons. Am J Pathol 1986; 122: 1-5.

42 Manson J, West JD, Thomson V, McBride P, Kaufman MH, Hope J. The prion protein gene:a role in mouse embryogenesis? Development 1992; 115: 117-122.

43 Brown HR, Goller NL, Rudelli RD. The mRNA encoding the scrapie agent protein is present in a variety of non-neuronal cells. Acta Neuropathol 1990; 80: 1-6.

44 Steward O, Banker GA. Getting the message from the gene to the synapse: sorting and intracellular transport of RNA in neurons. TINS 1992; 15: 180-186.

45 Holtzman DM, Bayney RM, Li Y, et al. Dysregulation of gene expression in mouse trisomy 16, an animal model of Downs syndrome. EMBO J 1992; 11: 619-627

46 Bolton DC, McKinley MP, Prusiner SB. Identification of a protein that purifies with the scrapie prion. Science 1982; 218: 1309-1311

47 Bolton DC, Bendheim PE, Marmorstein AD, Potemska A. Isolation and structural studies of the intact scrapie agent protein. Arch Biochem Biophys 1987; 258: 579-590.

48 Bendheim PE, Potemska A, Kascsak R, Bolton DC. Purification and partial characterisation of the normal cellular homologue of the scrapie agent protein. J Infect Dis 1988; 158: 1198-1208.

49 Stahl N, Borchelt DR, Prusiner SB. Differential release of cellular and scrapie prion proteins from cellular membranes by phosphatidylinositol-specific phospholipase C. Biochemistry 1990; 29; 5405-5412.

50 Sulkowski E. Aromatic palindrome motif in prion protein. FASEB J 1992; 6: 2363.

51 Endo T, Groth D, Prusiner SB, Kobata A. Diversity of oligosaccharide structures linked to asparagines of the scrapie prion protein. Biochemistry 1989; 28: 8380-8388.

52 Stahl N, Baldwin MA, Hecker R, Pan KM, Burlingame AL, Prusiner SB. Glycosylinositol phospholipid anchors of the scrapie and cellular prion proteins contain sialic acid. Biochemistry 1992; 31: 5043-5053.

53 Stahl N, Baldwin MA, Burlinghame AL, Prusiner SB. Identification of glycoinositol phosphlipid linked and truncated forms of the scrapie prion protein. Biochem 1990; 29: 8879-8884.

54 Hay B, Prusiner SB, Lingappa VR. Evidence for a secretory form of the cellular prion protein. Biochemistry 1987; 26: 8110-8115.

55 Caughey B, Race RE, Vogel M, Buchmeier MJ, Chesebro B. In vitro expression in eukaryotic cells of a prion protein gene cloned from scrapie-infected mouse brain. Proc Natl Acad Sci USA 1988; 85: 4657-4661.

56 Tagliavini F, Prelli F, Porro M, Salmona M, Bugiani O, Frangione B. A soluble form of prion protein in human cerebrospinal fluid. Biochem Biophys Res Commun 1992; 184: 1398-1404.

57 Hope J. The biochemistry, protein chemistry and molecular biology of BSE. J Am Med Assoc 1993: In press

58 Bazan FF, Fletterick RJ, McKinley MP, Prusiner SB. Predicted secondary structure and membrane topology of the scrapie prion protein. Protein Eng 1987; 1: 125-135.

59 Caughey BW, Dong A, Bhat KS, Ernst D, Hayes S, Caughey WS. Secondary structure analysis of the scrapie-associated protein PrP 27-30 in water by infrared spectroscopy. Biochemistry 1991; 30: 7672-7680.

60 Hay B, Barry RA, Lieberburg I, Prusiner SB, Lingappa VR. Biogenesis and transmembrane orientation of the cellular isoform of the scrapie prion protein. Mol Cell Biol 1987; 7: 914-920.

61 Lopez CD, Yost CS, Prusiner SB, Myers RM, Lingappa VR. Unusual topogenic sequence directs prion protein biogenesis. Science 1990; 248: 226-229.

62 Yost CS, Lopez CD, Prusiner SB, Myers RM, Lingappa VR. Non-hydrophobic extracytoplasmic determinant of stop transfer in the prion protein. Nature 1990; 343: 669-672.

63 Goldmann W, Hunter N, Benson G, Foster JD, Hope J. Different scrapie-associated fibril proteins (PrP) are encoded by lines of sheep selected for different alleles of the Sip gene. J Gen Virol 1991; 72: 2411-2417.

64 Laplanche JL, Chatelain J, Westaway D, et al. PrP polymorphisms associated with natural scrapie discovered by denaturing gradiant gel electrophoresis. Genomics 1993; 15: 30-37.

65 Hunter N, Goldmann W, Benson G, Foster J, Hope J. Swaledale sheep affected by natural scrapie differ significantly in PrP genotype frequencies from healthy sheep and those selected for reduced incidence of scrapie. J Gen Virol 1993; 74: 1025-1031.

66 Goldfarb LG, Petersen RB, Tabaton M, et al. Fatal familial insomnia and familial Creutzfeldt-Jakob disease: Disease phenotype determined by a DNA polymorphism. Science 1992; 258: 806-808.

67 Brenner HR, Herczeg A, Oesch B. Normal development of nerve-muscle synapses in mice lacking the prion protein gene. Proc R Soc [Lond] 1992; 250: 151-155.

British Medical Bulletin (1993) Vol. 49, No. 4, pp. 860–872
© The British Council 1993

Scrapie associated PrP accumulation and its prevention: insights from cell culture

B Caughey
Laboratory of Persistent Viral Diseases, Rocky Mountain Laboratories, National Institute for Allergy and Infectious Diseases, Hamilton, Montana 59840, USA

Transmissible spongiform encephalopathies (TSEs), Alzheimer's disease and other amyloidoses result in the accumulation of abnormally stable, potentially amyloidogenic proteins that appear to play central roles in disease pathogenesis. Scrapie-infected tissue culture cells have become well-developed models for studying how the TSE-specific protein, protease-resistant PrP, is made from its apparently normal precursor. The conversion of PrP to the protease-resistant state occurs on the plasma membrane or along an endocytic pathway to the lysosomes. The protease-resistant PrP has a much longer half-life than normal PrP and its accumulation in lysosomes may feature in TSE pathogenesis. Congo red and certain sulfated glycans potently inhibit protease-resistant PrP formation or stabilization in cell culture. These and other observations suggest that an interaction of PrP with glycosaminoglycans is critical in protease-resistant PrP accumulation and raises the possibility that therapeutic strategies for TSEs and other amyloidoses could be based on blocking (pre)amyloid-glycosaminoglycan interactions.

Despite the intriguing clues that have emerged in recent years, many fundamental issues in transmissible spongiform encephalopathy (TSE) research remain unresolved. These uncertainties include the precise nature of the transmissible TSE agents, the mechanisms of TSE pathogenesis, and strategies for treating these diseases. One factor that appears to play a role in both the transmission and pathogenesis of the TSEs is the abnormally protease-resistant and amyloidogenic isoform of the host encoded protein, PrP (for reviews, *see* other chapters in this issue). Hence, it is important to understand how the abnormal PrP arises in infected cells. Studies of this process have been aided greatly by the availability of cell cultures which replicate the infectious scrapie agent and produce the scrapie-associated, protease-resistant isoform of PrP (PrP-res)*.

Furthermore, the recent identification of potent inhibitors of PrP-res accumulation in such cultures has begun to define essential steps in PrP-res formation that are attractive targets to consider in the development of drug therapies for TSEs and other amyloidoses such as Alzheimer's disease.[1,2] The infection of cell cultures with scrapie and the metabolism of PrP isoforms in scrapie-infected cells have been reviewed recently.[3-5] Here I provide brief updated overviews of these subjects and follow with a more detailed discussion of the inhibitor studies and their apparent ramifications regarding mechanisms of amyloidogenesis.

CELL CULTURE MODELS OF SCRAPIE

PC12 cells

Rubenstein and coworkers have shown that PC12 rat pheochromocytoma cells that have been terminally differentiated into neuron-like cells with nerve growth factor can be readily infected with scrapie.[6,7] The scrapie agent replicates in the non-dividing PC12 cultures over a period of weeks to the highest specific infectivities available in tissue culture cell lines. Interestingly, the scrapie agent replication in these cultures is accompanied by decreases in the activities of enzymes involved in the cholinergic, but not the adrenergic, neurotransmitter pathways, suggesting a mechanism for clinical manifestations observed in TSEs.[8] Further studies have demonstrated that PC12 infection is strain specific and that the level of replication of a given agent strain correlates with the degree of alteration of the cholinergic pathway.[9] Both normal and protease-resistant forms of PrP have been observed in scrapie-infected PC12 cells (R Rubenstein and B Caughey, unpublished observations), but our understanding of PrP metabolism in this system remains limited.

Note: The scrapie-specific isoform of the PrP protein is known by many different names, most prominent among them being scrapie prion protein (PrP^{sc}: see Prusiner, this issue). However, since this name makes the unproven assumption that this protein is a component of the infectious agent or 'prion', we have preferred to call it protease-resistant PrP (PrP-res) which distinguishes it operationally from the normal, protease-sensitive PrP but makes no prejudgment regarding its relationship to the scrapie agent.

Mouse neuroblastoma (MNB) and HaB cells

Most of the current knowledge of normal and scrapie-associated PrP metabolism is derived from studies of MNB (neuro 2a or C1300)[10–12] and hamster-derived HaB[13] cells, which can maintain persistent scrapie agent infection while continuously dividing. Like the scrapie agent derived from brain tissue, MNB-derived agent was found to be resistant to nuclease and mild proteinase K treatments, but sensitive to exhaustive proteinase K treatments.[14] In what follows, we focus primarily on studies of PrP metabolism using MNB and HaB cells.

METABOLISM OF NORMAL AND SCRAPIE-ASSOCIATED PrP

The cause of the different chemical and physical properties of PrP-res and its normal protease-sensitive, detergent soluble isoform remains unknown. No general scrapie-specific covalent modifications of PrP have been identified that can account for the aberrant properties of PrP-res. However, studies with scrapie-infected cell cultures have identified dramatic differences in the metabolism of the two PrP isoforms which appear to shed light on TSE pathogenesis at the cellular level.

Normal PrP biosynthesis

Our early studies with MNB cells characterized the normal metabolic life-cycle of PrP.[11,15] As a membrane glycoprotein, PrP begins its metabolic cycle in the endoplasmic reticulum where a glycophosphatidylinositol anchor and high mannose glycans are rapidly attached. On the way to the cell surface via the Golgi apparatus, the high mannose glycan moieties are converted to complex or hybrid glycans. Ultimately, most of the PrP is anchored to the cell surface by the phosphatidylinositol moiety and can be removed with phospholipase or protease treatments.[15–17] However, some intracellular vesicular staining of normal PrP has been observed in both neuroblastoma cells[17] and neurons.[18] Once on the plasma membrane, PrP normally has a half-life of 3–6 h, with a small proportion released into the medium.[15,19–21] Soluble forms of PrP have now been identified in vivo as well.[22]

Scrapie-associated PrP biosynthesis

Unlike normal PrP, PrP-res is resistant to phospholipase and protease treatments of intact scrapie-infected cells or their membranes[17,23,24] and shows no sign of turnover within the cells.[20,21] The low turnover of PrP-res can explain its accumulation in non-dividing neurons of the central nervous system in vivo. The formation of PrP-res occurs relatively slowly[20,21] after its apparently normal (phospholipase- and protease-sensitive) PrP precursor reaches the cell surface.[21] Soon after its formation, PrP-res in MNB cells is exposed to lysosomal or endosomal proteases and truncated at the N-terminus.[25,26] Taken together, these studies indicated that the conversion of PrP to the protease-resistant state likely occurs at the plasma membrane or along an endocytic pathway to the lysosomes[21,25,27] (Fig. 1). Once formed, PrP-res appears to accumulate in lysosomes.[21,25,28]

These and other lines of evidence have elicited a proposal that the accumulation of PrP-res in lysosomes plays a role in TSE pathogenesis.[29] In light of this proposal, it is interesting to note that much of the PrP-res isolated from scrapie-infected mouse or hamster brain is not N-terminally truncated.[30,31] One explanation for this could be that lysosomal function is impaired at the clinical stages of disease in vivo.[25] In any case, although the truncation of PrP-res has been a useful indicator of metabolic events in vitro, it is not clear that proteolysis or any other covalent modification is important in PrP-res formation or the scrapie disease process. Thus, it remains possible that the difference between PrP-res and normal PrP is purely conformational or dependent upon an interaction of PrP with another molecule.[30]

Influence of glycosylation on PrP-res accumulation

Since PrP-res is a glycoprotein, one might expect that the glycan moieties would help protect PrP-res from proteases. However, the presence of glycans does not protect normal PrP from cellular proteolysis, as indicated by its short half-life.[4,15] Furthermore, there is evidence from the MNB and HaB cell systems that N-linked glycosylation is not necessary for PrP-res formation[32] and may actually disfavor PrP-res formation or stability.[21,25] Although PrP-res appears to be made from a normal PrP precursor, there is a striking predominance of the less glycosylated species in PrP-res as compared to normal PrP.[21] This suggests that the less glycosylated species are either selected preferentially by the process that generates PrP-res or are more stable within the cell once PrP-res is formed. Interestingly, one of the two potential N-linked glycosylation sites is located within what is predicted to be a long hydrophobic β-sheet region.[33] The addition of a hydrophilic glycan in such a position might have a profound effect on the folding of the PrP molecule and its propensity to form amyloidogenic aggregates.

Diversity in PrP biosynthesis

Studies of PrP from other sources have indicated that there is diversity in the way the PrP polypeptide is post-translationally modified. For instance, in mouse C127 cells expressing recombinant PrP, the array of metabolic intermediates were somewhat different than those observed in MNB cells.[19] Furthermore, chemical analyses of PrP-res derived from hamster brain tissue showed that PrP-res could have as many as 400 different glycan moieties.[34] Thus, it is likely that post-translational processing as well as other aspects of PrP metabolism might vary between cell types within a given host and tissue.[4] These variations may influence the tendency of PrP isoforms to form PrP-res and the susceptibility of a given cell type to infection with particular TSE agent strains. This, in turn, may influence the neuropathological and clinical manifestations of TSE strains.

Expression of recombinant PrPs in cell culture

Although the conversion of PrP to scrapie-associated PrP-res does not require an alteration in the primary amino acid sequence, it is clear that in host-specific variations in the PrP primary amino acid sequence have strong effects on TSE disease parameters (for review see other chapters in this issue). The ability to express recombinant PrP molecules in cell cultures has made it possible to begin in vitro studies of the potential effects of PrP gene variations on PrP metabolism, PrP-res formation, agent replication, agent strain, and host cell susceptibility to infection.[19,35–37]

CHEMICAL INHIBITION OF PROTEASE-RESISTANT PrP ACCUMULATION

Congo red inhibition

To aid further studies of: (a) the fundamental mechanism of PrP-res formation, (b) the relationship of PrP-res to pathogenesis and infectivity, and (c) potential therapies for the TSEs, we sought to identify selective inhibitors of PrP-res accumulation using the scrapie-infected MNB cell model. Congo red, a dye that has long been used as a diagnostic stain for amyloids,[38] was found to potently inhibit PrP-res accumulation in scrapie-infected MNB cells (Figs 1 & 2) without apparent effects on normal PrP metabolism.[1,2] Concurrently, the level of infectious scrapie agent in the cells was reduced.[38a] The mechanism for the inhibition of PrP-res and scrapie agent accumulation by Congo red has not been clearly established. However, since Congo red binds to PrP-res amyloid,[39] it is likely that this direct interaction interferes with a critical event in PrP-res formation or destabilizes the structure once it is formed.[1] Recent X-ray crystallography studies of Congo red bound to insulin amyloid showed that Congo red intercalates between globular insulin molecules at an interface formed by β-strands and that this mode of dye binding to amyloids may be general.[40] Thus amyloid-bound Congo red appears to be well-positioned to affect amyloid fibril stability. Other recent studies have shown that, although Congo red enhances the lateral aggregation of synthetic Alzheimer's β/A4 amyloid fibrils in vitro, it reduces their axial growth.[41] On the basis of some of the above observations, we and others proposed that Congo red or its derivatives may be of therapeutic value as anti-amyloids in vivo.[1,40] In fact, one early study had already shown that Congo red treatments could inhibit experimental, casein-induced amyloidosis in mice.[42]

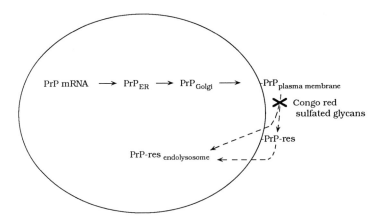

Fig. 1 Schematic diagram of the PrP-res biosynthetic pathway and its inhibition by Congo red and sulfated glycans in MNB cells.

Sulfated glycan inhibition

The fact that Congo red has two sulfonate groups suggested that its polyanionic character may be important in its inhibitory activity.[1,2] Interestingly, prophylactic administration of certain polyanions has been shown to prolong the life span of animals inoculated with scrapie.[43–49] Although there is evidence that the polyanions inhibit the early uptake and replication of the scrapie agent in the lymphoreticular system[43–48] or in nerve endings,[49] the therapeutic mechanism of these polyanions has not been defined at the cellular or molecular level. However, one consequence of the prophylactic treatment of scrapie-infected mice with pentosan polysulfate is a lack of PrP-res in brain tissue.[48] Given these observations, it seemed possible that a mechanism of action of the polyanions was the inhibition of PrP-res accumulation in scrapie-infected cells like that observed in cultured cells with Congo red.[1]

To explore this possibility, the effects of sulfated glycans on PrP-res metabolism were tested.[2] Pentosan polysulfate, like Congo red, potently

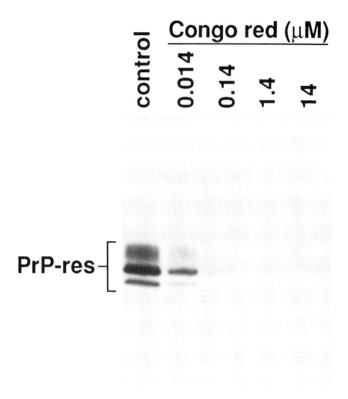

Fig. 2 Inhibition of PrP-res accumulation in cells grown in Congo red. Scrapie-infected MNB cells were seeded at a 1:20 dilution of a confluent culture and grown 5 days to confluence in the presence of the designated concentrations of Congo red. The PrP-res content in equivalent cell numbers was analyzed by immunoblot as described previously.[1] Reproduced with permission from a previous publication.[1]

inhibited the accumulation of PrP-res in these cells without apparent effects on the metabolism of the normal isoform. The inhibition was due primarily to prevention of new PrP-res accumulation rather than destabilization of pre-existing PrP-res and remained in effect long after removal of the inhibitors. A comparison of the activities of various sulfated glycans, non-sulfated polyanions, dextran and DEAE-dextran provided evidence that the density of sulfation and molecular size are factors influencing anti-PrP-res activity of sulfated glycans. The relative potencies of these compounds corresponded well with their previously determined anti-scrapie activities in vivo,[44–49] suggesting that the prophylactic effects of sulfated polyanions may in fact be due to inhibition of PrP-res accumulation. This may also be the case for amphotericin B,[50] but this drug is likely to work by a different biochemical mechanism than the sulfated polyanions because it is not polyanionic.

Potential mechanisms of inhibition of PrP-res accumulation by sulfated glycans and Congo red

Highly sulfated glycosaminoglycans (GAGs) are components of all naturally derived amyloid plaques, including those composed of PrP-res, and it has been proposed that such GAGs may be involved in the formation or stabilization of amyloid deposits.[51–54] A hypothetical adaptation of this type of proposal to PrP-res accumulation is diagrammed in Figure 3A. Since our inhibitors of PrP-res accumulation are GAGs, or can be viewed as analogs of GAGs, we proposed that these inhibitors can bind to PrP and competitively inhibit an interaction with a specific cellular sulfated GAG that is essential for PrP-res formation or metabolic stabilization (Fig.3B).[2] Implicit in this hypothesis is the idea that the inhibitors can bind PrP, but lack certain features required to facilitate PrP-res accumulation within cells by themselves. In any case, the fact that PrP-res accumulation is blocked by these exogenous GAGs or GAG analogs is consistent with the idea that endogenous GAGs play key functional roles in amyloidogenesis. Further functional evidence supporting this idea has come from studies showing that: (a) sulfate ions and Congo red can influence synthetic Alzheimer's β/A4 amyloid fibril formation[41]; and (b) GAGs can induce conformational shifts from α-helix to the apparent β-sheet structure that is predominant in amyloid fibrils (reviewed by Kisilevsky[55]), including those comprising PrP-res.[33] The observation that PrP-res 27-30 amyloid fibrils have substantially higher β-sheet and lower α-helix than was predicted theoretically suggested that a transformation from α-helix to β-sheet may be involved in PrP-res formation.[33] Recent studies with synthetic PrP peptides are consistent with this hypothesis.[56]

If, as is suspected, endogenous sulfated GAGs play an essential role in PrP-res accumulation, it is conceivable that differential GAG expression influences whether or not a given cell can accumulate PrP-res and, thus, be a 'clinical target' in TSEs. It is clear from genetic analyses that certain unidentified genes besides the PrP gene can have overriding effects on host susceptibility to TSE strains or the clinical course of TSE disease.[57,58] Genes controlling GAG expression and metabolism would seem to be good candidates to consider.

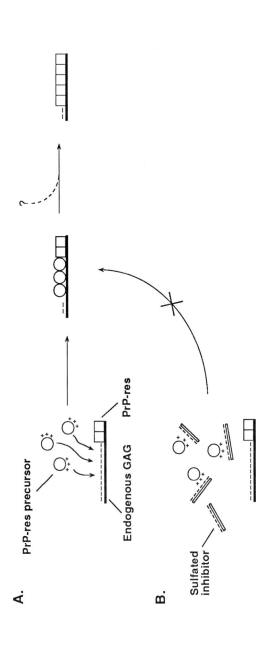

Fig. 3 A hypothetical mechanism for the role of endogenous GAG in PrP-res formation (**A**) and the inhibition of this process by sulfated glycans (**B**). Since endogenous sulfated GAGs are polyanionic, binding to cationic groups on the PrP-res precursor is assumed in this diagram. However, it is also conceivable that multivalent cations mediate the binding, in which case anionic groups on PrP could be involved. It is proposed that the sulfated glycan inhibitor (e.g., pentosan polysulfate) binds to the GAG binding site of PrP and thereby competitively inhibits PrP precursor binding to endogenous GAG. This, in turn, prevents PrP-res formation or metabolic stabilization. For simplicity, only one sequence of events is shown, however, alternative orders of addition of the reactants must also be considered. The ? refers to whatever it is in an infected cell that causes the conversion of PrP-sen to PrP-res, an event that we now suspect involves GAG.

KEY POINTS FOR CLINICAL PRACTICE

The inhibition of PrP-res accumulation by Congo red and certain sulfated glycans raises the possibility that therapies for the TSEs could be based on drugs related to these inhibitors. Several studies have already demonstrated that sulfated glycans can have substantial chemoprophylactic effects against scrapie in mice and hamsters. Since all naturally derived amyloids contain GAGs, it is tempting to speculate that the interaction of GAGs with a variety of amyloidogenic proteins might also be blocked by sulfated glycans, Congo red or related compounds. Application of Congo red and appropriate inhibitors of GAG-(pre)amyloid interactions in vivo might thereby result in reduced accumulation of amyloids associated with other diseases such as Alzheimer's disease or systemic amyloidoses.

ACKNOWLEDGEMENTS

I thank Richard Race, Suzette Priola, John Coe, Kathy Toohey, Kathy Brown and Pamela Caughey for critically reading this manuscript, and Gary Hettrick and Bob Evans for graphics assistance.

REFERENCES

1 Caughey B, Race RE. Potent inhibition of scrapie-associated PrP accumulation by Congo red. J Neurochem 1992; 59: 768-771.
2 Caughey B, Raymond GJ. Sulfated polyanion inhibition of scrapie-associated PrP accumulation in cultured cells. J Virol 1993; 67: 643-650.
3 Race R. The scrapie agent in vitro. Curr Top Microbiol Immunol 1991; 172: 181-193.
4 Caughey B. Cellular metabolism of normal and scrapie-associated forms of PrP. Sem Virol 1991; 2: 189-196.
5 Caughey B, Race R and Chesebro B. Effects of scrapie infection on cellular PrP metabolism. In: Prusiner SB, Collinge J, Powell J, Anderton B eds. Prion Diseases in Humans and Animals. Chichester: Ellis Horwood, 1992: 445-456.
6 Rubenstein R, Carp RI, Callahan SM. In vitro replication of scrapie agent in a neuronal model: infection of PC12 cells. J Gen Virol 1984; 65: 2191-2198.
7 Rubenstein R, Scalici CL, Papini MC, Callahan SM, Carp RI. Further characterization of scrapie replication in PC12 cells. J Gen Virol 1990; 71: 825-831.
8 Rubenstein R, Deng H, Scalici CL, Papini MC. Alterations in neurotransmitter-related enzyme activity in scrapie-infected PC12 cells. J Gen Virol 1991; 72: 1279-1285.
9 Rubenstein R, Deng H, Race RE, et al. Demonstration of scrapie strain diversity in infected PC12 cells. J Gen Virol 1992; 73: 3027-3031.
10 Race RE, Fadness LH, Chesebro B. Characterization of scrapie infection in mouse neuroblastoma cells. J Gen Virol 1987; 68: 1391-1399.
11 Race RE, Caughey B, Graham K, Ernst D, Chesebro B. Analyses of frequency of infection, specific infectivity, and prion protein biosynthesis in scrapie-infected neuroblastoma cell clones. J Virol 1988; 62: 2845-2849.
12 Butler DA, Scott MRD, Bockman JM, et al. Scrapie-infected murine neuroblastoma cells produce protease-resistant prion proteins. J Virol 1988; 62: 1558-1564.
13 Taraboulos A, Serban D, Prusiner SB. Scrapie prion proteins accumulate in the cytoplasm of persistently infected cultured cells. J Cell Biol 1990; 110: 2117-2132.

14 Neary K, Caughey B, Ernst D, Race RE, Chesebro B. Protease sensitivity and nuclease resistance of the scrapie agent propagated in vitro in neuroblastoma cells. J Virol 1991; 65: 1031-1034.

15 Caughey B, Race RE, Ernst D, Buchmeier MJ, Chesebro B. Prion protein (PrP) biosynthesis in scrapie-infected and uninfected neuroblastoma cells. J Virol 1989; 63: 175-181.

16 Stahl N, Borchelt DR, Hsiao K, Prusiner SB. Scrapie prion protein contains a phosphatidylinositol glycolipid. Cell 1987; 51: 229-240.

17 Caughey B, Neary K, Buller R, et al. Normal and scrapie-associated forms of prion protein differ in their sensitivities to phospholipase and proteases in intact neuroblastoma cells. J Virol 1990; 64: 1093-1101.

18 Piccardo P, Safar J, Ceroni M, Gajdusek DC, Gibbs CJ Jr. Immunohistochemical localization of prion protein in spongiform encephalopathies and normal brain tissue. Neurology 1990; 40: 518-522.

19 Caughey B, Race RE, Vogel M, Buchmeier MJ, Chesebro B. In vitro expression in eukaryotic cells of the prion protein gene cloned from scrapie-infected mouse brain. Proc Natl Acad Sci USA 1988; 85: 4657-4661.

20 Borchelt DR, Scott M, Taraboulos A, Stahl N, Prusiner SB. Scrapie and cellular prion proteins differ in the kinetics of synthesis and topology in cultured cells. J Cell Biol 1990; 110: 743-752.

21 Caughey B, Raymond GJ. The scrapie-associated form of PrP is made from a cell surface precursor that is both protease- and phospholipase-sensitive. J Biol Chem 1991; 266: 18217-18223.

22 Tagliavini F, Prelli F, Porro M, Salmona M, Bugiani O, Frangione B. A soluble form of prion protein in human cerebrospinal fluid: Implications for prion-related encephalopathies. Biochem Biophys Res Commun 1992; 184: 1398-1404.

23 Stahl N, Borchelt DR, Prusiner SB. Differential release of cellular and scrapie prion proteins from cellular membranes by phosphatidylinositol-specific phospholipase C. Biochemistry 1990; 29: 5405-5412.

24 Safar J, Ceroni M, Gajdusek DC, Gibbs CJ Jr. Differences in the membrane interaction of scrapie amyloid precursor proteins in normal and scrapie- or Creutzfeldt-Jakob disease-infected brains. J Infect Dis 1991; 163: 488-494.

25 Caughey B, Raymond GJ, Ernst D, Race RE. N-terminal truncation of the scrapie-associated form of PrP by lysosomal protease(s): implications regarding the site of conversion of PrP to the protease-resistant state. J Virol 1991; 65: 6597-6603.

26 Taraboulos A, Raeber AJ, Borchelt DR, Serban D, Prusiner SB. Synthesis and trafficking of prion proteins in cultured cells. Mol Biol Cell 1992; 3: 851-863.

27 Borchelt DR, Taraboulos A, Prusiner SB. Evidence for synthesis of scrapie prion protein in the endocytic pathway. J Biol Chem 1992; 267: 16188-16199.

28 McKinley MP, Taraboulos A, Kenaga L, et al. Ultrastructural localization of scrapie prion proteins in cytoplasmic vesicles of infected cultured cells. Lab Invest 1991; 65: 622-630.

29 Laszlo L, Lowe J, Self T, et al. Lysosomes as key organelles in the pathogenesis of prion encephalopathies. J Pathol 1992; 166: 333-341.

30 Hope J, Morton LJD, Farquhar CF, Multhaup G, Beyreuther K, Kimberlin RH. The major polypeptide of scrapie-associated fibrils (SAF) has the same size, charge distribution and N-terminal protein sequence as predicted for the normal brain protein (PrP). EMBO J 1986; 5: 2591-2597.

31 Bolton DC, Bendheim PE, Marmostein AD, Potempska A. Isolation and structural studies of the intact scrapie agent protein. Arch Biochem Biophys 1987; 258: 579-590.

32 Taraboulos A, Rogers M, Borchelt DR, et al. Acquisition of protease resistance by prion proteins in scrapie-infected cells does not require asparagine-linked glycosylation. Proc Natl Acad Sci USA 1990; 87: 8262-8266.

33 Caughey BW, Dong A, Bhat KS, Ernst D, Hayes SF, Caughey WS. Secondary structure analysis of the scrapie-associated protein PrP 27-30 in water by infrared spectroscopy. Biochemistry 1991; 30: 7672-7680.

34 Endo T, Groth D, Prusiner SB, Kobata A. Diversity of oligosaccharide structures linked to asparagines of the scrapie prion protein. Biochemistry 1989; 28: 8380-8388.

35 Scott MRD, Butler DA, Bredesen DE, Walchli M, Hsiao KK, Prusiner SB. Prion protein gene expression in cultured cells. Protein Eng 1988; 2: 69-76.

36 Scott MR, Kohler R, Foster D, Prusiner SB. Chimeric prion protein expression in cultured cells and transgenic mice. Protein Sci 1992; 1: 986-997.

37 Chesebro B, Wehrly K, Caughey B, Nishio J, Ernst D, Race R. Foreign PrP expression and scrapie infection in tissue culture cell lines. Dev Biol Stand 1993: (In press).

38 Glenner GG. Amyloid deposits and amyloidosis: the beta-fibrillosa (second of two parts). N Engl J Med 1980; 302: 1333-1343.

38aCaughey B, Ernst D, Race R. Congo red inhibition of scrapie agent replication. J Virol 1993: (In press).

39 Prusiner SB, McKinley MP, Bowman KA, et al. Scrapie prions aggregate to form amyloid-like birefringent rods. Cell 1983; 35: 349-358.

40 Turnell WG, Finch JT. Binding of the dye Congo red to the amyloid protein pig insulin reveals a novel homology amongst amyloid-forming peptide sequences. J Mol Biol 1992; 227: 1205-1223.

41 Fraser PE, Nguyen JT, Chin DT, Kirschner DA. Effects of sulfate ions on Alzheimer β/A4 peptide assemblies: implications for amyloid fibril-proteoglycan interactions. J Neurochem 1992; 59: 1531-1540.

42 Kagan DZ, Rozinova VN. Inhibition of amyloidogenesis by Congo red during experimental amyloidosis. Probl Tuberk 1974; 9: 72-74.

43 Kimberlin RH, Walker CA. The antiviral compound HPA-23 can prevent scrapie when administered at the time of infection. Arch Virol 1983; 78: 9-18.

44 Ehlers B, Rudolf R, Diringer H. The reticuloendothelial system in scrapie pathogenesis. J Gen Virol 1984; 65: 423-428.

45 Ehlers B, Diringer H. Dextran sulphate 500 delays and prevents mouse scrapie by impairment of agent replication in spleen. J Gen Virol 1984; 65: 1325-1330.

46 Farquhar CF, Dickinson AG. Prolongation of scrapie incubation period by an injection of dextran sulphate 500 within the month before or after infection. J Gen Virol 1986; 67: 463-473.

47 Kimberlin RH, Walker CA. Suppression of scrapie infection in mice by heteropolyanion 23, dextran sulfate, and some other polyanions. Antimicrob Agents Chemother 1986; 30: 409-413.

48 Diringer H, Ehlers B. Chemoprophylaxis of scrapie in mice. J Gen Virol 1991; 72: 457-460.

49 Ladogana A, Casaccia P, Ingrosso L, et al. Sulphate polyanions prolong the incubation period of scrapie-infected hamsters. J Gen Virol 1992; 73: 661-665.

50 Xi YG, Ingrosso L, Ladogana A, Masullo C, Pocchiari M. Amphotericin B treatment dissociates in vivo replication of the scrapie agent from PrP accumulation. Nature 1992; 356: 598-601.

51 Snow AD, Kisilevsky R, Willmer J, Prusiner SB, DeArmond SJ. Sulfated glycosaminoglycans in amyloid plaques of prion diseases. Acta Neuropathol 1989; 77: 337-342.

52 Guiroy DC, Gajdusek DC. Fibril-derived amyloid enhancing factor as nucleating agents in Alzheimer's disease and transmissible virus dementia. Disc Neurosci 1989; 5: 69-73.

53 Snow AD, Wight TN, Nochlin D, et al. Immunolocalization of heparan sulfate proteoglycans to the prion protein amyloid plaques of Gerstmann-Straussler Syndrome, Creuzfeldt-Jakob disease and scrapie. Lab Invest 1990; 63: 601-611.

54 Guiroy DC, Yanagihara R, Gajdusek DC. Localization of amyloidogenic proteins and sulfated glycosaminoglycans in nontransmissible and transmissible cerebral amyloidoses. Acta Neuropathol 1991; 82: 87-92.

55 Kisilevsky R. From arthritis to Alzheimer's disease: current concepts on the pathogenesis of amyloidosis. Can J Physiol Pharmacol 1987; 65: 1805-1815.

56 Gasset M, Baldwin MA, Lloyd DH, et al. Predicted α-helical regions of the prion protein when synthesized as peptides form amyloid. Proc Natl Acad Sci USA 1992; 89: 10940-10944.
57 Carlson GA, Kingsbury DT, Goodman PA, et al. Linkage of prion protein and scrapie incubation time genes. Cell 1986; 46: 503-511.
58 Race RE, Graham K, Ernst D, Caughey B, Chesebro B. Analysis of linkage between scrapie incubation period and the prion protein gene in mice. J Gen Virol 1990; 71: 493-497.

British Medical Bulletin (1993) Vol. 49, No. 4, pp. 873–912
© The British Council 1993

Transgenetics and cell biology of prion diseases: investigations of PrPSc synthesis and diversity

S B Prusiner
Departments of Neurology and Biochemistry and Biophysics, University of California, San Francisco, California, USA

Studies with Tg mice have contributed a wealth of new knowledge about the synthesis of prion particles and the pathogenesis of both the genetic and infectious forms of the prion diseases. Transgenetic studies argue persuasively that the 'species barrier' is due to differences in PrP gene sequences among mammals.

The study of prions has taken several unexpected directions over the past few years. The discovery that prion diseases in humans are uniquely both genetic and infectious has greatly strengthened and extended the prion concept. To date, 13 different mutations in the human prion protein (PrP) gene all resulting in non-conservative substitutions have been found to segregate with the inherited prion diseases and for many mutations genetic linkage has been established. Yet, the transmissible prion particle is composed largely, if not entirely, of an abnormal isoform of the prion protein designated PrPSc.[1] These findings argue that prion diseases should be considered pseudoinfections since the particles transmitting disease appear to be devoid of a foreign nucleic acid and thus differ from all known microorganisms as well as viruses and viroids. Because much information especially about scrapie of rodents has been derived using experimental protocols adapted from virology, we continue to use terms such as infection, incubation period, transmissibility and endpoint titration in studies of prion diseases.

An impressive amount of new knowledge about prions and the diseases caused by them has been accumulated over the past 4 years using transgenic (Tg) mice expressing foreign or mutant PrP genes. Tg mice now permit virtually all facets of prion diseases to be studied and have created a framework for future investigations. From such studies, we have gained information about the synthesis of prions, the control of scrapie incubation times, the determinants of neuropathology in prion diseases and the genetic mechanisms of prion diseases. Tg mice have also given us much new information about the mechanisms involved in the propagation of distinct isolates or 'strains' of prions.

Transgenetic investigations coupled with studies on the synthesis of PrP^{Sc} in cultured cells and on the molecular properties of PrP^{Sc} are beginning to provide a coherent picture of prion propagation and the pathogenesis of prion diseases. The structure and organization of the PrP gene suggested that PrP^{Sc} is derived from PrP^{C} or a precursor by a post-translational process. Studies with scrapie-infected cultured cells have provided much evidence that the conversion of PrP^{C} to PrP^{Sc} is a post-translational process that probably occurs in the endocytic pathway. The molecular basis of the PrP^{Sc} synthetic process remains to be elucidated, but extensive protein chemical studies suggest that this process is likely to involve a conformational change. Biophysical studies have produced new approaches to deciphering the structural transitions that PrP^{Sc} undergoes during its synthesis. The production of artificial prions and the construction of mice lacking both PrP alleles (Prn-p$^{0/0}$) provide novel strategies for investigating molecular biological events that feature in the prion diseases.

It seems likely that the principles learned from the study of prion diseases will be applicable to elucidating the causes of more common neurodegenerative diseases. Such disorders include Alzheimer's disease (AD), amyotrophic lateral sclerosis and Parkinson's disease. Since people at risk for inherited prion diseases can now be identified decades before neurologic dysfunction is evident, the development of an effective therapy is imperative. If PrP^{C} can be diminished in humans without deleterious effects as is the case for Prn-p$^{0/0}$ mice[2], then reducing the level of PrP mRNA with antisense oligonucleotides might prove an effective therapeutic manoeuvre in delaying the onset of CNS symptoms and signs.

The study of prion biology and diseases seems to be a new and emerging area of biomedical investigation. While prion biology has its roots in virology, neurology and neuropathology, its relationships to the disciplines of molecular and cell biology as well as protein chemistry have become evident only recently. Indeed, the results of all the studies described here support the hypothesis that prion diseases are disorders of protein conformation. Certainly, the possibility that learning how prions multiply and cause disease will open up new vistas in biochemistry and genetics seems likely.

TRANSGENIC MICE EXPRESSING SYRIAN HAMSTER (SHa) PrP GENES

Four lines of Tg mice expressing SHaPrP mRNA

To test the hypothesis that the 'species barrier' for transmission of prions between 2 different species of mammals is due to differences in the primary structure of PrP, 4 lines of Tg mice expressing SHaPrP[C] were constructed and propagated. Southern blot analysis of the 4 lines suggested that the transgenes are integrated at one chromosomal site in a tandem array as has been reported for many Tg mice harboring other foreign genes.[3] Northern blots showed that Tg(SHaPrP)69 mice with 2–4 copies of the transgene expressed the lowest levels of SHaPrP mRNA while Tg(SHaPrP)71 with a similar number of transgenes expressed slightly higher levels of SHaPrP mRNA. Tg(SHaPrP)81 mice with 30–50 copies of the transgene expressed substantially higher levels of SHaPrP mRNA. The hierarchy of SHaPrP mRNA levels for the 4 Tg lines was found which reflected the transgene copy number.[4]

The Tg(SHaPrP)20 line was produced in the same series of microinjections into (C57BL/6 x LT/Sv)F2 fertilized eggs that yielded Tg(SHaPrP)7 mice which carry ~60 copies of the transgene. Neither SHaPrP[C] nor SHaPrP mRNA were detectable in Tg(SHaPrP)20 mice. Digestion with Xbal yielded an aberrant 3-kb hybridizing fragment rather than the 3.8-kb fragment seen in Tg(SHaPrP)7 and in Syrian hamsters. Whether a rearrangement or deletion within the SHaPrP insert in Tg(SHaPrP)20 mice is responsible for the lack of expression is unknown.

The spectrum of incubation times

A range of scrapie incubation times varying from 277 ± 6.7 to 48 ± 1.0 days were recorded for the 4 Tg(SHaPrP)Mo lines expressing SHaPrP mRNA inoculated with SHa prions (Fig. 1). Tg(SHaPrP)69 mice with lowest steady-state levels of SHaPrP mRNA had the longest incubation times while Tg(SHaPrP)7 mice with the highest levels of SHaPrP mRNA had the shortest incubation times. The Tg(SHaPrP)71 and 81 mice had intermediate levels of SHaPrP mRNA and displayed incubation times of intermediate length. The Tg(SHaPrP)20 mice which failed to express SHaPrP mRNA have scrapie incubation times after inoculation with SHa prions exceeding 300 days. These observations demonstrate an inverse relationship between the level of transgene SHaPrP mRNA and the length of the incubation time after inoculation with SHa prions.

While non-Tg mice developed scrapie between 128 and 148 days after inoculation with mouse (Mo) prions, Tg(SHaPrP)69 and Tg71

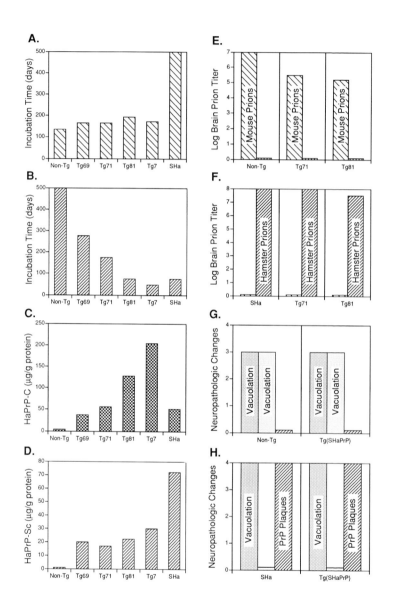

mice exhibited incubation times of 166 ± 4.7 and 165 ± 3.4 days, respectively. Even greater prolongation of the incubation times after Mo prion inoculation was seen with Tg(SHaPrP)81 and Tg7 mice where periods of 194 ± 3.5 and 173 ± 4.8 were observed, respectively. Tg(SHaPrP)20

Fig. 1 Transgenic (Tg) mice expressing Syrian hamster (SHa) prion protein exhibit species-specific scrapie incubation times, infectious prion synthesis and neuropathology.[4] **(A)** Scrapie incubation times in non-transgenic mice (Non-Tg) and 4 lines of Tg mice expressing SHaPrP and Syrian hamsters inoculated intracerebrally with ~10^6 ID_{50} units of Chandler Mo prions serially passaged in Swiss mice. The 4 lines of Tg mice have different numbers of transgene copies: Tg69 and 71 mice have 2 to 4 copies of the SHaPrP transgene, whereas Tg81 have 30 to 50 and Tg7 mice have >60. Incubation times are number of days from inoculation to onset of neurologic dysfunction. **(B)** Scrapie incubation times in mice and hamsters inoculated with ~10^7 ID_{50} units of Sc237 prions serially passed in Syrian hamsters and as described in (A). **(C)** Brain SHaPrP^C in Tg mice and hamsters. SHaPrP^C levels were quantitated by an enzyme-linked immunoassay. **(D)** Brain SHaPrP^{Sc} in Tg mice and hamsters. Animals were killed after exhibiting clinical signs of scrapie. SHaPrP^{Sc} levels were determined by immunoassay. **(E)** Prion titers in brains of clinically ill animals after inoculation with Mo prions. Brain extracts from Non-Tg, Tg71, and Tg81 mice were bioassayed for prions in mice (left) and hamsters (right). **(F)** Prion titers in brains of clinically ill animals after inoculation with SHa prions. Brain extracts from Syrian hamsters as well as Tg71 and Tg81 mice were bioassayed for prions in mice (left) and hamsters (right). **(G)** Neuropathology in non-Tg mice and Tg(SHaPrP) mice with clinical signs of scrapie after inoculation with Mo prions. Vacuolation in grey (left) and white matter (center); PrP amyloid plaques (right). Vacuolation score: 0 = none, 1 = rare, 2 = modest, 3 = moderate, 4 = intense. **(H)** Neuropathology in Syrian hamsters and transgenic mice inoculated with SHa prions. Degree of vacuolation and frequency of PrP amyloid plaques as described in (G). Adapted from Ref. 1.

mice developed scrapie 134 ± 3.1 days after inoculation with Mo prions consistent with their failure to express the SHaPrP transgene. These observations argue that expression of the SHaPrP transgene impedes Mo prion synthesis.

Species-specific inocula direct synthesis of SHa or Mo prions

Inoculation of Tg mice expressing SHaPrP genes with SHa prions resulted in the formation of SHa prions as determined by bioassay in hamsters. As shown in Figure 1, inoculation of either Tg(SHaPrP)71 or 81 mice with SHa prions produced high levels of SHa prions, but virtually no Mo prions were detected by bioassay. Conversely, inoculation with Mo prions generated substantial levels of Mo prions, but virtually no SHa prions were found. These findings argue that the origin of the prion inoculum determines whether SHa or Mo prions are produced by Tg(SHaPrP) mice which are capable of supporting the replication of either prion.

Our results also show that the scrapie prion titers in the brains of Tg mice were independent of the length of the incubation time. For example, Tg(SHaPrP)71 and 81 mice exhibited SHa prion titers of ~10^8 ID_{50}/g of brain yet the incubation time after inoculation with SHa prions for the Tg(SHaPrP)71 mice was 161 ± 1.3 days compared to incubation times of 75 ± 0.9 days for Tg(SHaPrP)81 mice.

Development of scrapie in non-Tg mice after inoculation with SHa prions is a stochastic process presumably due to the relative incompatibility between SHaPrP[Sc] and MoPrP[C].[3] Crossing the species barrier is a slow and inefficient process[5] where only a few non-Tg mice inoculated with SHa prions eventually develop scrapie after greatly extended incubation periods.[3] Other studies argue that these mice synthesize *de novo* Mo but not SHa prions.[3,6,7] Non-Tg mice inoculated with SHa prions sacrificed at the same time that their Tg littermates developed scrapie were found to have low or undetectable levels of SHa prions as determined by bioassay (Fig. 1). From earlier studies, non-Tg mice inoculated with SHa prions might be expected to have a residual titer as high as $\sim 10^6$ ID_{50} U/g of brain[8], yet the highest titer of SHa prions found by bioassays in hamsters was $\sim 10^3$ ID_{50} U/g of brain; generally the titer was <10 ID_{50} U/g of brain in these non-Tg control mice regardless of the SHa prion inoculum used. These experimental measurements demonstrate conclusively that infectious SHa prions are produced *de novo* in the brains of Tg(SHaPrP) mice inoculated with SHa prions but not in the brains of non-Tg littermate controls.

In additional control experiments, serial passage of Tg(SHaPrP)71 and 81 brain extracts from mice inoculated with SHa prions into Tg(SHaPrP)71 and 81 mice, respectively, produced incubation periods similar to those observed for SHa prions inoculated into these mice (Fig. 1). More importantly, two Tg(SHaPrP)71 Mo brain extracts inoculated into Tg(SHaPrP)81 mice produced clinical signs of scrapie in ~75 days. These results are consistent with bioassays in Syrian hamsters where brain extracts from clinically ill Tg(SHaPrP)71 and Tg 81 mice inoculated with SHa prions produced disease in hamsters in ~75 days.[3] Dilution of the extract $\sim 10^5$-fold increased the incubation time for Tg81 mice from 80 ± 2.6 to 119 ± 2.5 days showing that the length of the incubation time in Tg(SHaPrP) mice is dependent on the dose of SHa prions inoculated.

Synthesis of SHaPrP[C] and SHaPrP[Sc] in Tg mice

Western immunoblots showed a correlation between the translation product SHaPrP[C] and SHaPrP mRNA levels in the 4 Tg lines.[4] While the levels of SHaPrP[C] increased as the steady-state levels of SHaPrP mRNA rose in the 4 lines, the level of MoPrP[C] was unaltered.

Steady-state levels of SHaPrP[C] in the brains of 4 Tg(SHaPrP) Mo lines were determined by ELISA (Fig. 1). The levels of SHaPrP[C] as determined by ELISA are in reasonable agreement with those estimated by Western immunoblotting. For example, the levels of SHaPrP[C] in Tg(SHaPrP)69, 71 and Syrian hamsters appear similar by Western blotting and give values of 38, 56 and 52 μg SHaPrP/g protein by ELISA, respectively. The scrape incubation times after inoculation with SHa prions were inversely related to the SHaPrP[C] concentration in the brains of the four Tg(SHaPrP) lines (Fig. 1). When the data were fitted to an exponential function, a correlation coefficient of ~0.95 was found.[4]

Since the titers of SHa prions in the brains of Tg(SHaPrP)71 and 81 mice at the time of illness were similar, we surmised that it was likely that the levels of SHaPrP[Sc] would also be similar. Indeed, the levels of SHaPrP[Sc] in all 4 lines of Tg(SHaPrP) mice were similar in their brains at the time of illness (Fig. 1). These findings are in accord with earlier observations showing that the scrapie prion titer at the time of clinical illness is independent of the incubation time;[9-11] whereas, the concentration of PrP[Sc] is directly proportional to the prion titer.[12] As shown in Figure 1, SHaPrP[Sc] levels in the brains of Tg mice with clinical signs of scrapie ranged between 25 and 50% of those found in Syrian hamster brains. Differences in SHaPrP[Sc] levels of 2- to 4-fold would not be expected to be reflected as measurable changes in prion titers.

Neuropathology

Consistent with our observations that species-specific inocula dictate whether SHa or Mo prions are produced in Tg(SHaPrP) mice (Fig. 1), we found that the inocula also determine the distribution of spongiform change as well as the formation of PrP amyloid plaques. Tg(SHaPrP) mice inoculated with SHa prions developed an intense spongiform change confined to grey matter of the hippocampus, thalamus, cerebral cortex and brainstem sparing the white matter. Numerous PrP amyloid plaques reactive with the SHaPrP-specific monoclonal antibody (mAb) 13A5[13] were found in the subcallosal and periventricular regions. Interestingly, the mean size of the PrP amyloid plaques was proportional to the level of PrP transgene expression. The distribution of spongiform changes and the PrP amyloid plaques resembled those found in Syrian hamsters inoculated with SHa prions.[14]

Astrocytic gliosis was a prominent feature of the brains of all Tg (SHaPrP) mice developing clinical signs of scrapie. Neither the distribution nor extent of gliosis was altered by the scrapie inoculum.

Tg(SHaPrP)69, 71 and 81 mice inoculated with Mo prions had widespread spongiform change in both the grey and white matter but the degree of vacuolation was less than that found when the Tg(SHaPrP) mice were inoculated with SHa prions. Only a few PrP amyloid plaques were found in these Tg (SHaPrP) mice inoculated with Mo prions. These plaques reacted with SHa-specific monoclonal antibodies.[13] In non-Tg mice (*Prn^a*) inoculated with Mo prions, spongiform change in the grey and white matter is commonly seen. SHaPrP reactive plaques were not seen in non-Tg mice developing scrapie after inoculation with Mo prions.

TRANSGENIC MICE EXPRESSING Mo PrP-B GENES

Genetic linkage of PrP with scrapie incubation times

Studies of PrP genes (*Prn-p*) in mice with short and long incubation times demonstrated genetic linkage between a *Prn-p* restriction fragment length polymorphism and a gene modulating incubation times (*Prn-i*).[15] Other investigators have confirmed the genetic linkage and one group has shown that the incubation time gene *Sinc* is also linked to PrP.[16,17] *Sinc* was first described by Dickinson and colleagues 25 years ago;[18] whether the genes for PrP, *Prn-i* and *Sinc* are all congruent remains to be established. The PrP sequences of NZW (*Prn-p^a*) and I/Ln (*Prn-p^b*) mice with short and long scrapie incubation times, respectively, differ at codons 108 (L→F) and 189 (T→V).[19] While these amino acid substitutions argue for the congruency of *Prn-p* and *Prn-i*, experiments with *Prn-p^a* mice expressing *Prn-p^b* transgenes demonstrated a paradoxical shortening of incubation times[20] instead of a prolongation as predicted from (*Prn-p^a* × *Prn-p^b*) F1 mice which exhibit long incubation times that are dominant.[15,18] Whether this paradoxical shortening of scrapie incubation times in Tg(*Prn-p^b*) mice results from high levels of PrP^C-B expression remains to be established.[20]

Construction of *Prn-p^b* Tg mice

Because the long incubation time allele of *Prn-i* is dominant, we thought that the scrapie incubation times of *Prn-p^a* mice harboring *Prn-p^b* transgenes could clarify the relationship between *Prn-p* and *Prn-i*. To isolate a molecular clone appropriate for this experiment, it was necessary to define the 5′structure of the *Prn-p^b* gene. Previous analyses positioned an upstream exon or exons (designated 'exon 1') for the 5′untranslated (5′UT) sequence of the *Prn-p^b* mRNA at least 11.5 kb 5′of the PrP coding exon.[19] To map these exons, full-length PrP cDNAs were generated using single-sided specificity polymerase chain reaction (PCR).[21,22] Sequence analysis of these clones and a cognate genomic cosmid clone, cos6.I/LnJ-4, revealed that *Prn-p* mRNA 5′UT sequences are encoded by 2 exons.[20] Sequences 5′of the first exon show homology to the SHaPrP gene promoter[23] and are assumed to constitute the *Prn-p^b* promoter; expression studies detailed below are consistent with this assumption. The cos6. I/LnJ-4 clone encompasses ca. 6.0 kb of 5′and >12.5 kb 3′flanking sequences, respectively (Westaway et al., in preparation).

Three Tg founders derived from microinjection of the cos6.I/LnJ-4 insert, animals Tg(Prn-p^b)93, 94, and 117, were identified by BstE II digestion of a PCR-amplified fragment of the *Prn-p^b* open reading frame (ORF).[20] BstE II is diagnostic for the Thr to Val transition at codon 189. While the Tg(Prn-p^b)94 and 117 founders transmitted the *Prn-p^b* transgene in a Mendelian fashion, either low-copy or high-copy number transgene arrays were detected in 4 Tg(Prn-p^b)93 offspring out of a total of 50 animals scrutinized. We established 2 Tg(Prn-p^b)93 sublines, Tg(Prn-p^b)93L (low-copy) and Tg(Prn-p^b)93H (high-copy), which both transmit their transgene arrays in a Mendelian fashion. To confirm the results of PCR analysis, high molecular weight DNA samples from offspring of Tg93L and Tg93H, and from second generation offspring of the Tg94 and Tg117 founders were analyzed by Southern blotting (Fig. 1). All Tg animals harbor a ~17 kb Bst E II fragment diagnostic for the *Prn-p^b* gene (lanes 4–7) in addition to 5.6 and 3.4 kb fragments which correspond to the 5′and 3′fragments of the endogenous *Prn-p^a* gene. These fragment sizes are in reasonable agreement with estimates of 15.5, 5.7 and 3.5 kb.[19] The Tg(*Prn-p^b*)117 line is distinguished from the Tg(*Prn-p^b*)93H and 94 lines by the absence of a submolar 7.9 kb fragment and transgene copy numbers per haploid genome are 2, ~52, ~31 and ~36 copies for the Tg(*Prn-p^b*)93L, 93H, 94 and 117 lines, respectively.

Expression of transgene encoded mRNA and protein

Prn-p^b transgene mRNA expression was established by PCR analysis of brain cDNAs. cDNA was amplified with a 5′primer that lies within exon 2 and a 3′primer that lies within the exon 3 (the PrP coding exon), and the amplified cDNAs products were digested with BstE II to distinguish transcripts originating from the *a* and *b Prn-p* alleles. Brain RNA from non-Tg littermates and NZW mice generated cDNA-PCR products that approximate to the predicted size of 655 bp following BstE II digestion, diagnostic of the *a* allele.[20] An additional fragment approximating the predicted size of 738 bp, resistant to BstE II and diagnostic for the *b* allele, was seen in control *a/b* heterozygous mice and in all the Tg lines examined. Whereas the ratio of *a:b* cDNA fragments in Tg93L mice was comparable to that in *Prn-p^a* × *Prn-p^b* F1 mice, cDNA fragments diagnostic for the *b* allele predominated in the Tg(Prn-p^b)94 and 117 mice, indicating over expression of *Prn-p^b*. This interpretation was supported by Northern blot analyses of total *Prn-p* mRNA using an ORF-specific hybridization probe. The signals corresponding to the 2.5-kb *Prn-p* mRNA in Tg(Prn-p^b)93L RNA were slightly stronger than in control mice. Higher levels of *Prn-p* mRNA were evident in the Tg(*Prn-p^b*)94 and Tg117 lines.[20]

Antibodies that discriminate PrP-A and PrP-B are not available, precluding direct quantitation of transgene-encoded protein. Therefore a polyclonal rabbit anti-SHaPrP 27–30 antiserum, which strongly cross-reacts with MoPrP, was used to estimate total levels of PrP^C expression in the brains of Tg($Prn-p^b$) mice. All 4 Tg($Prn-p^b$) lines produced greater amounts of PrP^C than non-Tg mice, as assessed through ELISA of serial dilutions of membrane bound brain protein. Overexpression ranged from 2- to 4-fold, for Tg($Prn-p^b$)93L, to approximately 8-fold for Tg($Prn-p^b$)94 and 117 mice. No signal was exhibited on control blots processed using preimmune serum as the primary antibody. Of note, PrP^C expression in Tg($Prn-p^b$)94 mice is comparable to that found in Tg(SHaPrP)7 and 81 mice.[4]

Abbreviated scrapie incubation times in Tg($Prn-p^b$) mice

Tg animals and non-Tg littermate controls were inoculated with an isolate of Chandler murine scrapie agent that had been passaged in NZW mice.[24] Non-Tg animals exhibited typical scrapie incubation times of ca. 125–137 d, but, unexpectedly, all 4 Tg($Prn-p^b$) Mo lines exhibited significantly shorter incubation times (Table 1). There were no obvious differences in incubation times between male and female Tg mice. Incubation times measured from inoculation to onset of illness of 79, 75, and 78 days were exhibited by the Tg($Prn-p^b$)93H, 94 and 117 lines, respectively. The Tg($Prn-p^b$)93L line exhibited longer incubation periods of ca. 97 days, though still about 30 days shorter than non-Tg controls. The interval between the onset of clinical symptoms and death ranged from 6.9 days in Tg($Prn-p^b$)93H line to 17.2 days in the Tg93L line. All the Tg($Prn-p^b$) Mo lines showed clinical signs and characteristic pathological features of scrapie disease in Prn-p^a mice,[24] including spongiform degeneration and reactive astrocytic gliosis.[20] The spongy degeneration tended to be bilaterally symmetrical and focal, concentrated in the hippocampus and thalamus. There was a delicate spongy degeneration in the white matter. No amyloid plaques were detected with either the trichrome staining or by immunohistochemistry with PrP-directed antisera.

To assess the replication of prions in the brains of the Tg($Prn-p^b$) animals, homogenates were prepared from the brains of 3 clinically ill Tg($Prn-p^b$)94 animals and inoculated intracerebrally into CD-1 ($Prn-p^a$) mice. These CD-1 mice developed scrapie at ~143 d in all 3 experiments, similar to the incubation time observed for CD-1 passaged prions, ~138 d, indicating that selection for a more rapidly replicating prion variant had not occurred in the Tg($Prn-p^b$) mice.[20] The recipient CD-1 mice exhibited neuropathological changes typical of murine scrapie.

Table 1 Incubation times of Prn-p^b transgenic lines

Mice	Illness[a]	Death[b]
	Incubation times (days ± S.E.)	
Tg93L[c]	96.7 ± 3.0 (12)	107.1 ± 5.0 (3)
non-Tg[d]	125.3 ± 2.8 (16)	135.8 ± 3.3 (10)
Tg93H	79.4 ± 2.9 (14)	86.3 ± 3.0 (6)
non-Tg	129.9 ± 3.7 (9)	145.4 ± 5.7 (7)
Tg94	75.5 ± 1.8 (15)	83.4 ± 1.7 (10)
non-Tg	137.0 ± 2.1 (21)	145.9 ± 2.4 (15)
Tg117	78.5 ± 1.9 (13)	85.8 ± 2.7 (8)
non-Tg[e]	129.5 ± 4.6 (15)	140.5 ± 4.2 (11)

[a]Mice were inoculated intracerebrally with ~$10^7 ID_{50}$ units of RML extract prepared from the brains of NZW mice. In parentheses are the number of animals developing clinical signs of scrapie. [b]In parentheses are the number of mice dying of scrapie. Mice sacrificed for pathologic examination were excluded in these calculations. [c]One mouse with sickness and death times of 124 and 138 d, respectively, was presumably a mistyped non-Tg animal; however, no tissues were available for retyping. [d]One mouse with sickness and death times of 93 and 96 d, respectively, was presumably a mistyped Tg animal, but no tissues were available for retyping. [e]One mouse with sickness and death times of 77 and 85 d, respectively, was presumably a mistyped Tg animal; however, no tissues were available for retyping. Reprinted from Ref. 20.

TRANSGENIC MICE EXPRESSING GERSTMANN-STRÄUSSLER-SCHEINKER SYNDROME (GSS) MoPrP GENES

Inherited human prion diseases

Thirteen mutations in the human PrP gene (PRNP) on the short arm of chromosome 20 have been found to segregate in families with a variety of inherited prion diseases[25–35]; wherever the families of sufficient size and DNA samples have been available, significant genetic linkage between the PrP gene mutation and the development of CNS disease has been established. The finding of mutations in the PRNP gene which segregate with the inherited human prion diseases seems to be most compatible with the hypothesis that prions are composed only of PrP^{Sc} molecules. Besides familial Creutzfeldt-Jakob disease (CJD) and GSS, a new inherited human prion disease designated fatal familial insomnia (FFI) has recently been identified.[36,37] Mutant PrP^C molecules appear to undergo spontaneous conversion into PrP^{Sc}, the accumulation of which causes CNS degeneration. Whether all of the inherited human prion diseases involve PrP^{Sc} formation is unknown; the possibility that mutant PrP^C can also cause disease must also be considered.

GSS in humans was genetically linked to a mutation at codon 102 in the PrP gene which results in the substitution of leucine for proline[25,38,39] and is present in families with GSS from different ethnic backgrounds.[25,27,38] As noted above, 6 additional point mutations and

6 different octarepeat insertions have been found to segregate with the inherited human prion diseases; a correlation between specific PrP mutations and different clinical forms of familial prion diseases has been suggested.[40,41]

Construction of Tg(MoPrP-P101L) mice

Studies showing that SHaPrP transgenes modify virtually all aspects of experimental scrapie in mice suggested that the dominantly inherited GSS phenotype might be manifest in Tg mice expressing mutant PrP.[3,4] To test this hypothesis, MoPrP genes containing a codon 101 leucine substitution (homologous to codon 102 in PRNP) were microinjected into fertilized oocytes to produce Tg mice.[3] The microinjected DNA consisted of a chimeric murine cosmid constructed by exchanging the BamH I-Sal I fragment containing the open reading frame from a recombinant NZW genomic clone[19] for the corresponding fragment in an I/Ln mouse cosmid.[20] A ~100 nucleotide region flanking the codon 101 leucine was modified to yield DNA sequence homology to SHaPrP while retaining amino acid homology to MoPrP, thus enabling tail DNA of weanling mice to be screened with a ~60 nucleotide probe derived from this region. Mice containing MoPrP-P101L transgenes were detected by comparing intensities of the radiolabeled probe hybridized to approximately 20 µg of denatured tail DNA from weanling mice or control hamsters.

Three transgenic founder lines were initially created — Tg(MoPrP-P101L)174, Tg(MoPrP-P101L)180, and Tg(MoPrP-P101L)196. All animals were housed in a room in which no animals inoculated with scrapie prions had ever been kept; all second and third generation Tg mice were kept in new cages and drank from new water bottles not previously exposed to scrapie-infected animals. The haploid transgene copy numbers in each line were determined by comparison of the intensities of a radiolabeled 0.6 kb BstE II-EcoR I fragment near the 3′end of exon III (containing the open reading frame)[19,20] hybridized to mouse DNA of varying dilutions. Tg(MoPrP-P101L)174, 180 and 196 mice harbored approximately 60, 5 and 5 haploid transgene copies, respectively. The male Tg(MoPrP-P101L)174 founder mouse readily produced offspring, but the Tg(MoPrP-P101L)180 founder was sterile and the female Tg(MoPrP-P101L)196 founder was slow to produce progeny. PrP^C expression in Tg(MoPrP-P101L)174 brains was ~8-fold higher than controls as determined by intensities of immunoblots on nitrocellulose of varying dilutions of brain extracts. The ~60 nucleotide hamster-biased probe hybridized to 0.1 µg Tg brain RNA but not to 20 µg non-Tg brain RNA confirming expression of the transgene. The mutant transgenes were inherited in a manner consistent with a single autosomal site of insertion, since it was present in approximately half (87/176) of Tg(MoPrP-P101L)174 progeny and could be transmitted by males.

Spontaneous CNS degeneration in Tg(MoPrP-P101L) mice

Ninety-eight Tg(MoPrP-P101L)174 mice appeared healthy until symptoms of ataxia, lethargy, and rigidity developed between 7 and 39 weeks of age. The mean age of the 98 animals that developed neurologic dysfunction was 180 ± 6 days (± SEM). To date, the oldest Tg(MoPrP-P101L) mouse to develop disease was 287 days of age, and the youngest animal was 49 days old. The youngest mouse was the offspring of 2 Tg mice and may be homozygous for the MoPrP-P101L transgene. Once affected, the animals deteriorated over 3 to 36 days until death. Although initially it was a formal possibility that either the site of MoPrP-P101L transgene insertion alone was the cause of spontaneous neurodegeneration in Tg(MoPrP-P101L)174 mice, additional lines of Tg(MoPrP-P101L) mice that spontaneously develop CNS degeneration argue against the site of insertion being important.

Neurodegeneration and PrP amyloid plaques in Tg(MoPrP-P101L) mice

Clinically sick Tg(MoPrP-P101L)174 mice, both immersion-fixed and perfusion-fixed, had the same pathological features. Numerous 5 to 15 μm vacuoles (spongiform degeneration) were present in both the grey and white matter (Fig. 2B). Vacuoles in perfusion-fixed animals appeared to contain a pale staining, amorphous substance which was absent from most of the vacuoles in immersion-fixed animals; however, some vacuoles in the latter also contained this material. The vacuoles were found in most grey and white matter structures of the cerebral hemispheres and brainstem. There was a mild to moderate degree of reactive astrocytic gliosis in a patchy distribution in both grey and white matter. A prominent Bergmann radial gliosis was present in much of the molecular layer of the cerebellar cortex. The vacuolation and gliosis induced by inoculation of non-Tg CD-1 mice with scrapie prions (Fig. 2A) was virtually indistinguishable from that found in the uninoculated Tg(MoPrP-P101L) mice (Fig. 2B).

   Like GSS in humans, amyloid plaques were found in the brains of affected Tg(MoPrP-P101L) mice as shown by PAS staining (Fig. 2C); immunostaining demonstrated that these plaques are PrP positive (Fig. 2D). In our initial report, we stated that no plaques were found by the Gomori trichrome method or with PrP antiserum R073.[42] We probably failed to observe the plaques because they are relatively infrequent. PrP amyloid plaques are a constant feature of GSS in humans, but they

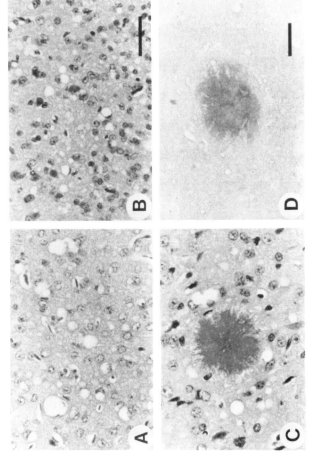

Fig. 2 Neuropathology of Tg(MoPrP-P101L) mice developing neurodegeneration spontaneously. (**A**) Vacuolation in cerebral cortex of a Swiss CD-1 mouse that exhibited signs of neurologic dysfunction. (**B**) Vacuolation in cerebral cortex of a Tg(MoPrP-P101L) mouse that exhibited signs of neurologic dysfunction with $\sim 10^6$ ID$_{50}$ units of RML scrapie prions. (**C**) Kuru-type PrP amyloid plaque stained with PAS in the caudate nucleus of a Tg(MoPrP-P101L) mouse that exhibited signs of neurologic dysfunction at 252 days of age. (**D**) PrP amyloid plaques stained with α-PrP antiserum (RO73) in the caudate nucleus of a Tg(MoPrP-P101L) mouse that exhibited signs of neurologic dysfunction. Bar in B also applies to A = 50 μm. Bar in D also applies to C = 25 μm.

are infrequent in familial CJD.[25,29,33,43–45] It is noteworthy that PrP amyloid plaques are relatively rare in mice inoculated with most isolates of Mo prions. Only the 87V 'strain' of prions induces large numbers of PrP amyloid plaques and these are confined to *Prn-p^b* mice.[46–48]

Even though PrP amyloid plaques were found which presumably contain PrP^{Sc} in the brains of Tg(MoPrP-P101L)174 mice, only very low levels of proteinase K-resistant prion proteins could be demonstrated by Western blots of brain extracts. Because Tg(MoPrP–P101L)174 mice express high levels of MoPrP(P101L)^C, we assumed that some or all of the low levels of protease-resistant PrP detected on Western blots were residual PrP^C rather than PrP^{Sc}.[49] With Tg(SHaPrP) mice, uncertainties about low levels of protease-resistant SHaPrP on immunoblots were resolved by ELISA using SHaPrP mAb[4] but no MoPrP mAb are currently available. Although the accumulation of PrP^{Sc} seems to be responsible for both clinical dysfunction and neuropathological lesions in scrapie, mutant MoPrP(P101L)^C may through an inborn error of PrP metabolism produce neurologic disease without the generation of infectivity.[40,44,50]

Transmission of CNS disease by extracts from Tg(MoPrP-P101L) 174 mice

To assess whether brains of affected Tg(MoPrP-P101L)174 mice synthesize infectious prions *de novo*, 10% (w/v) brain homogenates from clinically ill Tg(MoPrP-P101L)174 mice and from non-Tg controls were injected intracerebrally into Swiss CD-1, Tg(SHaPrP)7, Tg(MoPrP-B)117 and Tg(MoPrP-P101L)196 mice as well as Syrian golden hamsters. Subsequently, we learned that uninoculated Tg(SHaPrP)7 and Tg(MoPrP-B)117 mice develop spontaneous neurodegeneration after 300–500 days of age. This finding forced us to abandon studies with these 2 Tg lines but studies with the other 3 inoculated hosts seem valid. We found that 3/17 extracts prepared from ill Tg(MoPrP-P101L)174 mice produced neurologic disease in 9/112 Syrian hamsters between 221 and 441 days while 24 extracts from non-Tg controls failed to produce disease. 11/16 extracts transmitted CNS disease to 52/160 Tg(MoPrP-P101L)196 mice between 226 and 549 days. The Tg(MoPrP-P101L)196 mice expressing MoPrP(P101L)^C at low levels did not develop disease either spontaneously or after inoculation with 9 extracts prepared from non-Tg control brains. Neither 17 extracts prepared from clinically ill Tg(MoPrP-P101L)174 mice nor 14 extracts from non-Tg controls produced disease in 260 Swiss CD-1 mice that were observed for >600 days.

Murine model of inherited prion disease

Our clinical and neuropathological observations on spontaneous disease in Tg(MoPrP-P101L)174 mice support the hypothesis that the PrP codon 101 leucine change is the cause of their neurologic disease and, by inference, the PRNP codon 102 leucine mutation is responsible for GSS in humans. Although the neurologic disorder in Tg(MoPrP-P101L)174 mice is clinically and pathologically similar to scrapie, the low levels of protease-resistant PrP distinguish these animals from those developing scrapie after inoculation with prions.

The broad range in the age of onset and the duration of disease in Tg(MoPrP-P101L)174 mice is in contrast to the narrow range in the incubation period and disease duration observed in mice inoculated with prions.[15–17,51,52] However. it resembles that observed in human GSS[25,40,44,50,53] and argues that PrP primary structure is not the sole determinant of age of onset and disease duration. Genes both linked and unlinked to PrP can also have a major influence on incubation times.[15–17,51,52] Since Tg(MoPrP-P101L)174 mice were not inbred being derived from (C57BL/6 x SJL)F2 fertilized oocytes,[54] some of the variation may be due to modifier genes.[55–58]

The development of spontaneous spongiform neurodegeneration in Tg(MoPrP–P101L)174 mice established, for the first time, that a neurodegenerative process similar to a human disease could be genetically modeled in an animal. The argument that the leucine PrP variants in humans and Tg(MoPrP-P101L)174 mice are potent susceptibility genes for a ubiquitous, but as yet unidentified pathogen, remains a formal interpretation of our results.[59,60] However, multiple lines of investigation on the physical and biological properties of the infectious agent consistently converge upon PrP[Sc], and fail to reveal additional essential components.[61,62]

PROPAGATION OF ARTIFICIAL PRIONS IN Tg MICE EXPRESSING CHIMERIC Mo/SHa PrP GENES

Tg mice expressing chimeric PrP genes

We constructed several chimeric PrP gene cassettes, by replacing regions of the murine PrP ORF with corresponding sections of the Syrian hamster PrP ORF.[63] One chimeric construct, MHM2 PrP, has been previously described[63–65] and contains 2 amino acid substitutions from Syrian hamsters, a Leu to Met at position 108 and a Val to Met at position 111 (Fig. 3). MHM2 PrP appears to behave similarly to murine PrP; it forms recombinant MHM2 PrP[Sc] when expressed in murine neuroblastoma (N_2a) cells infected with RML isolate of mouse prions.[63,64] Another chimeric ORF, MH2M PrP, contains a total of 5 amino acid substitutions from Syrian hamsters. In addition to the two represented in MHM2 PrP, MH2M PrP contains an Iso to Met at position 138, a Tyr to Asn at position 154 and a Ser to Asn at position 169. The presence of 108 Met and 111 Met in both of these constructs provides an epitope for a Syrian hamster-specific monoclonal antibody, mAb 3F4,[66] which allows the recombinant proteins to be easily discriminated from endogenous murine PrP.[63,64] When expressed in scrapie-infected (Sc) N_2a cells, MH2M PrP also appears to be eligible for formation of PrP[Sc], but at much reduced efficiency relative to MHM2 PrP (M. Scott, unpublished). In contrast, SHaPrP does not form PrP[Sc] when expressed in these same cells.[63] Because of this, we considered that MH2M PrP might represent a new, artificial 'species' of PrP which would be intermediate between that of hamsters and mice.

To test this hypothesis, Tg mice expressing MHM2 PrP and MH2M PrP were constructed. The recombinant SHa/Mo PrP ORFs were transferred into the transgene expression vector cosSHa.Tet.[63] This vector was derived by manipulation of a 45-kb segment of SHa DNA which encompasses the entire SHaPrP gene and was designed to allow exact replacement of the ORF, without disruption of any neighbouring regions.[63] Following transfer of the recombinant ORFs into cosSHa.Tet, the recombinant transgenes were used to construct transgenic mice as described previously.[3] Of 3 founders originally constructed harboring the MH2M PrP transgene, only one, Tg(MH2M PrP)92, proved suitable for further analysis. One line expressed the recombinant protein at low levels, and the other could not be bred. The level of expression of the transgene product in the brains of Tg(MH2M PrP)92 mice is similar to that of Tg(SHaPrP)81, a Tg mouse line harboring the SHaPrP gene.[3,4] We also obtained 3 lines expressing MHM2 PrP designated Tg(MHM2 PrP)285, Tg(MHM2 PrP)294 and Tg(MHM2 PrP)321. Tg(MHM2 PrP)285 mice which contain similar levels of transgene product as Tg(SHaPrP)81 and Tg(MH2M PrP)92 mice. These Tg mice express 2- to 4-fold more PrP per mg of total brain protein than normal hamsters.[67]

Terminology

In order to define clearly the transmission history prion inocula, we created a scheme for naming the prions.[67] For example, the Sc237 prion isolate previously passaged in Syrian hamsters and inoculated into the same animals again are designated SHa(SHa(Sc237)) or abbreviated SHa(Sc237).[68] Passage of Sc237 prions from Syrian hamsters through Tg(MH2M PrP) mice twice and back into Syrian hamsters is denoted SHa(MH2M(MH2M(SHa(Sc237)))) or abbreviated SHa(MH2M(MH2M(Sc237))) where the host for the last passage is written first and the isolate designation is last. We prefer this expression since it places the most recent passage first and it is shorter than showing the passage history in a linear array:

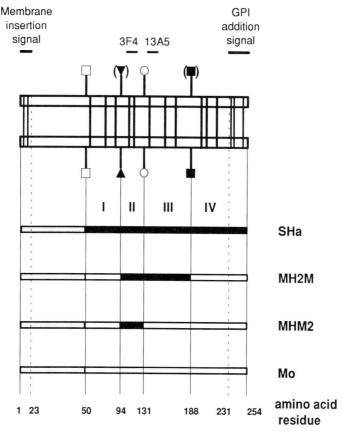

Fig. 3 Construction and expression of chimeric Mo/SHaPrP transgenes. Relationship of chimeric PrP constructs to SHa and MoPrP ORFs. The graphic at top is a schematic of the SHa and MoPrP ORFs. The approximate locations of amino acid sequence differences are depicted as vertical bars which correspond to Syrian hamster codons: 5, 14, 53, 71, 79, 108, 111, 138, 154, 169, 202, 204, 215, 232, 233 and 252. Those occurring in the 22-amino acid N-terminal signal peptide and within the glycoinositol phospholipid anchor signal are depicted within these lines. Also shown are the approximate locations of restriction enzyme cleavage sites used to construct chimeric molecules. These are, together with the location of their cleavage sites relative to the start of the SHaPrP ORF: □, OxaNI (151); ▼, KpnI (283); (open circles), BglI (392, this site is not unique within the SHaPrP and MoPrP ORFs); ■,BstEII (563). Parentheses indicate that enzyme sites do not exist in the native DNA sequence but were introduced by site-directed mutagenesis in such a way as to avoid disruption of the amino acid sequence. The graphic at the bottom depicts the relationship of various chimeric ORFs. Black regions were derived from SHaPrP, white regions from MoPrP. The region shown in gray is homologous between SHa and MoPrP. The names of the ORFs are shown at right. The amino acid positions of boundaries defined in this diagram are shown at bottom. Reprinted from Ref. 67.

SHa(Sc237)→MH2M→MH2M→SHa where the most recent passage is last.

Scrapie incubation times in mice expressing chimeric PrP[C]

By comparing Tg lines with similar levels of foreign PrP expression, we sought to minimize the influence of gene dosage on incubation time, which has been described for Tg(SHaPrP) mice.[4] When Tg(MH2M PrP)92 mice were inoculated with SHa(Sc237) or Mo(RML) prions, the animals developed scrapie at ~140 days.[67] In contrast, all 3 lines of Tg(MHM2 PrP) mice behaved like non-Tg mice and were resistant to infection with SHa(Sc237) prions, showing no evidence of disease at >350 days. Brains of Tg(MH2M PrP)92 animals inoculated with SHa(Sc237) prions contained large quantities of protease-resistant MH2M PrP[Sc], at levels similar to Tg(SHa PrP)81 mice, which develop scrapie at ~70 days following inoculation with SHa(Sc237) prions and Tg(SHa PrP)7 mice that develop scrapie at ~50 days after inoculation with SHa(Sc237) prions. The presence of MH2M PrP[Sc] suggests that MH2M (Sc237) prions are produced in these animals as well. That Tg(MH2M PrP) and Tg(MHM2 PrP) mice display markedly different susceptibility to infection with SHa(Sc237) prions argues that the larger region of identity with SHaPrP contained in MH2M PrP as compared to MHM2 PrP is apparently able to confer sensitivity to SHa prions. These studies and those reported previously[4] suggest that initiation of prion infection may require a homotypic interaction between PrP[Sc] in the infecting prion and PrP[C] synthesized by the host. Since MHM2 and MH2M PrP differ at only 3 amino acid locations, it seems reasonable to conclude that some or all 3 of these amino acid residues influence this putative interaction.

All of the Tg mouse lines were susceptible to infection with Mo(RML) prions and succumbed to the disease at 110–150 days. The presence of the endogenous MoPrP gene should ensure that these mice are permissive for Mo(RML) infection. In previous studies using Tg(SHaPrP) mice, however, expression of SHaPrP caused a prolongation of the incubation period after inoculation with Mo(RML) scrapie prions. The most pronounced effects were with lines expressing the highest levels of SHaPrP; those same lines exhibited the shortest incubation periods following inoculation with SHa(Sc237) prions.[4] In contrast to the Tg(SHaPrP) mice, Tg(MH2M PrP) and Tg(MHM2 PrP) mice exhibited shorter incubation times after inoculation with Mo(RML) prions compared to non-Tg littermate controls. This was especially evident in Tg(MHM2 PrP)294 mice, which express the highest levels of the chimeric PrP. Furthermore, the brains of Tg(MHM2 PrP)285 and Tg(MHM2 PrP)294 mice infected with Mo(RML) prions contained high levels of MHM2 PrP[Sc] when analyzed using a monospecific antiserum. The resistance to infection with SHa prions, the acceleration rather than inhibition of Mo(RML) prion replication, and the efficient formation of MHM2 PrP^{Sc} in Mo(RML) infected Tg(MHM2 PrP) mice all suggest that MHM2 PrP is similar to MoPrP, differing only by virtue of a fortuitous epitope 'tag'. In contrast, SHaPrP does not efficiently form SHaPrP^{Sc} following infection with Mo(RML) prions. Taken together these observations provide further evidence that the inhibition of Mo(RML) prion replication in Tg(SHaPrP) mice arises because SHaPrP^{C} in some unknown manner inhibits the conversion of MoPrP^{C} to MoPrP^{Sc}, perhaps via competitive inhibition.[4]

If MH2M PrP contains all of the SHa residues needed for these PrP molecules to behave as SHaPrP, then these mice should resemble Tg(SHaPrP) mice in all respects. After inoculation of Tg(MH2M PrP)92 mice with Mo(RML) prions, the incubation times were similar to those found in non-Tg littermate controls, with no evidence of the prolongation observed for Tg(SHaPrP) mice. Additionally, MH2M PrP^{Sc} was readily detected in the brains of Mo(RML) infected Tg(MH2M PrP)92 mice, in quantities similar to those observed in the brains of Tg(MHM2 PrP)285 inoculated with Mo(RML) prions. Protease-resistant SHaPrP^{Sc} was not observed in Tg(SHaPrP) mice infected with Mo prions as judged by measuring protease-resistant SHaPrP on immunoblots.[4] Thus Tg(MH2M PrP) mice clearly differ from Tg(SHaPrP) mice, and resemble Tg(MHM2 PrP) mice when inoculated with Mo prions. The incubation period of Tg(MH2M PrP)92 following inoculation with Mo(RML) prions was similar to that observed for Tg(MHM2 PrP)285 mice, which express similar levels of chimeric PrP. The chimeric MH2M PrP^{Sc} was indistinguishable in these animals whether they were inoculated with Mo(RML) or SHa(Sc237) prions.[67]

Chimeric prions with artificial properties

Previous studies with 3 species of hamsters showed that individual prion isolates have distinct properties which are highly dependent on the host.[69,70] Brain extracts of Tg(MH2M PrP)92 mice containing MH2M(Sc237) prions were serially passaged in Tg(MH2M PrP)92 and Syrian hamsters (Table 2). The incubation period for the homologous transmission shortened from ~140 days for the initial passage from hamsters to Tg(MH2M)92 to ~70 days. After a second passage of MH2M(MH2M(Sc237)) prions, the incubation was reduced to ~65 days (Table 2) but this is not a significant change.[67] As expected, MH2M PrP^{Sc} was detected in the brains of these animals after both passages. In contrast, when MH2M(Sc237) prions were transmitted to hamsters, the incubation period was ~120 days which is significantly protracted compared to a homologous passage of SHa(Sc237) prions in hamsters with an incubation period of ~70 days. After a second passage in Tg(MH2M PrP)92 mice, the MH2M(MH2M(Sc237)) inoculum gave an even longer incubation period when reintroduced into hamsters, lengthening to ~155 days. The presence of SHaPrP[Sc] in the recipient hamsters was confirmed by Western blotting.

Table 2 Incubation times for chimeric prions passaged in Tg(MH2M PrP)92 mice or Syrian hamsters

Inoculum	Host		Scrapie incubation times		
		(n/n_o)	Illness (days ± S.E.)	(n/n_o)[a]	Death (days ± S.E.)
SHa(Sc237)	Tg(MH2M PrP)92	34/34	133.8 ± 3.6	26/26	141.7 ± 4.4
MH2M (SHa(Sc237))	Tg(MH2M PrP)92	22/22	72.8 ± 0.7	12/12	85.3 ± 1.2
MH2M(MH2M (SHa(Sc237)))	Tg(MH2M PrP)92	10/10	63.9 ± 1.9	8/8	75.5 ± 2.9
SHa(Sc237)	Syrian hamsters	48/48	77 ± 1.1[b]	48/48	89 ± 1.7
MH2M (SHa(Sc237))	Syrian hamsters	23/23	116.0 ± 3.8	10/10	136.2 ± 3.5
MH2M(MH2M (SHa(Sc237)))	Syrian hamsters	6/6	161.0 ± 3.8	4/4	187.0 ± 2.4
SHa(MH2M (SHa(Sc237)))	Syrian hamsters	8/8	76.9 ± 0.6	4/4	84.8 ± 1.2

[a]The reduced number of animals in the death column reflects sacrifice of some animals for immunoblotting and neuropathology. [b]From Ref. 3.

The abbreviated incubation times of MH2M(Sc237) prions compared to SHa(Sc237) prions passaged in Tg(MH2M PrP)92 mice did not permanently alter the characteristic incubation time of the Sc237 isolate. Re-introduction into hamsters followed by serial transmission in hamsters, i.e. SHa(SHa(MH2M(Sc237))), produced incubation times of ~70 days which are characteristic of SHa(Sc237) prions. To characterize further the properties of (Sc237) prions passaged through Tg(MH2M PrP)92 mice and back into Syrian hamsters, the patterns of PrP[Sc] accumulation were determined by histoblotting.[71]

The distribution of PrP[Sc] in Syrian hamsters inoculated with MH2M(Sc237) prions passaged in Tg(MH2M PrP)92 mice was similar to that in Syrian hamsters inoculated with SHa(Sc237) prions. The only differences in the patterns of PrP[Sc] accumulation were in the intensity of immunostaining. For example, the hippocampus and medial hypothalamus were less intensely immunostained with SHa(Sc237) prions than with MH2M(Sc237) prions. The intensity and extent of PrP[Sc] deposition in the subependymal and subpial regions were reversed, i.e. more with SHa(Sc237) prions than with MH2M(Sc237) prions. Thus the histoblot patterns were qualitatively similar but different quantitatively.

Distinct prion isolates passaged in Tg(MH2M PrP)92 mice

Similar results were obtained when Tg(MH2M PrP)92 mice were inoculated with a second distinct isolate or 'strain' of Syrian hamster-adapted scrapie prions, 139H,[70,72] with the mice developing disease at ~110 days, slightly shorter than with Sc237.[67] Western blotting experiments confirmed the presence of MH2M PrP^{Sc} (data not shown). Interestingly, the SHa(139H) isolate showed a somewhat different behavior during serial transmission in Tg(MH2M PrP)92 mice. Passage of SHa(139H) prions in Tg(MH2M PrP)92 mice gave a slightly shorter incubation time of ~105 days on second passage. These incubation times contrast with those produced by the SHa(Sc237) isolate. On first passage in Tg(MH2M PrP)92 mice, SHa(Sc237) prions gave incubation times of ~140 days while second passage was ~70 days (Table 2). It will be important to learn whether the properties of the SHa(139H) isolate are permanently altered by repeated passage through Tg(MH2M PrP)92 mice by subsequent passaging back into Syrian hamsters.

We also serially passaged extracts from Tg(MH2M PrP)92 mice infected with Mo(RML) prions into Tg(MH2M PrP)92 mice. Although the significance of these data is clouded by the presence of endogenous MoPrP, some shortening of incubation period was detected during the homologous passage. Construction of Tg mice devoid of an endogenous MoPrP gene[2] will obviate this problem. Passage of MH2M(RML) prions into Syrian hamsters also produced a unique pattern of PrP^{Sc} deposition, as determined by histoblotting. The 3 most obvious differences in the distribution of PrP^{Sc} compared to that found with either SHa(Sc237) or MH2M(Sc237) prions were: (a) the intensity and thickness of PrP^{Sc} deposition in the region of the hippocampal fissure and the molecular layer of the dentate gyrus of the hippocampus; (b) the prominent subpial deposition of PrP^{Sc}, particularly in the molecular layer of the cerebral cortex; and (c) the absence of PrP^{Sc} deposition in the subependyma.

Contrasting neuropathology of prion isolates in Syrian hamsters

We observed other striking differences in the neuropathology of Syrian hamsters infected with MH2M(RML) or MH2M(Sc237) prions. With MH2M(Sc237) prions, a delicate vacuolation occurred in the hippocampus throughout the apical dendrite portion (stratum radiatum) of the pyramidal cells of the CA1 region.[67] These vacuoles varied in diameter from 5 to 15 μm and corresponded spatially with the small amount of PrP^{Sc} in that region. With MH2M(RML) prions, a similar very delicate vacuolation occurred in most of the stratum radiatum; however, intense spongiform degeneration with more vacuoles of greater size, up to 50 μm in diameter, occurred in the deeper layers of the CA1 region coincident with the intense PrP^{Sc} signal in the region of the hippocampal fissure. We have not seen this pattern before which supports the view that the properties of the MH2M(RML) isolate may be unique in hamsters.

In the cerebellum, additional differences in the distribution of vacuolation were seen. Scrapie caused by MH2M(SHa(Sc237)) prions was characterized by very large vacuoles with diameters as great as 60 μm in the deep cerebellar nuclei but none in the granule cell layer of the cerebellar cortex. In contrast, MH2M(Mo(RML)) prions caused 25 μm vacuoles in the granule cell layer of the cerebellar cortex but no vacuoles in the deep cerebellar nuclei.

PrP amyloid plaques in Tg(MH2M PrP)92 mice and Syrian hamsters

In Syrian hamsters inoculated with SHa(Sc237) prions, numerous amyloid plaques are found, particularly in the subcallosal region. These plaques stained strongly with α-PrP antiserum designated RO73, less strongly with the α-PrP mAb designated 13A5 and not at all with α-PrP mAb designated 3F4.[67] Whether this lack of staining with 3F4 is due to limited proteolysis where the N-terminal PrP residues containing the 3F4 epitope[65] are hydrolyzed or the epitope remains buried in situ even after denaturation remains to be established. Similarly, when SHa(Sc237) prions were inoculated into Tg(MH2M PrP)92 mice, kuru-type amyloid plaques developed which were strongly RO73 immunopositive.

Surprisingly, although passage of SHa(Sc237) prions in Tg(MH2M PrP)92 mice produced cerebral amyloid plaques, brain extracts from Tg(MH2M PrP)92 mice inoculated with SHa(Sc237) failed to produce amyloid plaques upon a second passage in Tg(MH2M PrP)92 mice or upon passage back into Syrian hamsters.[67] However, upon a second passage through Syrian hamsters the PrP amyloid plaques were found indicating that the properties of the Sc237 prions were changed by passage through Tg(MH2M PrP)92 mice.

No PrP amyloid plaques were found in the brains of Tg(MH2M PrP)92 mice inoculated with Mo(RML) prions. A few, weakly antigenic amyloid plaques were found in one of 3 Tg(MH2M PrP)92 mice inoculated with MH2M (RML) prions derived by a single passage in Tg(MH2M PrP)92 mice. However, the MH2M (RML) prions, when passaged in Syrian hamsters, produced multiple amyloid plaques which were RO73 immunopositive.

Homophilic interactions feature in prion propagation

The unique host range of MH2M prions, especially those derived by infection with SHa(Sc237) prions, has several important implications for understanding scrapie prion replication. Homologous transmissions, back into Tg(MH2M PrP)92 animals, are clearly favored, although the chimeric prions may also be passaged into Syrian hamsters and mice.[67] We conclude this by observing the lengthening and shortening of incubation period during homologous or heterologous transmissions (Table 2). This preference, for infection of animals expressing a homologous PrP, demonstrates that prion infection requires an interaction of PrP[Sc] molecules in the inoculum with the PrP[C] in cells of the host.

Further evidence for the unique tropism of MH2M(Sc237) prions was obtained following serial transmission to normal CD-1 mice. When Tg(SHaPrP) mice infected with SHa(Sc237) prions were serially passaged into mice, no evidence for transmission of the SHa prions was observed[4] In contrast, MH2M(Sc237) prions were able to infect mice efficiently, with an incubation period of ~200 days for the first passage (Table 2). As expected, mice inoculated with MH2M(Sc237) prions contain PrP[Sc] when analyzed by Western blot.

Extracts of brains from Tg(MH2M PrP) mice inoculated with Mo(RML) prions transmitted to Syrian hamsters in ~240 days.[67] Since Tg(MH2M PrP)92 mice contain an endogenous MoPrP gene, we would expect that the inocula will also contain MoPrP[Sc] in addition to MH2M PrP[Sc] which was observed by Western blotting. Unfortunately, no MoPrP-specific antibody exists which could be used to confirm this proposal. However, since previous studies have clearly shown that Mo(RML) prions cannot infect hamsters,[3, 4] it seems reasonable to conclude that MH2M(RML) prions are responsible for the transmission to hamsters observed in this experiment. It will be important to perform a detailed analysis of SHa(RML) prions in comparison to other known Syrian hamster prion isolates, such as Sc237 and 139H.[70] In addition, construction of Tg(MH2M PrP) mice in a background lacking an endogenous MoPrP gene[2] will clarify the results of transmission experiments using Mo(RML) prions, as well as those of other Mo prion isolates. A similar approach to study the other chimeric PrP gene (MHM2 PrP) described in this report, will presumably be required to establish the host range of MHM2 prions.

Prion replication and diversity

Although conversion of PrP[C] to PrP[Sc] might involve a conformational change and the transgenetic data reported here implicate homotypic interactions between PrP[C] and PrP[Sc] during prion replication, the diversity of scrapie prions[73–76] poses a conundrum. Some investigators invoke the participation of a hitherto unidentified nucleic acid genome to explain distinct isolates or 'strains' of prions. Since no scrapie-specific polynucleotide has been found and a wealth of data refutes the existence of such a molecule, alternative hypotheses merit consideration. The finding that the pattern of PrP^{Sc} accumulation in the CNS is characteristic for a particular prion isolate led us to propose a mechanism for the propagation of distinct prion isolates.[70] In this model, different scrapie strains would be either confined to or targetted to different cells depending on the disposition of covalent structures attached to the PrP backbone, the best candidate being the Asn-linked oligosaccharides. As we have shown here, small variations in the primary structure of PrP can create dramatic variations in the susceptibility of the host animal to scrapie prions presumably through alterations in the tertiary structure of PrP^{Sc}. Variations in the Asn-linked oligosaccharides might influence either the specificity of the homophilic interactions between PrP^C and PrP^{Sc} or the targetting of PrP^{Sc} to specific sets of neurons.

If different subpopulations of cells with distinct variations in covalent modifications of PrP exist, it follows that prions derived from these same cells could be more efficiently able to infect cells of the same cell type as those from which they were originally derived, due to the requirement for a specific interaction between PrP^C and PrP^{Sc}. This model yields an interesting prediction. The proposed interaction of PrP^C and PrP^{Sc} would be dependent both upon the PrP sequence as well as the putative structures responsible for 'strain'-specific behaviour. If this were true, it might be expected that the susceptibility of the host to infection with prions derived from another species would vary depending on the particular 'strain' being studied. This phenomenon is mirrored in experiments described here which indicate a marked difference in the relative efficiency of transmission of the Sc237 and 139H isolates between hamsters and Tg(MH2M PrP)92 mice. Indeed, it appears that Tg(MH2M PrP)92 mice are more susceptible to SHa(139H) prions than to SHa(Sc237). Adaptation of the Sc237 to the MH2M background required at least 2 serial transmissions, shortening from ~135 days to ~70 days, whereas the 139H isolate did not appreciably change its incubation period (~115 days) following the first passage. Although the data seem consistent, it is noteworthy that PrP^{Sc} synthesis can occur in absence of Asn-linked glycosylation in scrapie-infected cultured cells.[64] Since prion replication in the absence of Asn-linked glycosylation has not been demonstrated, further studies are needed to determine the molecular basis of the cellular trophism exhibited by prions. Since no other covalent modifications of PrP have been described which could effect this diversity, it is also conceivable that an as yet unrecognized tightly bound ligand might modify scrapie prion interaction with the host in a cell-specific manner.[77]

From these experiments, it appears likely that the Mo(RML) and SHa(Sc237) inocula probably represent different isolates or 'strains'.

This is suggested by the contrasting incubation periods and neuro-pathology observed when these isolates were transmitted to homologous hosts. Although Syrian hamsters are generally preferred as hosts for biochemical studies on scrapie prions, most studies on scrapie 'strains' have been performed in mice. Transgenic mice expressing MH2M PrP may contribute to the analysis of scrapie prion 'strains' by virtue of their ability to act as a 'bridge' across the species barrier between hamsters and mice, allowing murine scrapie 'strains' to be adapted to Syrian hamsters. Similar experiments, using chimeric PrP genes derived from other species, might facilitate the development of murine models for human prion diseases, scrapie of sheep and transmissible bovine spongiform encephalopathy.

These data demonstrate that it is possible to manipulate to proper-ties of scrapie prions, the clinical manifestation of the disease and the susceptibility of the host by changing the side chains of a few amino acids encoded by the PrP gene. In concert with biochemical studies on purified proteins, it may become feasible to reconcile the effects of PrP gene manipulation directly with the biochemical characteristics of the genetically engineered prion proteins, suggesting a new approach where 'artificial' prions with contrived properties may be used to unravel the complexities of scrapie replication.

TRANSGENIC MICE WITH ABLATED PrP GENES

Prn-p$^{0/0}$ mice develop normally

A molecular clone containing the third exon of the *Prn-p* gene was modified by removing 183 codons of PrP and substituting the neomycin phosphotransferase gene. This modified PrP gene was introduced into ES cells derived from agouti 129 mice[78] by electroporation and recom-binates were selected in the presence of G418.[2] These G418 resistant ES cells were injected into the blastocysts of 16–32 cell embryos and chimeric offspring identified by agouti coat color characteristic for the ES cell genotype. Chimeric mice were mated to C57BL6 mice and mice heterozygous for the *Prn-p* ablation were identified by hybridization of Neo and Prn-p probes to the PCR product of the hybrid *Neo/Prn-p* gene.

The heterozygous (Prn-p$^{0/+}$) ablated mice were mated to each other and offspring homozygous (Prn-p$^{0/0}$) for ablation of the Prn-p gene were born.[2] The absence of PrP expression was established by measure-ments of PrP mRNA and PrP^C. Development of the Prn-p$^{0/0}$ mice was normal and behavioral evaluation failed to show any differences among the wild-type (wt), Prn-p$^{0/+}$ and Prn-p$^{0/0}$ mice. Morphologic studies of brain, muscle and spleen also failed to show any differences among the 3 groups of mice. Similarly, the results of lymphocyte activation studies were also similar for all 3 groups; it had previously been suggested that PrP^C functions as a lymphocyte activation molecule because of its cell surface localization and changes in mitogenesis induced by α-PrP antibodies. That Prn-p$^{0/0}$ mice develop normally and remain healthy for >600 days argues that CNS dysfunction in scrapie results from the accumulation of PrP^{Sc} rather than an inhibition of PrP^C function.

Prn-p$^{0/0}$-mice are resistant to scrapie and fail to propagate prions

Wild–type (Prn-p$^{+/+}$), Prn-p$^{0/+}$ and Prn-p$^{0/0}$ mice were inoculated with Mo(RML) prions passaged in Swiss CD-1 mice.[79] By 184 days after inoculation, all of the Prn–p$^{+/+}$ littermates developed clinical signs of scrapie while the Prn-p$^{0/0}$ mice remain alive and well at more than 350 days after inoculation. Prn-p$^{0/0}$ mice sacrificed at intervals after inoculation failed to show evidence of significant prion titers by bioassay of brain and spleen extracts inoculated into CD-1 mice while Prn-p$^{+/+}$ littermates showed propagation of prions to high levels in brain. The results of these studies are in accord with a wealth of data which argue that PrP^{Sc} is necessary for both transmission of prion infectivity and pathogenesis of disease.

SYNTHESIS OF PrP^{Sc} IS A POST-TRANSLATIONAL PROCESS

PrP^{Sc} synthesis in cultured cells

Metabolic labeling studies of scrapie-infected cultured cells have shown that PrP^C is synthesized and degraded rapidly while PrP^{Sc} is synthesized slowly by a post-translational process (Fig. 4).[80–83] These observations are consistent with earlier findings showing that PrP^{Sc} accumulates in the brains of scrapie-infected animals while PrP mRNA levels remain unchanged.[8] Furthermore, the structure and organization of the PrP gene made it likely that PrP^{Sc} is formed during a post-translational event.[23]

Both PrP isoforms appear to transit through the Golgi apparatus where their Asn-linked oligosaccharides are modified and sialylated.[84–88] PrP^C is presumably transported within secretory vesicles to the external cell surface where it is anchored by a glycosyl phosphaditylinositol (GPI) moiety.[89–91] In contrast, PrP^{Sc} accumulates primarily within cells where it is deposited in cytoplasmic vesicles, many of which appear to be secondary lysosomes.[83,92–95]

Whether PrP^C is the substrate for PrP^{Sc} formation or a restricted subset of PrP molecules are precursors for PrP^{Sc} remains to be established. Several experimental results argue that PrP molecules destined to become PrP^{Sc} exit to the cell surface as does PrP^C [89] prior to their conversion into PrP^{Sc}.[82,83,93] Interestingly, the GPI anchors of both PrP^C and PrP^{Sc}, which presumably feature in directing the subcellular

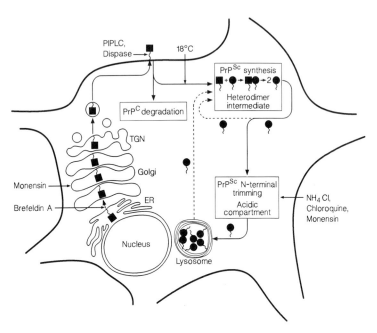

Fig. 4 Pathways of prion protein synthesis and degradation in cultured cells. PrP^{Sc} is denoted by circles; squares designate PrP^{C} and the PrP^{Sc} precursor, which may be indistinguishable. Rectangular boxes denote as yet unidentified subcellular compartments. Prior to becoming protease resistant, the PrP^{Sc} precursor transits through the plasma membrane and is sensitive to dispase or PIPLC added to the medium. PrP^{Sc} synthesis probably occurs in a compartment accessible from the plasma membrane, such as caveolae or endosomes; PrP^{Sc} formation is blocked at 18°C. PrP^{Sc} synthesis probably occurs through the interaction of PrP^{Sc} precursor with existing PrP^{Sc}; the dotted lines denote possible feedback pathways for the reflection of PrP^{Sc} in the active site. Acidic pH within vesicles is not obligatory for PrP^{Sc} synthesis. One to 2 h after PrP^{Sc} formation, it is N-terminally trimmed by an acidic protease; PrP^{Sc} then accumulates primarily in secondary lysosomes. The inhibition of PrP^{Sc} synthesis by brefeldin A demonstrates that the endoplasmic reticulum (ER)-Golgi is not competent for its synthesis and that transport of PrP down the secretory pathway is required for the formation of PrP^{Sc}. Reprinted from Ref. 93.

trafficking of these molecules, are sialylated (Fig. 4).[90] It is unknown whether sialylation of the GPI anchor participates in some aspect of PrP^{Sc} formation.

Brefeldin A inhibits PrP^{Sc} synthesis

Studies with brefeldin A (BFA) indicate that PrP^{Sc} synthesis does not occur in the ER-Golgi and that transport down the secretory pathway is required for this synthesis.[93] Experiments with monensin demonstrate that PrP^{Sc} precursor transverses the *mid*-Golgi in the same time frame as PrP^C. These PrP molecules continue along the secretory pathway to the cell surface where they are bound by a glycosylinositol phospholipid anchor.[82,83] A minority of these PrP molecules are then converted to PrP^{Sc}, presumably either in the endocytic pathway or on the plasma membrane. Brefeldin A is the first compound found to inhibit the synthesis of PrP^{Sc}.

Digestions with phosphatidylinositol-specific phospholipase C (PIPLC) and dispase inhibit PrP^{Sc} synthesis

Those PrP molecules that are destined to become PrP^{Sc} appear transiently on the cell surface and can be released with PIPLC[82, 83] or hydrolyzed by dispase.[83] The synthesis of PrP^{Sc} was dramatically reduced when nascent PrP^C was digested with PIPLC at 18°C, but digestion of nascent PrP^{Sc} with PIPLC at 37°C did not reproducibly diminish the synthesis of PrP^{Sc} by more than a factor of 2. Digestion of nascent PrP^C with dispase significantly reduced the synthesis of PrP^{Sc}, and this phenomenon could be partially prevented by delaying the exposure of cells to dispase. While trypsin digestion (2 mg/ml for 20 min at 37°C) of nascent PrP^C did on occasion cause a large decrease in PrP^{Sc} synthesis as reported by others,[82] these conditions were so harsh that we could not determine if the reduction in PrP^{Sc} synthesis was due to digestion of cell surface protein or to nonspecific effects of the treatment, such as the dislodging and reattachment of the cells.[83] Dispase proved to be a more gentle protease that did not dislodge cells from culture vessels.

Is PrP^{Sc} derived from a specific precursor pool?

Whether PrP^{Sc} is synthesized from a subset of PrP molecules or all PrP^C molecules are eligible for conversion remains to be established. Less than 10% of the radiolabeled nascent PrP molecules that have been synthesized by the end of a 1 h metabolic radiolabeling pulse are converted into PrP^{Sc}.[83] At present, we and other have not been able to identify any differences between those PrP molecules which are destined to become PrP^{Sc} and the pool of PrP^C molecules.[80,82,83] Both the PrP^{Sc} precursor molecules and PrP^C can be released from the surface of cells by PIPLC digestion or hydrolyzed by dispase. Furthermore, both PrP^C and those PrP molecules destined to become PrP^{Sc} appears to be susceptible to cellular degradation.

Synthesis of PrPSc from unglycosylated PrP

Although most of the difference in the mass of PrP 27–30 predicted from the amino acid sequence and that observed after post-translational modification is due to complex-type oligosaccharides, these sugar chains are not required for PrPSc synthesis in scrapie-infected cultured cells based on experiments with the Asn-linked glycosylation inhibitor tunicamycin and site-directed mutagenesis studies.[64] ScN2a cells produce 3 species of PrPSc that differ in their degree of N-linked glycosylation.[64] Since the formation of any particular PrPSc glycoform could not be uncoupled from another, all 3 species of PrPSc seem to traverse the same biosynthetic pathway. Studies with cultured cells showed that unglycosylated PrP produced in the presence of tunicamycin was converted to unglycosylated PrPSc,[64] but unglycosylated PrPC is not readily detected at the cell surface.[81] Recombinant PrP molecules lacking consensus sites for N-linked glycosylation were not detected on the cell surface,[88] but could be converted to unglycosylated PrPSc in ScN2a cells.[64] Although these results suggest that unglycosylated PrP need not transit to the cell surface before conversion into PrPSc, we could not eliminate the possibility that a small fraction of PrP was transported to the cell surface in these experiments and was converted to PrPSc upon re-entry into the cell. Alternatively, in the presence of tunicamycin, PrP may be transported directly from the endoplasmic reticulum or Golgi to the endocytic pathway where it may be converted to PrPSc prior to entering the lysosomes.[64,96]

Where does PrP acquire protease resistance?

Since infectious prions are composed largely, if not entirely, of PrPSc molecules,[1,4] it is important to identify the site of PrPSc synthesis and define the molecular events involved in this process. Our observations argue that PrPSc synthesis occurs within the endocytic pathway.[83] Exogenous prions could initiate infection by entry through the endocytic pathway to stimulate the conversion of PrPC molecules from cell surface to PrPSc.

Multiple lines of evidence suggest that PrP may acquire protease resistance in the endocytic pathway. First, when ScN2a cells were exposed to dispase immediately after the labeling pulse, no PrPSc was formed during the chase at 37°C (Fig. 4).[83] In contrast, when ScN2a cells were chased for 2 h at 37°C prior to dispase exposure, some PrP became inaccessible to the dispase in the media and subsequently acquired resistance to proteinase K. Second, when ScN2a cells were chased at 18°C but not at 37°C, PrP was released by PIPLC digestion and PrPSc synthesis was abolished.[83] In our studies, PIPLC catalyzed the release of PrPC from the cell surface relatively slowly; thus, we found that long digestions with PIPLC at 18°C were required to remove those molecules destined to become PrP^{Sc}.[83] At 37°C, radiolabeled PrP molecules probably transit to the surface and are endocytosed too rapidly for PIPLC digestion to be completely effective. As noted above, our results with both PIPLC and trypsin differ from those reported by others[82] and the basis for these discrepancies is unknown. Third, the formation of PrP^{Sc} in ScN$_2$a cells was inhibited when the chase was performed at 18°C, and PrP remained largely accessible to PIPLC throughout a long 18°C chase.[83] As predicted from the work of other investigators, endocytosis and vesicular compartmentalization of membrane glycoproteins was retarded at 18°C in ScN$_2$a cells. Fourth, if ScN$_2$a cells were held at 37°C for 1–2 h of chase prior to shifting to 18°C, then some PrP^{Sc} was formed at 18°C.[83] Presumably, some PrP was endocytosed at 37°C and acquired protease resistance via a process that is less temperature dependent.

Inhibition of PrP^{Sc} synthesis at 18°C

Many investigators have observed that the endosomal transport of membrane glycoproteins to lysosomes is inhibited at 18°C.[97–104] ScN$_2$a cells were found to behave in similar manner by demonstrating that endocytosis of FITC-WGA occurred at 18°C but the formation of well-defined cytoplasmic vesicles was greatly inhibited as compared to 37°C.[83] Thus, it seems likely that exposure to 18°C inhibited endosome function in ScN$_2$a cells as reported for other types of cells and that PrP^{Sc} acquires protease resistance in the endocytic pathway.

Numerous studies have shown that most membrane glycoproteins are transported to lysosomes via endosomes, which act as receptacles for plasma membrane proteins that are destined for degradation or recycling.[96,101,105,106] After endosomes have received membrane glycoproteins from endocytic vesicles they appear to mature as they change from 'early' to 'late' endosomes before delivery of their contents to lysosomes.[96]

Many membrane proteins are degraded after endocytosis and transit through endosomes to lysosomes.[99–101,104,107] Although PrP^{Sc} accumulates in cytoplasmic vesicles, many of which are secondary lysosomes,[108] recent studies argue that PrP^{Sc} is formed prior to entry into lysosomes. First, while lysosomotropic amines block the digestion of the N-terminal 90 amino acids of PrP^{Sc}, they do not interfere with the formation of PrP^{Sc}.[93,95] Second, lysosomotropic amines do not alter substantially the degradation of PrP^C suggesting that it might be degraded before reaching lysosomes. Third, kinetic studies indicate that PrP^{Sc} acquires protease resistance approximately 1 h before exposure to lysosomal proteases and digestion of the N-terminus.[93]

Subcellular site of PrP^{Sc} synthesis

Several caveats force our conclusions to be tentative with respect to the site at which PrP^C is converted to PrP^{Sc}. First, although it is likely that PIPLC and dispase prevent PrP^{Sc} synthesis by digestion of PrP^C at the cell surface, we cannot exclude the entry of these enzymes into cells prior to digestion of PrP^C. Second, we cannot exclude the possibility that PrP^C is converted at the cell surface into PrP^{Sc}. Perhaps, PrP enters the endocytic pathway as a result of an event that initiates PrP^{Sc} synthesis at the cell surface to produce a molecule that resists PIPLC and dispase digestion, but has not yet acquired all the properties of PrP^{Sc}. Third, multiple routes of PrP^C trafficking during conversion into PrP^{Sc} might occur[64]. Fourth, we do not know how either PrP^C or the PrP^{Sc} precursor enters the endocytic pathway. Some GPI-anchored proteins are internalized via cholesterol-rich membrane patches called caveolae.[109,110] Alternatively, PrP^C could enter the endocytic pathway via free-flow endocytosis.[111] While each of these issues requires further resolution, the current studies argue that the conversion of PrP^C into PrP^{Sc} is likely to occur in the endocytic pathway.

Identification of topogenic sequences in PrP

Cell-free translation studies have demonstrated 2 forms of PrP: a transmembrane form which spans the bilayer twice at the transmembrane (TM) and amphipathic helix domains and a secretory form.[112,113] The stop transfer effector (STE) domain controls the topogenesis of PrP. That PrP contains both a TM domain and a GPI anchor poses a topologic conundrum. It seems likely that membrane-dependent events feature in the synthesis of PrP^{Sc} especially since brefeldin A, which selectively destroys the Golgi stacks[114], prevents PrP^{Sc} synthesis in scrapie-infected cultured cells.[93] For many years, the association of scrapie infectivity with membrane fractions has been appreciated[115]; indeed, hydrophobic interactions are thought to account for many of the physical properties displayed by infectious prion particles.[116,117]

CONFORMATIONAL TRANSITIONS IN PRION SYNTHESIS

Since infectious prions are composed largely, if not entirely, of PrP^{Sc} molecules, the propagation of prions must involve the production of nascent PrP^{Sc}. Much evidence argues that the synthesis of infectious prions involves the conversion of PrP^C into PrP^{Sc} [1] and that formation of PrP^{Sc} is a post-translational process occurring in the endocytic pathway.[80,82,83]

Search for post-translational chemical modifications to determine whether the synthesis of PrP^{Sc} involves chemical modification of PrP^C,

PrPSc was enzymatically cleaved into peptide fragments and each peptide was analyzed by mass spectrometry and Edman sequencing.[118] The amino acid sequence was identical to that deduced from the translated genomic sequence and the only post-translational chemical modifications were Asn-linked oligosaccharides and a GPI anchor. Although no candidate chemical modification has been found that could distinguish PrPC from PrPSc,[118] there is considerable evidence that these isoforms may differ in their conformations.[62,108,119–121]

Synthetic PrP peptides form amyloids

By comparing the amino acid sequences of 11 mammalian and one avian prion proteins, structural analyses predicted 4 α-helical regions in PrP (J-M Gabriel, F Cohen, RA Fletterick and SB Prusiner, in preparation).[122] Peptides corresponding to these regions of the SHaPrP were synthesized and contrary to predictions, 3 of the 4 spontaneously formed amyloids as shown by electron microscopy and Congo red staining.[123] By infrared spectroscopy, these amyloid peptides were found to exhibit a secondary structure comprised largely of β-sheets. The first of the predicted α-helices is the 14-residue peptide corresponding to codons 109–122; this peptide and the overlapping 15-residue sequence 113–127 both form amyloid. The most highly amyloidogenic peptide is the sequence AGAAAAGA corresponding to PrP codons 113–120. This peptide is in a region of PrP that is conserved across all known species. Two other predicted α-helices corresponding to codons 178–191 and 202–218 form amyloids and exhibit considerable β-sheet structure when synthesized as peptides.

These findings with synthetic PrP peptides suggested the possibility that the conversion of PrPC to PrPSc involves the transition of one or more putative PrP α-helices into β-sheets. Infrared spectroscopy of PrP 27–30 showed a high β-sheet content[124] which decreased when PrP 27–30 was denatured and scrapie infectivity diminished concomitantly.[119] These structural investigations of synthetic PrP peptides and the correlations between PrP 27–30 secondary structure and scrapie infectivity offer a structural model for the conversion of PrPC to PrPSc as well as the replication of infectious prion particles involving a transition from β-sheets in PrP.

Mapping conformational dependent PrP domains using chimeric PrP transgenes

By combining the experimental approaches described above, it should be possible to refine significantly our knowledge of the events that feature in the synthesis of PrPSc and pathogenesis of prion diseases. The differences in amino acid sequence between MHM2 and MH2M PrP transgenes which account for the altered specificity are located within the second putative α-helix H2, and the region connecting H2 with the third α-helix, H3. However, the putative α-helix H1 is thought to be of primary importance in the conversion of PrP^C into PrP^{Sc} by adopting a β-sheet conformation in PrP^{Sc}.[119,125] Further studies, using different chimeric PrP genes with additional substitutions, may allow mapping of all the amino acid substitutions which alter prion/host specificity by influencing PrP structure.

CONCLUSION

Studies with Tg mice have contributed a wealth of new knowledge about the synthesis of prion particles and the pathogenesis of both the genetic and infectious forms of the prion diseases. Transgenetic studies argue persuasively that the 'species barrier' is due to differences in PrP gene sequences among mammals. Furthermore during the propagation of prions, PrP^C and PrP^{Sc} form a complex as PrP^C molecules are converted into PrP^{Sc}. This complex or replication intermediate involves a homophilic interaction between the substrate PrP^C and the pathogenic PrP^{Sc} molecule. Physical and chemical analyses of PrP^{Sc} contend that the conversion of PrP^C into PrP^{Sc} involves a conformational change. Spectroscopic and electron microscopic studies suggest that the post-translational synthesis of PrP^{Sc} involves an increase in β-sheet content.

Transgenetic studies have established that the PrP gene can drastically modify the length of the scrapie incubation time. Investigations with Tg mice have also demonstrated that the pattern of PrP^{Sc} accumulation as well as the distribution of neuropathologic lesions are dependent upon the PrP^{Sc} molecules which are synthesized. Both neuronal vacuolation and astrocytic gliosis appear to be a consequence of PrP^{Sc} deposition. Furthermore, PrP amyloid plaques are dependent on the PrP sequence as well as the 'strain' of prion which initiates the infection.

The foregoing studies on the synthesis and distribution of PrP^{Sc} have given new insights into the replication of scrapie prion 'strains' or isolates. Each isolate appears to induce a unique pattern of PrP^{Sc} deposition which suggests that each isolate may replicate in a distinct set of cells. The molecular basis of this cellular trophism remains to be established but has been suggested that it may reside either in the N-linked oligosaccharides of PrP^{Sc} or the tertiary structure of PrP^{Sc}.

The modeling of GSS in Tg(GSSMoPrP-P101L) mice argues that PrP gene mutations in humans cause prion diseases. These results are in accord with studies showing that nucleotide changes which result in non-conservative amino acid substitutions are genetically linked to the development of an inherited prion disease. These findings also offer an explanation for the sporadic prion diseases such as CJD: a somatic mutation of the PRNP gene rather than exogenous infection may initiate the formation of PrP^{Sc}.

All of these studies taken together offer a compelling view that prions are composed largely, if not entirely of PrP^{Sc} molecules. In addition, prion diseases seem to be diseases of protein conformation and arise through either infectious or genetic mechanisms.

ACKNOWLEDGEMENTS

I thank M. Baldwin, D. Borchelt, G. Carlson, F. Cohen, C. Cooper, S. DeArmond, R. Fletterick, D. Foster, J-M. Gabriel, M. Gasset, R. Gabizon, D. Groth, L. Hood, K. Hsiao, V. Lingappa, M. McKinley, W. Mobley, B. Oesch, D. Riesner, M. Scott, A. Serban, N. Stahl,A. Taraboulos, M. Torchia, C. Weissmann, and D. Westaway for their help in these studies. Special thanks to Lorraine Gallagher who assembled this manuscript. Supported by grants from the National Institutes of Health (NS14069, AG08967, AG02132 and NS22786) and the American Health Assistance Foundation, as well as by gifts from Sherman Fairchild Foundation, Bernard Osher Foundation and National Medical Enterprises.

REFERENCES

 1 Prusiner SB. Molecular biology of prion diseases. Science 1991; 252: 1515–1522.
 2 Büeler H, Fischer M, Lang Y, et al. The neuronal cell surface protein PrP is not essential for normal development and behavior of the mouse. Nature 1992; 356: 577–582.
 3 Scott M, Foster D, Mirenda C et al. Transgenic mice expressing hamster prion protein produce species-specific scrapie infectivity and amyloid plaques. Cell 1989; 59: 847–857.
 4 Prusiner SB, Scott M, Foster D, et al. Transgenetic studies implicate interactions between homologous PrP isoforms in scrapie prion replication. Cell 1990; 63: 673–686.
 5 Pattison IH. Experiments with scrapie with special reference to the nature of the agent and the pathology of the disease. In: Gajdusek DC, Gibbs CJ Jr, Alpers MP, eds. Slow, Latent and Temperate Virus Infections, NINDB Monograph 2. Washington DC: US Government Printing, 1965: 249–257.
 6 Bockman JM, Prusiner SB, Tateishi J, Kingsbury DT. Immunoblotting of Creutzfeldt-Jakob disease prion proteins: host species-specific epitopes. Ann Neurol 1987; 21: 589–595.
 7 Pattison IH, Jones KM. Modification of a strain of mouse–adapted scrapie by passage through rats. Res Vet Sci 1968; 9: 408–410.
 8 Oesch B, Westaway D, Wälchli M, et al. A cellular gene encodes scrapie PrP 27–30 protein. Cell 1985; 40: 735–746.
 9 Kimberlin R, Walker C. Characteristics of a short incubation model of scrapie in the golden hamster. J Gen Virol 1977; 34: 295–304.
10 Kimberlin RH, Walker CA. Pathogenesis of mouse scrapie: effect of route of inoculation on infectivity titres and dose–response curves. J Comp Pathol 1978; 88: 39–47.
11 Prusiner SB. Prions and neurodegenerative diseases. N Engl J Med 1987; 317: 1571–1581.
12 McKinley MP, Bolton DC, Prusiner SB. A protease-resistant protein is a structural component of the scrapie prion. Cell 1983; 35: 57–62.
13 Barry RA, Prusiner SB. Monoclonal antibodies to the cellular and scrapie prion proteins. J Infect Dis 1986; 154: 518–521.

14 DeArmond SJ, Mobley WC, DeMott DL, Barry RA, Beckstead JH, Prusiner SB. Changes in the localization of brain prion proteins during scrapie infection. Neurology 1987; 37: 1271–1280.

15 Carlson GA, Kingsbury DT, Goodman PA, et al. Linkage of prion protein and scrapie incubation time genes. Cell 1986; 46: 503–511.

16 Hunter N, Hope J, McConnell I, Dickinson AG. Linkage of the scrapie-associated fibril protein (PrP) gene and Sinc using congenic mice and restriction fragment length polymorphism analysis. J Gen Virol 1987; 68: 2711–2716.

17 Race RE, Graham K, Ernst D, Caughey B, Chesebro B. Analysis of linkage between scrapie incubation period and the prion protein gene in mice. J Gen Virol 1990; 71: 493–497.

18 Dickinson AG, Meikle VMH, Fraser H. Identification of a gene which controls the incubation period of some strains of scrapie agent in mice. J Comp Pathol 1968; 78: 293–299.

19 Westaway D, Goodman PA, Mirenda CA, McKinley MP, Carlson GA, Prusiner SB. Distinct prion proteins in short and long scrapie incubation period mice. Cell 1987; 51: 651–662.

20 Westaway D, Mirenda CA, Foster D, et al. Paradoxical shortening of scrapie incubation times by expression of prion protein transgenes derived from long incubation period mice. Neuron 1991; 7: 59–68.

21 Frohman MA, Dush MK, Martin GR. Rapid production of full-length cDNAs from rare transcripts: amplification using a single gene-specific oligonucleotide primer. Proc Natl Acad Sci USA 1988; 85: 8998–9002.

22 Loh EY, Elliott JF, Cwirla S, Lanier LL, Davis MM. Polymerase chain reaction with single–sided specificity: analysis of T cell receptor δ chain. Science 1989; 243: 217–220.

23 Basler K, Oesch B, Scott M, et al. Scrapie and cellular PrP isoforms are encoded by the same chromosomal gene. Cell 1986; 46: 417–428.

24 Carlson GA, Westaway D, DeArmond SJ, Peterson-Torchia M, Prusiner SB. Primary structure of prion protein may modify scrapie isolate properties. Proc Natl Acad Sci USA 1989; 86: 7475–7479.

25 Hsiao K, Baker HF, Crow TJ, et al. Linkage of a prion protein missense variant to Gerstmann-Sträussler syndrome. Nature 1989; 338: 342–345.

26 Hsiao KK, Westaway DA, Prusiner SB. An amino acid substitution in the prion protein of ataxic Gerstmann-Sträussler syndrome. Am J Hum Genet 1988; 43: A87.

27 Doh–ura K, Tateishi J, Sasaki H, Kitamoto T, Sakaki Y. Pro->Leu change at position 102 of prion protein is the most common but not the sole mutation related to Gerstmann-Sträussler syndrome. Biochem Biophys Res Commun 1989; 163: 974–979.

28 Owen F, Poulter M, Lofthouse R, et al. Insertion in prion protein gene in familial Creutzfeldt-Jakob disease. Lancet 1989; 1: 51–52.

29 Collinge J, Harding AE, Owen F, et al. Diagnosis of Gerstmann-Sträussler syndrome in familial dementia with prion protein gene analysis. Lancet 1989; 2: 15–17.

30 Goldgaber D, Goldfarb LG, Brown P, et al. Mutations in familial Creutzfeldt-Jakob disease and Gerstmann-Sträussler-Scheinker's syndrome. Exp Neurol 1989; 106: 204–206.

31 Goldfarb LG, Mitrova E, Brown P, Toh BH, Gajdusek DC. Mutation in codon 200 of scrapie amyloid protein gene in two clusters of Creutzfeldt-Jakob disease in Slovakia. Lancet 1990; 336: 514–515.

32 Goldfarb L, Korczyn A, Brown P, Chapman J, Gajdusek DC. Mutation in codon 200 of scrapie amyloid precursor gene linked to Creutzfeldt-Jakob disease in Sephardic Jews of Libyan and non–Libyan origin. Lancet 1990; 336: 637–638.

33 Hsiao KK, Cass C, Schellenberg GD, et al. A prion protein variant in a family with the telencephalic form of Gerstmann-Sträussler-Scheinker syndrome. Neurology 1991; 41: 681–684.

34 Gabizon R, Meiner Z, Cass C, et al. Prion protein gene mutation in Libyan Jews with Creutzfeldt-Jakob disease. Neurology 1991; 41: 160 (Abstr).

35 Ripoll L, Laplanche J-L, Salzmann M, et al. A new point mutation in the prion protein gene at codon 210 in Creutzfeldt-Jakob disease. Neurology 1993; (in press).

36 Medori R, Tritschler H-J, LeBlanc A, et al. Fatal familial insomnia, a prion disease with a mutation at codon 178 of the prion protein gene. N Engl J Med 1992; 326: 444–449.

37 Goldfarb LG, Petersen RB, Tabaton M, et al. Fatal familial insomnia and familial Creutzfeldt-Jakob disease: disease phenotype determined by a DNA polymorphism. Science 1992; 258: 806–808.

38 Hsiao KK, Doh-ura K, Kitamoto T, Tateishi J, Prusiner SB. A prion protein amino acid substitution in ataxic Gerstmann-Sträussler syndrome. Ann Neurol 1989; 26: 137.

39 Kretzschmar HA, Kufer P, Riethmuller G, DeArmond SJ, Prusiner SB, Schiffer D. Prion protein mutation at codon 102 in an Italian family with Gerstmann-Sträussler-Scheinker syndrome. Neurology 1991; 42: 809–810.

40 Hsiao K, Prusiner SB. Inherited human prion diseases. Neurology 1990; 40: 1820–1827.

41 Brown P. The phenotypic expression of different mutations in transmissible human spongiform encephalopathy. Rev Neurol 1992; 148: 317–327.

42 Serban D, Taraboulos A, DeArmond SJ, Prusiner SB. Rapid detection of Creutzfeldt-Jakob disease and scrapie prion proteins. Neurology 1990; 40: 110–117.

43 Gerstmann J, Sträussler E, Scheinker I. Über eine eigenartige hereditär-familiäre erkrankung des zentralnervensystems zugleich ein beitrag zur frage des vorzeitigen lokalen alterns. Z Neurol 1936; 154: 736–762.

44 Masters CL, Gajdusek DC, Gibbs CJ Jr. Creutzfeldt-Jakob disease virus isolations from the Gerstmann-Sträussler syndrome. Brain 1981; 104: 559–588.

45 Ghetti B, Tagliavini F, Masters CL, et al. Gerstmann-Sträussler-Scheinker disease. II. Neurofibrillary tangles and plaques with PrP-amyloid coexist in an affected family. Neurology 1989; 39: 1453–1461.

46 Bruce ME, Dickinson AG, Fraser H. Cerebral amyloidosis in scrapie in the mouse: effect of agent strain and mouse genotype. Neuropathol Appl Neurobiol 1976; 2: 471–478.

47 Bruce ME, Fraser H. Amyloid plaques in the brains of mice infected with scrapie: morphological variation and staining properties. Neuropathol Appl Neurol 1975; 1: 189–202.

48 Fraser H, Bruce ME. Argyrophilic plaques in mice inoculated with scrapie from particular sources. Lancet 1973; 1: 617.

49 Hsiao KK, Scott M, Foster D, Groth DF, DeArmond SJ, Prusiner SB. Spontaneous neurodegeneration in transgenic mice with mutant prion protein of Gerstmann-Sträussler syndrome. Science 1990; 250: 1587–1590.

50 Tateishi J, Ohta M, Koga M, Sato Y, Kuroiwa Y. Transmission of chronic spongiform encephalopathy with kuru plaques from humans to small rodents. Ann Neurol 1979; 5: 581–584.

51 Dickinson AG, Meikle VM. A comparison of some biological characteristics of the mouse-passaged scrapie agents, 22A and ME7. Genet Res 1969; 13: 213–225.

52 Carlson GA, Goodman PA, Lovett M, et al. Genetics and polymorphism of the mouse prion gene complex: the control of scrapie incubation time. Mol Cell Biol 1988; 8: 5528–5540.

53 Baker HF, Ridley RM, Crow TJ. Experimental transmission of an autosomal dominant spongiform encephalopathy: Does the infectious agent originate in the human genome? Br Med J 1985; 291: 299–302.

54 Brinster RL, Allen JM, Behringer RR, Gelinas RE, Palmiter RD. Introns increase transcriptional efficiency in transgenic mice. Proc Natl Acad Sci USA 1988; 85: 836–840.

55 Ridley RM, Frith CD, Crow TJ, Conneally PM. Anticipation in Huntington's disease is inherited through the male line but may originate in the female. J Med Genet 1988; 25: 589–595.

56 Haldane JBS. The relative importance of principal and modifying genes in determining some human diseases. J Genet 1941; 41: 149–157.

57 Laird CD. Proposed genetic basis of Huntington's disease. Trends Genet 1990; 6: 242–247.
58 Allen ND, Norris ML, Surani MA. Epigenetic control of transgene expression and imprinting by genotype-specific modifiers. Cell 1990; 61: 853–861.
59 Weissmann C. Prions: sheep disease in human clothing. Nature 1989; 338: 298–299.
60 Kimberlin RH. Scrapie and possible relationships with viroids. Semin Virol 1990; 1: 153–162.
61 Prusiner SB. Scrapie prions. Annu Rev Microbiol 1989; 43: 345–374.
62 Prusiner SB. Chemistry and biology of prions. Biochemistry 1992; 31: 12278–12288.
63 Scott MR, Köhler R, Foster D, Prusiner SB. Chimeric prion protein expression in cultured cells and transgenic mice. Protein Sci 1992; 1: 986–997.
64 Taraboulos A, Rogers M, Borchelt DR, et al. Acquisition of protease resistance by prion proteins in scrapie-infected cells does not require asparagine-linked glycosylation. Proc Natl Acad Sci USA 1990; 87: 8262–8266.
65 Rogers M, Serban D, Gyuris T, Scott M, Torchia T, Prusiner SB. Epitope mapping of the Syrian hamster prion protein utilizing chimeric and mutant genes in a vaccinia virus expression system. J Immunol 1991; 147: 3568–3574.
66 Kascsak RJ, Rubenstein R, Merz PA, et al. Mouse polyclonal and monoclonal antibody to scrapie-associated fibril proteins. J Virol 1987; 61: 3688–3693.
67 Scott M, Groth D, Foster D, Torchia M, et al. Propagation of prions with artificial properties in transgenic mice expressing chimeric PrP genes. Cell 1993; (submitted).
68 Prusiner SB, Baldwin M, Collinge J, et al. Classification and nomenclature of viruses: Prions. Arch Virol 1993; (in press).
69 Lowenstein DH, Butler DA, Westaway D, McKinley MP, DeArmond SJ, Prusiner SB. Three hamster species with different scrapie incubation times and neuropathological features encode distinct prion proteins. Mol Cell Biol 1990; 10: 1153–1163.
70 Hecker R, Taraboulos A, Scott M, et al. Replication of distinct prion isolates is region specific in brains of transgenic mice and hamsters. Genes Dev 1992; 6: 1213–1228.
71 Taraboulos A, Jendroska K, Serban D, Yang S-L, DeArmond SJ, Prusiner SB. Regional mapping of prion proteins in brains. Proc Natl Acad Sci USA 1992; 89: 7620–7624.
72 Kimberlin RH, Walker CA, Fraser H. The genomic identity of different strains of mouse scrapie is expressed in hamsters and preserved on reisolation in mice. J Gen Virol 1989; 70: 2017–2025.
73 Dickinson AG, Fraser H. An assessment of the genetics of scrapie in sheep and mice. In: Prusiner SB, Hadlow WJ, eds. Slow Transmissible Diseases of the Nervous System, Vol. 1. New York: Academic Press, 1979: 367–386 .
74 Bruce ME, Dickinson AG. Biological evidence that the scrapie agent has an independent genome. J Gen Virol 1987; 68: 79–89.
75 Kimberlin RH, Cole S, Walker CA. Temporary and permanent modifications to a single strain of mouse scrapie on transmission to rats and hamsters. J Gen Virol 1987; 68: 1875–1881.
76 Dickinson AG, Outram GW. Genetic aspects of unconventional virus infections: the basis of the virino hypothesis. In: Bock G, Marsh J, eds. Novel Infectious Agents and the Central Nervous System. Ciba Foundation Symposium 135. Chichester, UK: John Wiley and Sons, 1988: 63–83.
77 Weissmann C. A 'unified theory' of prion propagation. Nature 1991; 352: 679–683.
78 McMahon AP, Bradley A. The Wnt–1 (int–1) proto-oncogene is required for development of a large region of the mouse brain. Cell 1990; 62: 1073–1085.
79 Büeler H, Aguzzi A, Sailer A, et al. Mice devoid of PrP are resistant to scrapie. Cell 1993; (submitted).
80 Borchelt DR, Scott M, Taraboulos A, Stahl N, Prusiner SB. Scrapie and cellular prion proteins differ in their kinetics of synthesis and topology in cultured cells. J Cell Biol 1990; 110: 743–752.
81 Caughey B, Race RE, Ernst D, Buchmeier MJ, Chesebro B. Prion protein biosynthesis in scrapie–infected and uninfected neuroblastoma cells. J Virol 1989; 63: 175–181.

82 Caughey B, Raymond GJ. The scrapie-associated form of PrP is made from a cell surface precursor that is both protease- and phospholipase-sensitive. J Biol Chem 1991; 266: 18217–18223.
83 Borchelt DR, Taraboulos A, Prusiner SB. Evidence for synthesis of scrapie prion proteins in the endocytic pathway. J Biol Chem 1992; 267: 6188–6199.
84 Bolton DC, Meyer RK, Prusiner SB. Scrapie PrP 27-30 is a sialoglycoprotein. J Virol 1985; 53: 596–606.
85 Manuelidis L, Valley S, Manuelidis EE. Specific proteins associated with Creutzfeldt-Jakob disease and scrapie share antigenic and carbohydrate determinants. Proc Natl Acad Sci USA 1985; 82: 4263–4267.
86 Haraguchi T, Fisher S, Olofsson S, et al. Asparagine-linked glycosylation of the scrapie and cellular prion proteins. Arch Biochem Biophys 1989; 274: 1–13.
87 Endo T, Groth D, Prusiner SB, Kobata A. Diversity of oligosaccharide structures linked to asparagines of the scrapie prion protein. Biochemistry 1989; 28: 8380–8388.
88 Rogers M, Taraboulos A, Scott M, Groth D, Prusiner SB. Intracellular accumulation of the cellular prion protein after mutagenesis of its Asn-linked glycosylation sites. Glycobiology 1990; 1: 101–109.
89 Stahl N, Borchelt DR, Hsiao K, Prusiner SB. Scrapie prion protein contains a phosphatidylinositol glycolipid. Cell 1987; 51: 229–240.
90 Stahl N, Baldwin MA, Hecker R, Pan K–M, Burlingame AL, Prusiner SB. Glycosylinositol phospholipid anchors of the scrapie and cellular prion proteins contain sialic acid.
Biochemistry 1992; 31: 5043–5053.
91 Safar J, Ceroni M, Piccardo P, et al. Subcellular distribution and physicochemical properties of scrapie associated precursor protein and relationship with scrapie agent. Neurology 1990; 40: 503–508.
92 Taraboulos A, Serban D, Prusiner SB. Scrapie prion proteins accumulate in the cytoplasm of persistently-infected cultured cells. J Cell Biol 1990; 110: 2117–2132.
93 Taraboulos A, Raeber AJ, Borchelt DR, Serban D, Prusiner SB. Synthesis and trafficking of prion proteins in cultured cells. Mol Biol Cell 1992; 3: 851–863.
94 McKinley MP, Taraboulos A, Kenaga L, et al. Ultrastructural localization of scrapie prion proteins in cytoplasmic vesicles of infected cultured cells. Lab Invest 1991; 65: 622–630.
95 Caughey B, Raymond GJ, Ernst D, Race RE. N-terminal truncation of the scrapie-associated form of PrP by lysosomal protease(s): implications regarding the site of conversion of PrP to the protease-resistant state. J Virol 1991; 65: 6597–6603.
96 Stoorvogel W, Strous GJ, Geuze HJ, Oorschot V, Schwartz AL. Late endosomes derive from early endosomes by maturation. Cell 1991; 65: 417–427.
97 Griffiths G, Hoflack B, Simons K, Mellman I, Kornfeld S. The mannose 6-phosphate receptor and the biogenesis of lysosomes. Cell 1988; 52: 329–341.
98 Salzman NH, Maxfield FR. Fusion accessibility of endocytic compartments along the recycling and lysosomal endocytic pathways in intact cells. J Cell Biol 1989; 109: 2097–2104.
99 Hare JF, Huston M. Degradation of surface-labeled hepatoma membrane polypeptides: Effect of inhibitors. Arch Biochem Biophys 1984; 233: 547–555.
100 Hare JF. Dissection of membrane protein degradation mechanisms by reversible inhibitors. J Biol Chem 1988; 263: 8759–8764.
101 Dunn WA, Hubbard AL, Aronson NN Jr. Low temperature selectively inhibits fusion between pinocytic vesicles and lysosomes during heterophagy of ^{125}I-asialofetuin by the perfused rat liver. J Biol Chem 1980; 255: 5971–5978.
102 Weigel PH, Oka JA. Temperature dependence of endocytosis mediated by the asialoglycoprotein receptor in isolated rat hepatocytes. J Biol Chem 1981; 256: 2615–2617 103 Marsh M, Bolzau E, Helenius A. Penetration of Semliki Forest virus from acidic prelysosomal vacuoles. Cell 1983; 32: 931–940.
104 Wolkoff AW, Klausner RD, Ashwell G, Harford J. Intracellular segregation of asialoglycoproteins and their receptor: A prelysosomal event subsequent to dissociation of the ligand-receptor complex. J Cell Biol 1984; 98: 375–381.

105 Marsh M, Helenius A. Adsorptive endocytosis of Semliki Forest virus. J Mol Biol 1980; 142: 439–454.
106 Willingham MC, Pastan I. The receptosome: an intermediate organelle of receptor-mediated endocytosis in cultured fibroblasts. Cell 1980; 21: 67–77.
107 Steinman RM, Mellman IS, Muller WA, Cohn ZA. Endocytosis and the recycling of plasma membrane. J Cell Biol 1983; 96: 1–27.
108 McKinley MP, Meyer R, Kenaga L, et al. Scrapie prion rod formation in vitro requires both detergent extraction and limited proteolysis. J Virol 1991; 65: 1440–1449.
109 Rothberg KG, Ying Y, Kolhouse JF, Kamen BA, Anderson RGW. The glycophospholipid linked folate receptor internalizes folate without entering the clathrin coated pit endocytic pathway. J Cell Biol 1990; 110: 637–649.
110 Anderson RGW, Kamen BA, Rothberg KG, Lacey SW. Potocytosis: sequestration and transport of small molecules by caveolae. Science 1991; 255: 410–411.
111 Tooze J, Hollinshead M. Tubular early endosomal networks in AtT20 and other cells. J Cell Biol 1991; 115: 635–653.
112 Yost CS, Lopez CD, Prusiner SB, Meyers RM, Lingappa VR. A non-hydrophobic extracytoplasmic determinant of stop transfer in the prion protein. Nature 1990; 343: 669–672.
113 Lopez CD, Yost CS, Prusiner SB, Myers RM, Lingappa VR. Unusual topogenic sequence directs prion protein biogenesis. Science 1990; 248: 226–229.
114 Doms RW, Russ G, Yewdell JW. Brefeldin A redistributes resident and itinerant Golgi proteins to the endoplasmic reticulum. J Cell Biol 1989; 109: 61–72.
115 Gibbons RA, Hunter GD. Nature of the scrapie agent. Nature 1967; 215: 1041–1043.
116 Prusiner SB, Groth DF, Cochran SP, Masiarz FR, McKinley MP, Martinez HM. Molecular properties, partial purification, and assay by incubation period measurements of the hamster scrapie agent. Biochemistry 1980; 19: 4883–4891.
117 Gabizon R, Prusiner SB. Prion liposomes. Biochem J 1990; 266: 1–14.
118 Stahl N, Baldwin MA, Teplow DB, et al. Structural analysis of the scrapie prion protein using mass spectrometry and amino acid sequencing. Biochemistry 1993; (in press).
119 Gasset M, Baldwin MA, Fletterick RJ, Prusiner SB. Perturbation of the secondary structure of the scrapie prion protein under conditions associated with changes in infectivity. Proc Natl Acad Sci USA 1993; 90: 1–5.
120 Prusiner SB, McKinley MP, Bowman KA, et al. Scrapie prions aggregate to form amyloid-like birefringent rods. Cell 1983; 35: 349–358.
121 Meyer RK, McKinley MP, Bowman KA, Braunfeld MB, Barry RA, Prusiner SB. Separation and properties of cellular and scrapie prion proteins. Proc Natl Acad Sci USA 1986; 83: 2310–2314.
122 Cohen FE, Abarbanel RM, Kuntz ID, Fletterick RJ. Turn prediction in proteins using a pattern–matching approach. Biochemistry 1986; 25: 266–275.
123 Gasset M, Baldwin MA, Lloyd D, et al. Predicted α-helical regions of the prion protein when synthesized as peptides form amyloid. Proc Natl Acad Sci USA 1992; 89: 10940–10944.
124 Caughey BW, Dong A, Bhat KS, Ernst D, Hayes SF, Caughey WS. Secondary structure analysis of the scrapie-associated protein PrP 27–30 in water by infrared spectroscopy. Biochemistry 1991; 30: 7672–7680.
125 Gasset M, Baldwin M, Nguyen J, et al. Reversible conformational changes in the scrapie prion protein induced by transition metals and chemical modification. J Mol Biol 1993; (submitted).

British Medical Bulletin (1993) Vol 49. No. 4, pp. 913–931

Genetic control of nucleation and polymerization of host precursors to infectious amyloids in the transmissible amyloidoses of brain

D C Gajdusek
Laboratory of Central Nervous System Studies, National Institute of Neurological Disorders and Stroke, National Institutes of Health, Bethesda, Maryland, USA

In recent years we have become aware that the unconventional or atypical slow virus diseases of kuru-Creutzfeldt-Jakob syndrome (CJD), Gerstmann Sträussler syndrome (GSS) and scrapie-bovine spongiform encephalopathy (BSE) are cerebral amyloidoses.[1-10] As with most amyloidoses, the spontaneous *de novo* generation of amyloid fibrils is under genetic control, although in many susceptible hosts all individuals are susceptible to even a minimal intracerebral infective dose; thus, for such inoculation there is no genetic control other than the species barrier.

Transmissible and infectious amyloidoses of brain, as with all amyloidoses, require three stages of fibrillar polymerization of the amyloid subunit into insoluble, semi-solid arrays or microfibrils which coalesce or agglutinate (aggregate) into structures of diverse morphology: SAFs and kuru plaques. The first is preliminary processing of the precursor into the amyloid subunit or monomer (C-terminal truncation, removal of the N-terminal signal peptide, and release from the inositol-stearic acid membrane anchor); the second is nucleation-induced configurational change in the subunit into a cross β-pleated configuration; and the third is the formation of oligomers or polymers – usually dimers, tetramers, octamers or hexadecamers – which may polymerize to produce electron microscopically visible fibrils (SAFs) and coalesce into kuru plaques.

All β-pleated proteins can also form vitreous-like solid arrays displaying extensive periodicity but which are not true three-dimensional crystals. They are, rather, semisolid, amorphous, vitreous or mucilaginous pseudocrystals, thick emulsions, or gels which are insoluble precipitates in the hydrophilic media of the milieu interieur. On heating, drying, or aging these may increase their hydrogen bonding and decrease their hydration to assume increasingly a β-pleated structure, even in the case of some proteins with α-helical structure.[11] This is the heart of amyloidology and the basis of much of the biochemical alteration of proteins of cuisine and of aging of leather, parchment, rubber, natural fabrics, and even cartilage and the lens of the eye.

GENETIC CONTROL OF GENERATION OF INFECTIOUS AMYLOIDS IN CREUTZFELDT-JAKOB DISEASE SYNDROMES

Eight point mutations, each changing an amino acid, have been found to cause familial CJD or its GSS and familial fatal insomnia (FFI) variants. Most GSS families display an amino acid replacement of proline by leucine at codon 102.[12–15] Two Japanese GSS families have the same proline to leucine change but at codon 105.[16] In two families with atypical GSS there is instead a replacement of alanine by valine at codon 117.[17,18] One GSS family has a codon 198 mutation replacing phenylalanine by serine;[19] and one other GSS family has a codon 217 mutation replacing glutamine by arginine.[20,21] The more common type of familial CJD has a codon 200 mutation which replaces glutamic acid with lysine.[12, 22–25] This has now been found in over 60 families with over 100 cases of CJD.[26,27] However, in a large Finnish kindred with CJD[28] there is a replacement of aspartic acid by asparagine at codon 178[29,30] and there are Dutch, French, Hungarian, British, and American CJD families also with a codon 178 point mutation: 8 families in all with 97 CJD cases[27,31–36] (Fig. 1).

There is a Japanese family with a mutation in codon 145 which changes the codon to a stop codon. This so-called amber mutation produces a disease with a clinical course resembling Alzheimer's disease.

Seven different insert mutations, which are insertions of additional copies of an octapeptide repeat in the region normally containing 5 repeating octapeptide-coding sequences between codons 51 and 90 of the precursor gene, also cause CJD in various modified clinical expressions. There are 2-fold, 4-fold, 5-fold, 6-fold, 7-fold, 8-fold, 9-fold octapeptide repeats in different families.[38–44] Two families with five repeats have been identified, all others have been found in only one family. Thus, we know seven different insertional mutations in eight families which are responsible for the alteration of the normal precursor protein into the infectious amyloid form (Fig. 1).

At codon 129 we have a nonpathogenic point mutation with substitution of valine for methionine which is a silent polymorphism in the

Infectious Amyloidoses of Brain

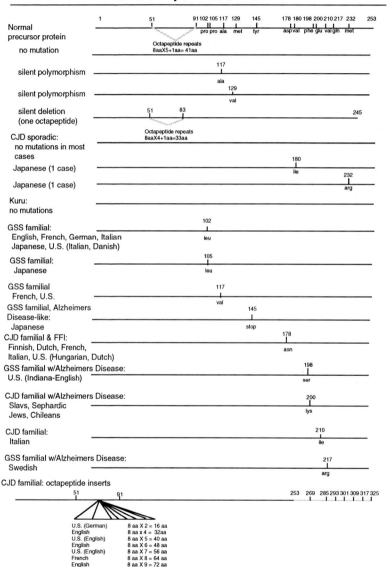

Fig. 1 21 different mutations in the gene specifying the host precursor molecule of CJD amyloid: 11 cause amino acid (aa) changes, 1 produces a stop codon, 1 a base change in the codon with no amino acid change, 7 are octapeptide inserts and 1 an octapeptide deletion. 8 causing an amino acid change (102, 105, 117, 178, 198, 200, 210, 211) and 1 a stop codon (145) are found in families of diverse ethnic origins with familial CJD and its GSS and FFI variants. 3 are silent polymorphisms: the codon 129 substitution of valine for methionine (which is found in about 20% of the normal population); a base mutation in codon 117 causing no amino acid change and an octapeptide deletion (in about 20% of the population). 7 additional mutations in families with CJD are insertions of octapeptide repeats into a region where there are already 5 copies of the same repeat. In a US family there are 2 copies of the octapeptide (8aa x 2 = 16aa) inserted, bringing the total to 7 copies; in a British family there are 4 copies of the octapeptide (8aa x 4 = 36aa) inserted, bringing the total to 9 copies; in a second US family there are 5 copies of the octapeptide (8aa x 5 = 40aa) inserted, bringing the total to 10 copies; in another British family there are 6 copies (8aa x 6 = 48aa) inserted, bringing the total to 11 copies; in a US family from England there are 7 copies (8aa x 7 = 56aa) inserted, bringing the total to 12 copies; in a French family there are 8 copies (8aa x 8 = 64aa) inserted, bringing the total to 13 copies; in another British family there are 9 copies (8aa x 9 = 72aa) inserted, bringing the total to 14 copies.

general population.[22] Another silent polymorphism is a point mutation at codon 117 of GCA to GCG which causes no amino acid change. Finally, we find some normal subjects carry four instead of five copies of the octapeptide normally at codon 41–91.[7] Two amino acid-changing point mutations have been found in sporadic cases of CJD in Japan.[16] Several other sporadic CJD cases have been fully sequenced and no mutations have been found.

Familial forms of CJD account for only about 5% of all cases. More than 90% are truly sporadic and only about 1% have been shown to be iatrogenic from direct inoculation of the patient with infected material from a CJD patient. For all other cases a chain of infection cannot be established, nor do they appear to be familial. At present the best explanation for the regular incidence of sporadic nonfamilial CJD around the world is the *de novo* creation of the CJD amyloid infectious agent by a rare, spontaneous event occurring at a frequency of one per million population per annum, the surprisingly uniform worldwide incidence of CJD.[5] If one of the point mutations of familial CJD is present this configurational change occurs with about a million-fold higher likelihood. One corollary of this paradigm is that the replication of the infectious amyloid caused by inoculations of a different species does not 'breed true'. The point mutation is not copied in the amyloid formed in the new host, although it, in turn, is also infectious. The new CJD amyloid has the amino acid sequence of the precursor protein in the newly inoculated host. CJD from patients with the 102, 117, 178, 200 and 210 codon mutations have all been transmitted to monkeys or chimpanzees which do not carry these point mutations, nor do the infectious proteins made in these experimentally infected hosts contain those point mutations. The process of conformational change may well be an induced nucleation and homotaxic pattern-setting for crystalline or fibril growth. The further elucidation of this transformation to β-pleated insoluble, protease-resistant and infectious configuration will require the full structural comparison of infectious and non-infectious forms of the molecule, using NMR, the synchrocyclotron, circular dichroism spectroscopy, infrared spectroscopy and high-resolution electron microscopy.

De novo spontaneous generation of the infectious form from the full-length CJD amyloid precursor may account for most sporadic CJD. It occurs to cause sporadic CJD as a rare stochastic event in one individual per million population base per annum (the worldwide incidence rate of CJD). In familial CJD, GSS and FFI these many point mutations (amino acid substitutions, a new stop codon or octapeptide inserts) have increased the likelihood of this spontaneous configurational change about 10^6-fold.

It appears likely that a coordinate-covalent or covalent alteration in the precursor may be induced which endows the infectious nucleant with great stability.[45,46,46a] We thus have reason to anticipate that the infectious form of the scrapie amyloid precursor may eventually be induced *in vitro*, even from synthetic polypeptides. These studies are underway, and monkeys and other animals inoculated with fibrils formed *in vitro* from synthetic peptides homologous to CJD pathogenic mutation-containing regions of the CJD amyloid precursor gene are under observation.

Autonucleation with induction of configurational change in the full-length infectious amyloid precursor protein is the basic process of scrapie replication. We have suggested that fibril amyloid-enhancing factor is a scrapie-like infectious agent,[5] operating by an analogous self-induction of configurational change, much as small fibrils of tropocollagen nucleate and pattern-set the polymerization of collagen monomers into specific fibril networks.[47]

ORAVSKE KURU

Mitrová [48] who followed the high incidence of CJD throughout Slovakia for more than two decades has identified a new focus of CJD in high incidences in several villages of Orava in the Western foothills of the High Tatra mountains near the Polish border. In 1980, she identified an unusually high incidence of CJD in the rural Lucenec area of south central Slovakia with many cases also across the border in Hungary.[49] During the past decade cases have been found in increasing frequency from the most sparsely populated rural sheep-raising area of Slovakia.[48,50] Here an epidemic of CJD has developed during the 1980s with some 30 cases occurring in patients born and reared in a dozen small villages with a total population of under 15 000. This yields an incidence over 1000 per million population per year in contrast to the worldwide incidence of 1 per million per year. The most intensely involved villages of Zuberec and Habovka with a total population of under 2000 have had over 20 cases of CJD in the past 3 years. The incidence in the villages has thus reached over 3000 times higher than in the rest of the world in such cities as Paris, London, New York, Sydney, Santiago or Shanghai, or any other large cities, and it is yet 100 times higher than that among the Sephardic Jews in Israel. Members of the same family who were 20–30 years different in age become sick at nearly the same time. This suggested a common source of infection rather than genetically determined etiology, as also did the new 'epidemic' of appearance of CJD in the 1980s. We suspected an accident causing massive contamination of the population with sheep scrapie, which the Orava farmers have long recognized in their sheep as *klusavka*. For these reasons at first we believed that this outbreak might not be explained genetically.

However, we have now sequenced DNA from 9 of the Orava and 6 of the Lucenec CJD brains and all have shown the substitution of lysine for glutamic acid at codon 200. 4 of the 11 healthy adult first-order relatives studied have the same mutation.[12] CJD had not been known in Orava before the 1970s.[48] The epidemic started with a few cases in the late 1970s and has developed into an escalating epidemic in the late 1980s. We have found some family members with the mutation although they are healthy and over 70 years of age. We are now look-ing for the cofactor that turns on the expression of the mutation, or a factor which in the past inhibited the post-translational configuration change of the precursor to amyloid. Thus, the new question is not what has caused the Orava outbreak – it is the codon 200 glutamic acid to lysine point mutation – but rather what has prevented its expression in previous generations so that it has accumulated as a frequent silent nonpathogenic polymorphism, only expressing itself as a pathogenic mutation in these people in the past 15 years.

THE CJD GENETIC MARKER FOR THE WANDERING JEWS OF THE DIASPORA

On discovering the codon 200 glutamine to lysine point mutation re-sponsible for the high-incidence foci of CJD in both Lucenec and Orava regions of Slovakia and widely disseminated in Slavic peoples of East-ern Europe, we screened a large number of sporadic and familial CJD brain specimens from our archive of frozen brain accumulated over the past 30 years.[24] This led us to discover the mutation in Greek CJD patients who were Sephardic Jews and quickly we found the mutation in Sephardic Jews who had some diagnosis of CJD in France from Tunisia and in Sephardic Jews with CJD in Israel, both Libyan-born and Israeli-born. Ashkenazic Jewish CJD patients did not have the codon 200 glutamic to lysine point mutation.[24]

We are thus now investigating other Circum-Mediterranean Sephardic Jews with CJD and with particular attention to the Iberian Peninsula, particularly Spain where in 1492 the Catholic monarchs, Ferdinand and Isabella, forced the quick conversion of large numbers of Sephardic Jews to Catholicism. Many of the remainder fled and gave rise to the large Sephardic Jewish group in Greece where we have found the mutation. Of those remaining in Spain and converted to Catholicism, many emigrated in the 15th century to the New World. We have now found that in Chile, the proportion of familial cases among the CJD patients is several-fold higher than elsewhere, and these patients and their family members have the 200 codon glutamine to lysine substitution.[26,27,35]

THE CJD POINT MUTATION FOR THE LARGE FINNISH PEDIGREE OF FAMILIAL CJD

One of the largest familial CJD pedigrees (Finnish) is that published in 1979 by Haltia et al[30] which we have now investigated and found therein none of the point mutations previously known in familial CJD or GSS, but instead a codon 178 replacement of aspartic acid by asparagine.[29] We have now found this codon 178 mutation in Dutch, French, Hungarian and US cases of familial CJD.[31,36] Furthermore, in Italian, French, and US families it causes a clinical variant of CJD, familial fatal insomnia (FFI).

Thus the paradigm from the amyloidosis literature of any one of several amino acid substitutions in the precursor molecule causing an enormously increased likelihood of its post-translational conversion to an amyloid configuration and its polymerization and deposition in the form of amyloid fibrils in various tissues has proved amazingly predictive in unravelling the pathogenesis of familial CJD and GSS and also of β-amyloid deposition in normal aging, Alzheimer's disease and Down's syndrome.

VARIETIES OF PHENOTYPIC EXPRESSION DETERMINED BY DIFFERENT MUTATIONS IN THE CJD AMYLOID PRECURSOR GENE

The pattern of clinical disease produced by the different mutations in different families is extremely uniform in some and quite variable in other families. It ranges from classical GSS in most families with codon 102, 105, and 117, and mutations to classical CJD with codon 178 and codon 200 mutations and the various insertions of 2, 4, 5, 6, 7, 8 or 9 octapeptide repeats. However, familial fatal insomnia (FFI) has been the clinical form of the disease in several families with codon 178 mutations whereas the clinical form of CJD without insomnia in other families with the same mutation. We have reported that presence of the valine polymorphism at codon 129 together with the 178 mutation on the same chromosome causes FFI, whereas the classical CJD-type disease appears in families with the more common methionine pleomorphism at codon 129 on the codon 178 mutated chromosome.

The age of onset is earlier and the duration of clinical disease is longer in codon 178 CJD than in codon 200 CJD, and in codon 200 disease the EEG usually shows the characteristic CJD spike and slow-wave periodicity. No such EEG change is found in the codon 178 CJD patients. Even the incubation period for clinical disease in intracerebrally inoculated squirrel, spider and capuchin monkeys differs for codon 178 and codon 200 cases of CJD, being considerably longer in codon 200 than for codon 178 cases.

Many other distinguishing phenotypical expressions of the pathogenic mutations have now been recorded. These include an Alzheimer's disease-type clinical course in the 145 stop codon mutation with no βA4 amyloid deposits in the amyloid plaques. On the other hand, the codon 198 and 217 have produced an Alzheimer's disease-like clinical course and also a combined CJD and Alzheimer's disease type neuropathology with both the CJD amyloid and the βA4 amyloid plaques.

TRANSTHYRETIN AMYLOIDOSES OF FAMILIAL AMYLOIDOTIC POLYNEUROPATHY (FAP) AS A PARADIGM FOR THE GENETIC CONTROL OF TRANSMISSIBLE AND NON-TRANSMISSIBLE BRAIN AMYLOIDOSES

Of most pertinence to our problem of the unconventional viruses, which are infectious amyloids, have been the transthyretin amyloidoses of familial amyloidotic polyneuropathies (FAP).[6,7,10,51] Patients are members of several hundred families scattered around the world in which the disease is an autosomal dominant trait. The onset of the clinical disease may occur at different ages and leads to the destruction of peripheral nerves by progressive deposition of amyloid in the perineurium. The human transthyretin gene has been cloned and its full sequence of 6.9 kb composed of four exons and three introns is known. Its encoding gene is located on chromosome 18.[52,53]. Transthyretin in its pure and crystalline form is a soluble prealbumin of 14kD molecular weight with 127 amino acids. Its secondary, tertiary, and quarternary structures have been determined by X-ray crystallography. It is a symmetrical tetramer of 55 kD made of 4 subunits showing extensive β-pleated sheet structure.[54–57] Thus, it is amyloidogenic by structural chemical considerations.

Members of different affected families have a mutation resulting in one amino acid substitution in the precursor that increase the statistical mechanical likelihood of the molecule falling into the amyloid conformation by a factor of about 10^4–10^6. There is no one specific mutation causing the disease in all families. Thus, in over 100 investigated families more than 30 different mutations have been detected (Fig. 2). The transthyretin amyloid may be deposited in the anterior chamber of the eye to cause familial amyloidotic blindness, in the heart to cause amyloidotic cardiopathy, or asymptomatically in the intestinal wall, as well as around peripheral nerves to cause FAP. The FAP is thus caused by precipitation of amyloid formed from the transthyretin precursor, with any of a set of point mutation each causing a single amino acid replacement which increases the likelihood of amyloid formation. This amyloid is not a replicating infectious molecule. Without one of these point mutations it is difficult to change the transthyretin polypeptide by concentration and nucleation into the amyloid configuration. With these single amino acid substitutions amyloid formation occurs spontaneously as a much more likely stochastic event, even extracellularly and *in vitro*.

In spite of the amyloidogenicity of the normal transthyretin by structural and chemical considerations, spontaneous amyloid formation does not occur in the absence of a facilitating mutation causing an amino acid substitution until the ninth decade, with the rare sporadic appearance of senile cardiac decompensation with cardiac amyloidosis. In these patients in their 80s the full-length molecule without any mutation is the amyloid subunit. There are also several silent polymorphisms in the population with point mutations causing non-pathogenic single amino acid substitutions (Fig. 2).

The codon 30 point mutation with proline replaced by methionine has been expressed in transgenic mice which develop deposits of human amyloid containing the methionine-30 mutation similar to depositions in FAP, but also in the intestine and other tissues, and they pass this trait to their offspring.[58,59]

TRANSTHYRETIN AMYLOIDOSES OF FAMILIAL AMYLOIDOTIC POLYNEUROPATHY (FAP)
Mutations Increasing Likelihood of Host Precursor Falling Into Amyloid Configuration

NORMAL	6	10	30	33	36	42	45	49	50	58	60	77	84	90	111	114	116	122	127
	gly	cys	val	phe	ala	glu	ala	thr	ser	leu	thr	ser	ile	his	leu	tyr	tyr	val	

FAMILIAL AMYLOIDOTIC POLYNEUROPATHY

	position	residue
Dutch, German, Greek, Italian, Japanese, Portuguese, Spanish, Swedish, Turkish	30	met
Jewish	33	ile
Greek, USA	36	pro
Japanese family KA	42	gly
Italian-Irish	45	thr
Italian	49	ala
Jewish	49	gly
Japanese family HY	50	arg
German USA:MD	58	his
Appalachian USA:WVA	60	ala
German USA:IL	77	tyr
Swiss USA:IN	84	ser
Italian-Sicilian	90	asn
Danish	111	met
Japanese family TK	114	cys

NORMAL: SILENT POLYMORPHISM

	position	residue
British	6	ser
German-Portuguese	90	asn
French-Canadian	116	val
USA: Scandinavian	122	ile

Fig. 2 16 different amino acid substitutions caused by point mutations in the gene specifying the transthyretin prealbumin precursor molecule in over 20 families of various ethnic origins are shown. 4 of these families are normal without FAP and the mutation is a silent non-pathogenic polymorphism in these. On codon 49 are 2 different amino acid substitutions, in a Jewish and Italian family, respectively. Codon 90 (asparagine replaces histamine) mutation has apparently caused FAP in the Italian Sicilian family, but not in the German, Portuguese families. There are over 20 additional such point mutations reported in the recent literature as responsible for different symphonies of pleomorphic clinical expression of familial amyloidotic polyneuropathy, familial amyloidotic blindness, and familial amyloidotic cardiopathy.

ANALOGIES WITH TRANSMISSABLE DEMENTIAS (CJD, GSS) SUGGEST THAT TRANSTHYRETIN AMYLOIDOSES OF FAP AND OTHER AMYLOIDOSES MAY ALSO BE TRANSMISSIBLE AND INFECTIOUS

The close parallel between multiple amino acid-changing mutations, each enormously facilitating the conversion to amyloid of the precursor protein which usually fails to spontaneously fall into amyloid configuration, except as a rare event (1 per million population per annum, the world-wide incidence of sporadic CJD) in the absence of any mutation in the precursor, and the transthyretin amyloidoses of FAP, determined by any one of many different point mutations, strongly suggests that FAP may also be transmissible. It will be difficult to demonstrate this in experimental animals since long-term observation will be essential and since subtle clinical signs, rather than flagrant, fatal disease should be expected. This will also have to be controlled by histopathological search for amyloid deposits in the perineurium and in other tissues. Amyloidoses based on other precursors may likewise be transmissible under the proper experimental conditions. This might be demonstrated using transgenic mice expressing the human precursors.

NUCLEATING INDUCTION OF CONFIGURATIONAL CHANGE IN HOST PRECURSORS AND POLYMERIZATION TO FIBRILS AS A GENERAL PHENOMENON IN AMYLOIDOGENESIS

We have recently demonstrated spontaneous generation of congophilic amyloid fibrils using synthetic polypeptides corresponding to sequences encoded by normal and mutant familial CJD alleles in the regions of codon 178 and codon 200. The 178 mutant and normal peptides formed fibrils with distinct morphological characteristics and differing aggregation tendencies from fibrils formed from the 200 mutant or normal peptides. The mutant peptides produce more filaments and denser masses of aggregate filaments than the unmutated peptides. Furthermore, mixtures of the normal with the mutant peptides for either codon region produce denser masses of fibrils than either peptide alone.[32]

The amyloid deposits of FAP contain both the mutated and the unmutated molecules, the mutated having nucleated and induced the β-pleating and co-polymerization of the unmutated molecules in the heterozygous patients (A. F. de Frietas, University of Oporto, personal communications).

Frangione has shown that the amyloid deposits in the vascular wall in hereditary cerebral hemorrhage with amyloidosis, Dutch type (HCHWA-D) contain both the codon 695 (glutamine substituted for glutamic acid) – mutated amyloid βA4 protein and the unmutated molecule with the normal βA4 sequence. The heterozygous patients are obviously polymerizing both the amyloid βA4 protein derived from the normal brain amyloid precursor protein (APP) and the mutated βA4 protein. He and his colleagues have synthesized polypeptides of the first 28 amino acids of the βA4 protein with and without the codon 695 mutation of HCHWA-D and studied the dynamics of fibril poly-merization with each. The synthetic 28-amino acid polypeptide with the mutation forms amyloids much faster than the polypeptide without the mutation. However, if both synthetic polypeptides are placed together in solution, the mutated polypeptide accelerates amyloid fibril formation by the unmutated polypeptide. Frangione uses the phrase accelerated instructive fibrillogenesis for this nucleating phenomenon of facilitation or induction of amyloidogenesis by a different amyloid.[60]

We are probably seeing the same phenomenon in the conversion of insulin-associated proteins to an amyloid in insulin-amyloid deposits in the amyloidosis of late diabetes. The same amyloid induction may also be occurring in the simultaneous appearance of βA4 amyloid and τ-amyloid in the neurofibrillary tangles of Alzheimer's disease, Down's syndrome and normal aging brain.

FIBRIL AMYLOID-ENHANCING FACTOR IN EXPERIMENTAL AA AMYLOIDOSIS MAY BE A SCRAPIE-LIKE NUCLEATING INFECTIOUS PROTEIN

Amyloid-enhancing factor[61-67] is a low-molecular weight glycoprotein found in tissues containing AA amyloid, which accelerates the laying down of AA amyloid in tissues in experimentally induced AA amyloi-dosis in mice and hamsters, shortening the lag time to 2 days from several weeks. It apparently serves as a nucleus for fibril formation and deposition[66] in animals with high serum level of acute phase re-actant AA amyloid precursor produced by the non-specific activation of inflammatory response with injections of casein, silver nitrate or lipopolysaccharide.[68,69]

Fibril amyloid-enhancing factor[66] is an example of pattern-setting induction of amyloid formation and polymerization, which is basically a nucleation process such as is required in all fibril polymerization. Such configurational change in the host precursor protein to the β-pleated infectious amyloid form occurs in the case of the transmissible agents of kuru-CJD-GSS-scrapie-transmissible mink encephalopathy-BSE. In these infections with infectious amyloid proteins a pattern-setting configurational change is induced in the host precursor. Thus, we suggest that the fibril amyloid-enhancing factor is a scrapie- (or kuru-CJD-GSS-) like agent, which induces a change in its own precursor to produce more of itself by copying its altered configuration. This pattern-setting nucleation we have mistaken for viral replication. It may be that we need to broaden our concept of a virus as have the computer virologists.[5,47]

ALZHEIMER'S DISEASE

The universal brain amyloidoses which everyone begins to get in old age and which is neuropathologically evident in all human brains from the ninth decade through the century is caused by amyloid deposits formed from a 42- or 43-amino acid (aa) peptide (βA4) proteolytically cleaved from the 80 kD brain amyloid precursor protein (APP). This precursor is a transmembrane protein the amyloid subunit from which extends from the center of the transmembrane region to the 15th extracellular amino acid. It is normally processed with a high rate of turnover with cleavage in the extracellular segment thereby preventing the formation of the amyloidogenetic 42-43 aa βA4 peptide. All metabolic interferences, environmental or genetic, with the high rate of turnover, lead to the possibility of cleavage resulting in this amyloidogenic peptide. This is the same process which, when accelerated from environmental factors or from point mutations on the precursor or on other chromosomes, specifying still unidentified proteins which must be either enzymes, chaperonins or binding proteins, or other rate-influencing molecules, is the cause of Alzheimer's disease. In Down's syndrome overproduction of the precursor appears to be enough to lead to formation of the βA4 peptide.

Familial Alzheimer's disease (FAD) families with pathological mutants of the APP gene account for only 3–5% of the familial Alzheimer's disease (FAD) families, whereas FAD accounts for 10–20% of all Alzheimer's disease, 80–90% of Alzheimer's disease being sporadic. The majority of FAD families with early onset appear to have a point mutation now localized on chromosome 14, whereas the late-onset FAD families appear to have a mutation less firmly localized on chromosome 19.

Figure 3 presents the mutations thus far identified on the βA4 amyloid precursor protein (APP) and shows clearly the mounting parallel with the infectious brain amyloids of the spongiform encephalopathies (Fig. 1). Both these transmissible and non-transmissible brain amyloidoses now demonstrate close similarities to the paradigm of the transthyretin amyloidoses of familial amyloidotic polyneuropathy (Fig. 2) in which some 40 pathogenic point mutations have now been found.

THE SEMANTIC WORD WARS OF SLOW VIROLOGISTS AND AMYLOIDOLOGISTS

The amyloidologists assiduously avoid the terminology of microbiology in their discipline. We, from microbiology, have entered their field through the infectious amyloids of the subacute spongiform viral encephalopathies (SSVEs) of kuru-CJD-GSS-scrapie-BSE. Thus, we have used the term replication, and the concepts of virulence and host range and incubation period, in describing phenomena for which they use other words and phrases. Various authors have exhausted the thesaurus to find terminology different from that used by their competing colleagues to describe the production of configurational change of host precursor proteins to β-pleated structure and the polymerization of amyloid fibrillogenesis:

    nucleation
    induction
    augmentation
    enhancement
    facilitation
    acceleration
    instruction
    heterodimer formation

Since the unconventional and atypical viruses of SSVE (kuru-CJD-GSS-scrapie-BSE) have been identified as infections amyloid molecules, our laboratory has slowly switched to designating them to infectious amyloids instead of unconventional viruses. Others have accepted the term prions for these agents. We prefer to draw on the important and informative paradigms of amyloidology which have directed much of our thinking over the past decade. I have facetiously pointed out that the founders of virology define a virus as an obligate parasite of submicroscopic dimensions requiring the informational and energy

Brain Amyloid of Aging (ßA4)

	670 671 673	692 695	713 717	(695) (751)
Normal precursor protein	ala met lys	ala glu	ala val	770
Normal Aging no mutations				
Familial Alzheimers Disease sporadic, no mutations				
Familial Alzheimers Disease w/chromosome 14 mutations Early onset, no mutations				
Familial Alzheimers Disease w/chromosome 19 mutations Late onset, no mutations				
Downs Syndrome no mutations				
silent polymorphism	673 thr			
silent polymorphism			713 thr	
silent polymorphism			713 val	
Familial Alzheimers Disease Swedish (double mutation)	670 671 asn leu			
HCHWA-D Dutch		692 gly		
HCHWA-D Dutch		693 gln		
Familial Alzheimers Disease English, Japan, USA			717 ile	
Familial Alzheimers Disease English			717 phe	
Familial Alzheimers Disease English			717 gly	

Fig. 3 11 point mutations on the βA4 amyloid precursor protein of normal aging and Alzheimer's disease: three different amino acid substitutions at the same codon 717 all cause familial Alzheimer's disease (FAD) in rare British, Japanese and US families. A double mutation at codon 670 and 671 cause FAD in a Swedish family. 2 adjacent mutations on codons 692 and 693 each cause hereditary cerebral hemorrhage with amyloidosis – Dutch type (HCHWA-D) in a different Dutch family. A mutation on codon 673 and two different amino acid changes on codon 713 are silent polymorphisms. Sporadic Alzheimer's disease and Down's syndrome patients show no mutations on the βA4 amyloid precursor protein. Only 3% of FAD have one of the 5 mutations causing the disease in rare families. Most of the early-onset FAD families have a mutation on chromosome 14 and late-onset FAD families appear to have a mutation on chromosome 19 but neither of these are associated with any mutation on the βA4 amyloid precursor protein gene.

systems of the host for replication: this embraces viroids, virules, virettes, nucleating agents of industrial infections, and computer viruses.

REFERENCES

1 Gajdusek DC. Unconventional virus infections as cerebral amyloidoses. In : Court LA, Dormont D, Brown P, eds. Unconventional virus diseases of the central nervous system. Proceedings of Conference, Paris, December 2–6, 1986. Commissariat a l'Energie Atomique (CEA), Service de Documentation, Fontenay-aux-Roses, France, 1986; 641-659.

2 Gajdusek DC. Transmissible and non-transmissible amyloidoses: autocatalytic post-translational conversion of host precursor proteins to β-pleated configurations. J Neuroimmunol 1988; 20: 95-110.

3 Gajdusek DC. Etiology versus pathogenesis: the causes of post-translational modifications of host specified brain proteins to amyloid configuration. In: Sinet PM, Lamour Y, Christen Y, eds. Genetics and Alzheimer's disease. Proceedings of a meeting held by the Foundation IPSEN pour la Recherche Thérapeutique, Paris, March 25. Berlin: Springer-Verlag, 174-176, 1988.

4 Gajdusek DC. Fantasy of a 'virus' from the inorganic world: pathogenesis of cerebral amyloidoses by polymer nucleating agents and/or 'viruses'. In: Neth R, Gallo RC, Greaves MF et al, eds. Modern trends in human leukemia VIII. New York: Springer-Verlag, 1989; 481-499.

5 Gajdusek DC. Subacute spongiform encephalopathies: transmissible cerebral amyloidoses caused by unconventional viruses, Ch 20. In: Fields BN, Knipe DM, Chanock RM et al, eds. Virology, 2nd edn, New York: Raven Press, 1990; 2289-2324.

6 Gajdusek DC. Genetic control of de novo conversion to infectious amyloids of host precursor proteins: Kuru-CJD-scrapie. In: Proceeding of Paul Ehrlich Institute Scientific Conference on 'Concepts in Biomedical Research'. New York: Springer-Verlag, 1991.

7 Gajdusek DC. Transthyretin amyloidoses of familial amyloidotic polyneuropathy as a paradigm for the genetic control of de novo generation of Creutzfeldt-Jakob disease infectious amyloid by a spontaneous change in the configuration of the host precursor protein. In: Bradley R, Savey M, Marchant BA, eds. Sub-acute spongiform encephalopathies. Current Topics of Veterinary and Animal Science, Vol. 55, Dordrecht: Kluwer Academic, 1991; 91-114.

8 Gajdusek DC. The transmissible amyloidoses: genetic control of spontaneous generation of infectious amyloid proteins by nucleation of configurational change in host precursors kuru-CJD-scrapie-BSE. Eur J Epidemiol 1991; 7: 567-577.

9 Gajdusek DC, Gibbs CJ Jr. Brain amyloidoses: precursor proteins and the amyloids of transmissible and non-transmissible dementias: scrapie-kuru-CJD viruses as infectious

polypeptides or amyloid-enhancing factors. In: Goldstein AL, ed. Biomedical advances in aging. New York: Plenum, 1990; 3-24.

10 Gajdusek DC, Beyreuther K, Brown P et al. Regulation and genetic control of brain amyloid. Brain Res Rev 1991; 16: 83-114.

11 Safar J, Roller PP, Ruben GC, Gajdusek DC, Gibbs CJ Jr. Secondary structure of proteins associated in thin films. Biopolymers 1993; 33: 1461-1476.

12 Goldgaber D, Goldfarb LG, Brown P et al. Mutations in familial Creutzfeldt-Jakob disease and Gerstmann-Sträussler syndrome. Exp Neurol 1989; 106: 204-206.

13 Hsiao KK, Baker HF, Crow TJ et al. Linkage of prion protein missense variant to Gerstmann-Sträussler syndrome. Nature 1989; 338: 342-345.

14 Hsiao KK, Doh-ura K, Kitamoto T, Tateishi J, Prusiner SB. A prion protein amino acid substitution in ataxic Gerstmann-Sträussler syndrome. Ann Neurol 1990; 26: 137.

15 Kretzschmar HA, Kufer P, Riethmüller G, DeArmond S, Prusiner SB, Schiffer D. Prion protein mutation at codon 102 in an Italian family with Gerstmann-Sträussler-Scheinker syndrome. Neurology 1992; 42: 809-810.

16 Kitamoto T, Ohta M, Doh-ura K, Hitash S, Tarao Y, Tateishi J. Novel miss-variants of prion protein in Creutzfeldt-Jakob disease or Gertsmann-Sträussler syndrome. Biochem Biophys Res Commun 1993 (In press).

17 Doh-ura K, Tateishi J, Sasaki H, Kitamoto T, Sakaki Y. Protein change at position 102 of prion protein gene is the most common but not the sole mutation related to Gerstmann-Sträussler syndrome. Biochem Biophys Res Commun 1989; 163: 974-979.

18 Hsiao KK, Cass C, Schellenberg G et al. A prion protein variant in a family with a teleacepholic form of Gerstmann-Sträussler-Scheinker syndrome. Neurology 1990; 41: 681-684.

19 Hsiao KK, Cass C, Conneally PM et al. Atypical Gerstmann-Sträussler-Scheinker syndrome with neurofibrillary tangles: no mutation in the prion protein open-reading-frame in a portion of the Indiana kindred. Neurobiol Aging 1990; 11: 3, 302.

20 Hsiao KK, Dloughy SR, Farlow MR et al. Mutant prion proteins in Gerstmann-Sträussler-Scheinker disease with neurofibrillary tangles. Nature Genetics 1992; 1: 68-71.

21 Dloughy SI, Hsiao K, Farlow MR et al. Linkage of the Indiana kindred of Gerstmann-Sträussler-Scheinker disease to the prion protein gene. Nature Genetics 1992; 1: 64-67.

22 Goldfarb LG, Brown P, Goldgaber D et al. Creutzfeldt-Jakob disease and kuru patients lack a mutation consistently found in Gerstmann-Sträussler-Scheinker syndrome. Exp Neurol 1990; 108: 247-250.

23 Goldfarb LG, Brown P, Goldgaber D et al. Identical mutation in unrelated patients with Creutzfeldt-Jakob disease. Lancet 1990; 336: 174-175.

24 Goldfarb LG, Korczyn AO, Brown P, Chapman J, Gajdusek DC. Mutation in codon 200 of scrapie amyloid precursor gene linked to CJD in Sephardic Jews. Lancet 1990; 336: 637.

25 Goldfarb LG, Mitrov E, Brown P, Toh BH, Gajdusek DC. Mutation in codon 200 of scrapie amyloid protein gene in two clusters of Creutzfeldt-Jakob disease in Slovakia. Lancet 1990; 336: 514-515.

26 Brown P, Gálvez S, Goldfarb LG et al. Familial Creutzfeldt-Jakob disease in Chile is associated with the codon 200[Asn] mutation of the codon 200 mutation of the PRNP amyloid precursor gene on chromosome 20 amyloid precursor gene. J Neurol Sci 1992; 112: 65-67.

27 Goldfarb LG, Brown P, Mitrov E et al. Creutzfeldt-Jakob disease associated with the PRNP codon 200[lys] mutation: an analysis of 45 families. Eur J Epidemiol 1991; 7: 477-486.

28 Haltia M, Kovanen J, van Crevel H, Bots GTAM, Stefanko S. Familial Creutzfeldt-Jakob disease. J Neurol Sci 1979; 42: 381-389.

29 Goldfarb LG, Haltia M, Brown P et al. New mutation in scrapie amyloid precursor gene (at codon 178) in Finnish Creutzfeldt-Jakob kindred. Lancet 1991; 337: 425.

30 Haltia M, Kovanen J, Goldfarb LG, Brown P, Gajdusek DC. Familial Creutzfeldt-Jakob disease in Finland: epidemiological, clinical, pathological and molecular genetic studies. Eur J Epidemiol 1991; 7: 494-500.
31 Nieto A, Goldfarb LG, Brown P et al. Mutation in codon 178 of amyloid precursor gene occurs in Creutzfeldt-Jakob disease families of diverse ethnic origins. Lancet 1991; 337: 622-623.
32 Goldfarb LG, Brown P, Haltia M et al. Synthetic peptides corresponding to different mutated regions of the amyloid gene in familial Creutzfeldt-Jakob disease show enhanced in vitro formation of morphologically different amyloid fibrils. Proc Natl Acad Sci USA; 1993; 90: 4451-4454.
33 Brown P, Goldfarb LG, Cathala F et al. The molecular genetics of familial Creutzfeldt-Jakob disease in France. J Neurol Sci 1991; 105: 240-246.
34 Brown P, Goldfarb LG, Gajdusek DC. The new biology of spongiform encephalopathy: infectious amyloidoses with a genetic twist. Lancet 1991; 337: 1019-1022.
35 Brown P, Goldfarb LG, Gibbs CJ Jr, Gajdusek DC. The phenotypic expression of different mutations in transmissible familial Creutzfeldt-Jakob disease. Eur J Epidemiol 1991; 7: 469-476.
36 Brown P, Goldfarb LG, Kovanen J et al. Phenotypic characteristics of familial Creutzfeldt-Jakob disease associated with the codon 178[Asn] PPNP mutation. Ann Neurol 1992; 31: 282-285.
37 Kitamoto T, Iizuka R, Tateishi J. An amber mutation of prion protein in Gertsmann-Sträussler syndrome with mutant PrP plaques. Biochem Biophys Res Commun 1993 (In press).
38 Brown P, Goldfarb LG, McCombie WR et al. Atypical Creutzfeldt-Jakob disease in an American family with an insert mutation in the PRNP amyloid precursor gene. Neurology 1992; 42: 422-427.
39 Goldfarb LG, Brown P, McCombie WR et al. Transmissible familial Creutzfeldt-Jakob disease associated with five, seven, and eight extra octapeptide coding repeats in the PRNP gene. Proc Natl Acad Sci USA 1991; 88: 10926-10930.
40 Goldfarb LG, Brown P, Vrbovska A et al. An insert mutation in the chromosome 20 amyloid precursor gene in a Gerstmann-Sträussler-Scheinker family. J Neurol Sci 1992; 111: 189-194.
41 Goldfarb LG, Brown P, Little BW et al. A new (2-repeat) octapeptide coding insert mutation in Creutzfeldt-Jakob disease, Neurology 1993 (In press).
42 Owen F, Poulter M, Lofthouse R et al. Insertion in prion protein gene in familial Creutzfeldt-Jakob disease. Lancet 1989; i: 51-52.
43 Owen F, Poulter M, Collinge J, Crow T. Codon 129 changes in the prion protein gene in Caucasians. Am J Hum Genetics 1990; 46: 1215-1216.
44 Owen F, Poulter M, Shah T et al. An in-frame insertion in the prion protein gene in familial Creutzfeldt-Jakob disease. Mol Brain Res 1990; 7: 273-276.
45 Safar J, Wang W, Padgett MP et al. Molecular mass, biochemical composition and physicochemical behavior of the infectious form of the scrapie precursor protein monomer. Proc Natl Acad Sci USA 1990; 87: 6373-6377.
46 Safar J, Roller PP, Gajdusek DC, Gibbs CJ Jr. Conformational transitions, dissociation, and unfolding of scrapie amyloid (prion) proteins, J Biol Chem 1993 (In press).
46a Safar J. Infectious amyloid, prions, unconventional viruses and disease, review. Neurobiology of Aging 1993 (In press).
47 Guiroy DC, Gajdusek DC. Fibril-derived amyloid enhancing factors as nucleating agents in Alzheimer's disease and transmissible virus dementia. In : Brown P, Bolis L, Gajdusek DC eds. Molecular genetic mechanisms in neurodegenerative disorders. Discussions Neurosci 1988; 5: 69-73.
48 Mitrov E. Analytical epidemiology and risk factors of CJD. In: Court LA, Dormont D, Brown P, Kingsbury DT, eds. Unconventional virus diseases of the central nervous system. Paris: Commissanat l'Energie Atomique, Service de Documentation, 1990.

49 Mitrov E. Focal accumulation of Creutzfeldt-Jakob disease in Slovakia. In: Boese A, ed. Search for the cause of multiple sclerosis and other chronic disease of the central nervous system. Weinheim Verlag Chemie, 1980: 356-366.

50 Mitrov E, Brown P, Hroncov D, Tatara M, Zil k J. Focal accumulation of CJD in Slovakia: retrospective investigation of a new rural familial cluster. Eur J Epidemiol 1991: 7: 487-489.

51 Costa PP, de Freitas AF, Saraiva MJM, eds. Familial amyloidotic polyneuropathy and other transthyretin related disorders. Archives de Medicina, Porto. 1990; 414 + xxvi.

52 Sasaki H, Yoshioka N, Takagi Y, Sakaki Y. Structure of the chromosomal gene for human serum prealbumin. Gene 1985; 37: 191-197.

53 Tsuzuki T, Mita S, Maede S, Araki S, Shimada KJ. Structure of the human preablumin gene. Biol Chem 1985; 260: 12224-12227.

54 Blake CFF, Swan IDA, Rerat C, Berthou J, Laurent A, Rerat B. An X-ray study of the subunit structure of prealbumin. J Mol Biol 1971; 61: 217-224.

55 Blake CFF, Geisow MJ, Swan IDA, Rerat C, Rerat B. Structure of human plasma prealbumin at 2.5 A resolution: a preliminary report on the polypeptide chain conformation, quaternary structure and thyroxine binding. J Mol Biol 1974; 88: 1-12.

56 Blake CCF, Oatley SJ. Protein-DNA and protein-hormone interactions in prealbumin: a model of the thyroid hormone nuclear receptor? Nature 1977; 268: 115-120.

57 Blake CCF, Geisow MJ, Oatley SJ, Rerat B, Rerat C. Structure of preablumin: secondary, tertiary and quaternary interactions determined by Fourier refinement at 1.8 A. J Mol Biol 1978; 121: 339-356.

58 Wakasugi S, Inomoto T, Yi S et al. A potential animal model for familial amyloidotic polyneuropathy through introduction of human mutant transthyretin gene into mice. In: Takashi I, Shakuro A, Fumike O, Shozo K, Eiro T, eds. Amyloid and amyloidoses. London: Plenum Press, 1988: 393-398.

59 Yi S, Tadahashi K, Tashiro F, Wakasugi S, Yamamura K, Araki S. Pathological similarity to human familial amyloidotic polyneuropathy (FAP) type 1 in transgenic mice carrying the human mutant transthyretin gene. Abstract No. 07/5 in Program and Abstracts of the VIth International Symposium on Amyloidosis, Oslo, Norway, August 5-9, 1990; 58.

60 Frangione B, Wisniewski T, Ghiso J. Accelerated instructive fibrillogenesis. J Cell Biochem 1992; Suppl 16E: 200 Abst.

61 Axelrad MA, Kisilevsky R. Biological characterization of amyloid enhancing factor. In: Glenner GG, Costa PP, de Freitas AF eds. Amyloid and amyloidosis. Amsterdam: Excerpta Medica, 1980: 527-533.

62 Axelrad MA, Kisilevsky R, Wilmer J, Chen SJ, Skinner M. Further characterization of amyloid-enhancing factor. Lab Invest 1982; 47: 139-146.

63 Hol PR, van Andel ACJ, van Ederen AM, Draüyer J, Gruys E. Amyloid enhancing factor in hamster. Br J Exp Pathol 1985; 66: 689-697.

64 Janigan DT. Pathogenetic mechanisms in protein-induced amyloidosis. Am J Pathol 1969; 55: 379-393.

65 Janigan DT, Druet RL. Experimental murine amyloidosis in X-irradiated recipients of spleen homogenates or serum from sensitized donors. Am J Pathol 1968; 52: 381-390.

66 Niewold TA, Hol PR, van Andel ACJ, Lutz ETG, Gruys E. Enhancement of amyloid induction by amyloid fibril fragments in hamster. Lab Invest 1987; 56: 544-549.

67 Ranlov P. The adoptive transfer of experimental mouse amyloidosis by intravenous injection of spleen cell extracts from casein-treated syngeneic donor mice. Acta Pathol Microbiol Scand 1967; 70: 321-335.

68 Cohen AS. The constitution and genesis of amyloid. Int Rev Exp Pathol 1965; 4: 159-243.

69 Janigan DT. Experimental amyloidoses. Am J Pathol 1965; 47: 159-171.

British Medical Bulletin (1993) Vol. 49, No. 4, pp. 932–959
©The British Council 1993

Epidemiology and control of bovine spongiform encephalopathy (BSE)

R Bradley
J W Wilesmith
Central Veterinary Laboratory, New Haw, Addlestone, Surrey, UK

BSE is a new disease of cattle. The first clinical case
occurred in April 1985 but the existence of a new disease
was first confirmed microscopically in November 1986.
Epidemiological studies show that cattle suddenly
became effectively exposed to a scrapie-like agent in
ruminant-derived feed in the form of meat and bone meal
in 1981/2. Most cases have occurred in Holstein Friesian
dairy cattle and have been exposed as calves. There is
no evidence that cattle to cattle transmission sufficient to
maintain the epidemic occurs. The principle animal health
control measures are bans on the feeding of ruminant
derived protein to ruminant animals and on the use of
specified bovine offals (SBO) for feeding to any species of
animal or birds. Human health is protected by compulsory
slaughter and destruction of suspect animals, and a ban
on the use of their milk, and by prohibiting the use of SBO
in food. The SBO are those tissues which, in clinically
healthy cattle incubating BSE, might conceivably harbour
infectivity. The effectiveness of the bans is supported by
recent evidence of a decline in the cattle epidemic. There
is no evidence that BSE is a zoonosis.

Until 1985 only 6 transmissible spongiform encephalopathies had occurred, 3 in man and 3 in animals (Table 1). From April 1985, quite
unexpectedly, a very low incidence of an unusual neurological disease
of cattle was seen by a few veterinary practitioners in Great Britain.
Though distinctive and unfamiliar none of these incidents resulted in
published reports at the time. Initially such cattle died or were killed
without any microscopic study of the brain. The epidemiological evi-

dence accumulated in the course of the epidemic indicates that, even at that time, but unsuspected by anyone, a large number of British dairy cattle were being exposed to, and infected with, the agent that was responsible for the subsequent epidemic of bovine spongiform encephalopathy (BSE).

Table 1 Naturally occurring transmissible spongiform encephalopathies to 1985

Host	Disease		Reported distribution
Man	Kuru		Papua New Guinea
	Creutzfeldt-Jakob Disease (CJD)	– Iatrogenic – Sporadic – Familial	Worldwide
	Gerstmann-Straussler (-Scheinker) Syndrome (GSS)	– Familial	Worldwide but extremely rare
Sheep Goats	Scrapie		Sheep scrapie - widely distributed, but not reported in Argentina, Australia, New Zealand, Uruguay and some other countries
Mule Deer, Elk	Chronic Wasting Disease (CWD)		North America
Farmed Mink	Transmissible Mink Encephalopathy (TME)		North America Europe

The unrecognised herald of the first BSE case in 1986 was a nyala (*Tragelaphus angasi*), an African herbivorous ungulate in a British zoo. This animal showed unusual nervous signs and was killed. The fixed brain was sent to the Pathology Department of the Central Veterinary Laboratory Weybridge (CVL) where spongiform encephalopathy was confirmed.[1] A few months later, 2 cows exhibiting signs similar to those observed earlier by a few alert practitioners were investigated in greater detail and submitted for necropsy at the local Veterinary Investigation Centre (VIC) of the Ministry of Agriculture, Fisheries and Food (MAFF). No significant gross lesions were found but brains were fixed and submitted to the CVL for neuropathological examination. Here a scrapie-like spongiform encephalopathy was found, reported and named bovine spongiform encephalopathy (BSE).[2] Because the tissue had been fixed, no immunoblotting for the disease-specific isoform of PrP, or examination for disease specific brain fibrils, could be undertaken. However such methods were employed in later cases, with positive results.[2,3] Initially 2 scenarios were envisaged. Either these 2 cases were scientific curiosities, as are many submissions to the CVL Pathology Department each year, or we were threatened by an epidemic of unknown size but which could prejudice the export of live cattle and cattle products. This possibility was foreseen at an early stage and plans laid accordingly.

From November 1986 onwards more cases of suspect BSE were intermittently presented and confirmed. An increasing amount of epidemiological data was collected by staff at the VICs, but not in a planned way. By June 1987 it was clear that the initial cases were not isolated curiosities, that an epidemic was a possibility and that there was a need for a focussed and substantial epidemiological input. The first part of this paper describes the epidemiological investigation which continues to this day, and reports the current status of the epidemic, the effect of the control measures which have been taken and its likely future progress.

In June 1987 the only statutory controls having any relevance to the epidemiological investigation into BSE or limiting the spread of infection were those governing cattle identification and movement[4-6] and those governing the use of certain offals in food products under the Meat Products and Spreadable Fish Products Regulations 1984.[7] Briefly the first required that all cattle be permanently identified by ear number, that movements from and to premises be recorded and the records kept for a minimum of 3 years. The second defines meat to include, in addition to skeletal muscle, head meat, tail meat, diaphragm, heart, liver, kidney, pancreas and thymus. The Regulations also prohibit the use of certain specified offals – brain, spinal cord, spleen, oesophagus, stomach, small and large intestines, rectum, lungs, testicles, udder and feet – in uncooked meat products. Thus the risk of human exposure to scrapie-like agents, which concentrate in some of these tissues, was limited long before BSE had been discovered. Clearly, since the Regulations had not been drafted to prevent human exposure to BSE, this protection was incomplete, and more comprehensive measures were introduced by the Bovine Offal (Prohibition) Regulations 1989.[8]

The second part of this paper will deal with the control measures implemented to protect animal and public health in regard to BSE. Some of these resulted from analysis of epidemiological data (the ruminant feed ban for example); some from advice from the independent expert Working Party on Bovine Spongiform Encephalopathy chaired by Sir Richard Southwood FRS, and others from advice from the Consultative Committee on Research and its successor the Spongiform Encephalopathy Advisory Committee, both chaired by Dr DAJ Tyrrell FRS.

In the international arena, and especially in the European Community (EC), account had to be taken of the differing BSE risk factors, differences in law (meat in the EC for example, is defined as any part of an animal suitable for human consumption), and differences in social habits in regard to butchering and cooking.

INITIAL EPIDEMIOLOGICAL STUDIES IN GREAT BRITAIN

From June 1987, when the formal epidemiological study was launched, until June 1988 BSE was not a notifiable disease, so information about each current (or past) incident was provided voluntarily, usually via the private veterinary practitioner to the local VIC. The flow of information was encouraged by a nationwide request to practising veterinary surgeons for cooperation. Investigations were purely scientific, and the cadre of veterinary officers in the Veterinary Field Service (VFS) (who are responsible for dealing with statutory aspects of animal disease) were not involved and so devoid of clinical experience of BSE. Once the decision had been taken to make the disease notifiable veterinary officers of the VFS had to be trained in the clinical aspects of disease recognition. This was achieved by preparing and distributing a video recording of various cases, discussion with colleagues at CVL and in the VICs and 'on job' experience.

Case definition

Clinically suspect cases are defined as cattle presenting signs consistent with, or representative of, the syndrome collectively described by Wells et al,[2] Cranwell et al[9] and Gilmour et al.[10]

Confirmed cases (and all major interpretations, decisions and predictions have been based only on this group) are defined as those exhibiting the cardinal features of spongiform encephalopathy in the brain, as described by Wells et al.[2,11] The procedures now used to confirm BSE have reduced the extent of the neuropathological examination without significantly affecting case definition. These procedures are described in detail by Bradley and Matthews.[12] Veterinary neuropathologists involved in statutory or voluntary cattle disease surveillance in the EC or in other countries have been trained in these procedures at 2 EC-funded workshops held at CVL in 1990 and in 1991, and in a third privately funded workshop held at CVL in 1992.

Collection of data

A comprehensive questionnaire completed by veterinarians from the State Veterinary Service is used to collect data required for epidemiological analysis. The questionnaire was modified in December 1987 when data had been assembled from 192 herds. Denominators to calculate national incidence rates and herd size distribution were obtained from agricultural censuses.

Was BSE a new disease?

Practising veterinary surgeons and herd owners were asked about the possible occurrence of clinical cases of BSE prior to November 1986, and at least 3 herds were identified in which cases could have occurred with a reasonable degree of certainty as far back as April 1985, but not before. Thus BSE does appear to be a new disease. This conclusion is supported by examining the age specific incidence data by year (Fig. 1), making allowance for a degree of adult exposure (most cases appear to result from infection acquired in calfhood). With the passage of time, from 1987 onwards, the annual age specific incidence increased in animals aged 6 years and older, as a result of the animals with longer than average incubation periods being detected later. Had BSE been a hitherto unreported, but regularly occurring disease, the age specific incidence data would not have been expected to change with time in this way.

In order to provide a further insight into whether BSE occurred before 1985, brains from adult cattle which died from 1980-1986 inclusive, held in archive in various laboratories and pathology departments in the UK, are being re-examined by MAFF with the benefit of 1993 knowledge. No cases have so far been found in cattle which died or were killed before 1985.

Aetiology of BSE

Analyses of data from questionnaires was reported by Wilesmith et al.[13] This revealed that disease was confined to adult cattle and that there was no association with the following factors:

● Imported animals or animal products
● Use of vaccines, pharmaceutical products or agricultural chemicals
● Direct contact with live sheep
● Sex, stage of lactation/pregnancy, breed or season.

The only factor common to all cases was the use of commercial concentrate feed either as finished calf pellets or cow cake or as protein supplements used in home mixed rations. These non-forage, prepared feeds could have contained one or both of two animal derived products, namely tallow (fat) and meat and bone meal (MBM). Both are derived by rendering of carcase waste, largely from abattoirs and butchers. The basic rendering process is one of mixing and crushing, to reduce particle

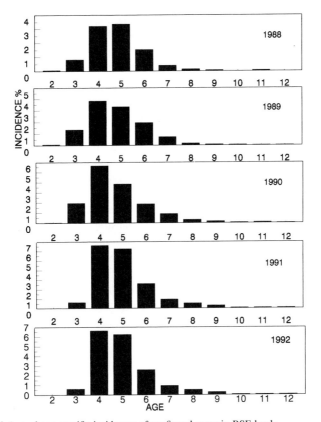

Fig. 1 Annual age specific incidences of confirmed cases in BSE herds.

size, cooking and then pressing, centrifuging or applying hydrocarbon solvents to remove the tallow.

The geographical variation in incidence (higher in the south and lower in the north of England and in Scotland) was not consistent with the distribution and use of tallow. MBM, on the other hand, is produced, distributed and used in cattle rations in a parochial fashion which relates much better to the distribution of disease, as will be explained later. Scrapie-like agents are intimately associated with cell membranes, particularly those of nervous tissue. They are closely associated with, if not composed only or partly of, a disease-specific isoform of a partially protease-resistant host-coded protein (PrP), and would be expected to co-partition with the greaves/meat and bone meal rather than with the tallow. Thus the hypothesis was developed that the cause of the BSE epidemic was the sudden exposure of a susceptible cattle population in 1981–1982 to sufficient quantities of a scrapie-like agent in prepared feed containing ruminant-derived MBM to produce clinical disease in 1985–1986 following a modal incubation period of 4–5 years (range 2 years to beyond the normal lifetime of cattle).

This exciting hypothesis provoked further detailed studies of the ways animal waste was disposed of including a thorough study[14] of the rendering systems used in Great Britain to identify reasons why BSE did not occur until 1985, despite MBM having been fed to cattle for decades.

Meantime, BSE was confirmed to be a member of the group of diseases known as the sub-acute, transmissible spongiform encephalopathies by the finding of the bovine homologue of sheep scrapie PrP in brain extracts of confirmed cases of BSE,[3] and by the successful transmission of scrapie-like disease to mice[15] and subsequently cattle[16] by parenteral inoculation of brain material derived from clinically affected cattle from 4 widely separated geographical locations.

Three alternative hypotheses were put forward to explain the occurrence of BSE in Great Britain.[14]

- An increase in exposure of cattle to the scrapie agent from sheep
- An increase in exposure of cattle to a cattle-adapted strain of scrapie
- Exposure to a novel strain of scrapie from sheep

The last hypothesis would have produced a propagative epidemic, unless one postulates sudden simultaneous mutation of scrapie agent in a large number of widely geographically dispersed sheep. The epidemic curve was not typical of a propagative disease occurrence, but had the features of a common source epidemic with all affected animals being index cases. This hypothesis is therefore inconsistent with the epidemiological findings, and can be discounted.

The first 2 hypotheses are consistent with the epidemiological findings and though each is tenable the evidence suggests that a sheep origin is more likely than a cattle origin. Firstly, there is no evidence that even a single case of BSE occurred anywhere in the world, including in Great Britain, before 1985. Second, the employment of Occam's razor (William of Occam c1290–1349). Nevertheless, the possibility of a bovine source cannot be completely dismissed.

SOME OF THE MAIN EPIDEMIOLOGICAL FEATURES

These are summarised in the following figures and tables with comments as appropriate.

Incidence by herd type (Table 2)

There is a much higher incidence in dairy than in beef suckler herds. This difference is attributed to the systems of management. Calves in the latter type of herd are suckled for several months, generally without supplementary feed. In contrast dairy calves are taken from their dams soon after birth and then fed artificially on reconstituted dried milk, with access to protein-rich concentrate feed which could include MBM at inclusion rates of around 5 %.

Table 2 Confirmed BSE incidence by herd type

Dairy herds	45.6%
Suckler herds	9.9%
Herds with breeding animals affected	27.5%
% Herds unaffected by BSE	72.5%

July 1993

Incidence by breed (Table 3)

Most cases of BSE occur in the Holstein Friesian breed. This is not because of a genetic pre-disposition, but merely reflects the relative numerical size of the breed compared with other dairy breeds.

Table 3 Distribution of confirmed cases in dairy herds by breed

Breed	% Cases confirmed	% Distribution of breed in Britain
Holstein Friesian	91.5	89.7
Channel Island	3.7	3.4
Ayrshire	3.9	2.2

Incidence by sex

Of the total of affected cattle (100 568) the vast majority are females (100 260). This is because of the disproportionately low numbers of adult entire males (bulls) in the cattle population due to the widespread use of artificial insemination.

The number of cases in bulls (292) reflects the numerical size of the population. Entire bulls reared for beef are usually killed for beef at 12–14 months old, and castrated males (steers) at around 2 years of age. BSE is unlikely to occur in animals as young as this. There have been 16 cases confirmed in steers. These, however, were animals with an unusual history. For example, one was a steer kept at a laboratory for experimental reasons unconnected with BSE, given feed including MBM which was 4 years old when signs of BSE developed. Another was a 'poor-doer' on a commercial farm which took 4 years to 'finish' and developed BSE before being sent for slaughter.

Herd size (Fig. 2)

The risk of BSE occurring in a herd increases with increase in herd size. This is attributed to the greater risk attached to purchasing an infected ration as a result of a larger number of batches of feed being bought.

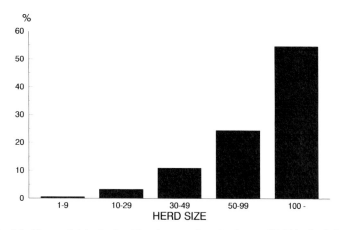

Fig. 2 Incidence of dairy herds with at least one homebred case of BSE by herd size.

Cases per herd (Fig. 3)

Over 40% of herds where BSE has occurred have had but one case, and 75% have four or less. In the majority of herds the occurrence of BSE is not a significant economic problem. However a very small number of herds have multiple cases, sometimes affecting an entire age cohort.

This is more of a financial and management problem, but fortunately has very rarely persisted into subsequent cohorts. These data support the view that cattle to cattle transmission either does not occur, or is rare and an insignificant factor in the maintenance of the epidemic.

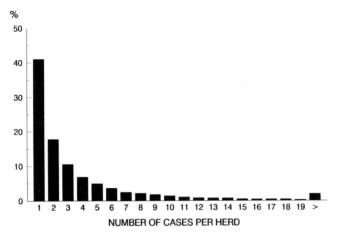

Fig. 3 Distribution of herds by number of suspect and confirmed cases of BSE per herd at 12 April 1991.

Within herd incidence (Fig. 4)
This has remained fairly constant at around 2% over the course of the epidemic. This also supports the notion that cattle to cattle transmission is unimportant.

Age specific incidence (*see* Fig. 1)
These data support the proposition that most cases of BSE are the result of calfhood exposure. The decline in incidence in the younger age classes (as shown in the height of the histogram for the 2 year old age class from 1991 and the 3 year old age class from 1992) is attributable to the introduction in July 1988 of the ban on feeding ruminant derived proteins to ruminants. The data also supports the concept that BSE was a 'new' disease, the modal age of occurrence and probably the modal length of the incubation period being 4–5 years.

Epidemic curve (Fig. 5)
This is the truest depiction of the course of the epidemic with time that is possible. Each case is confirmed and backdated to the date of

942 EPIDEMIOLOGY AND CONTROL OF BSE

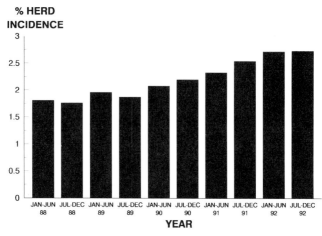

Fig. 4 Within herd incidence of BSE.

onset of clinical signs. There will be some error because of seasonal observations. No other histograms including those depicting numbers of BSE suspects by date of reporting or numbers of cases confirmed by date of confirmation have any scientific relevance; they will not be considered further in this paper.

The epidemic curve appeared to be levelling off in 1989 until July when a substantial increase in incidence occurred which was maintained until 1993. This increase is attributed predominantly to the recycling via MBM of infected cattle tissue derived from infected cattle from 1984 until the practice ceased as a result of the imposition of the ruminant feed ban in July 1988.

Purchased versus homebred cattle (Fig. 6)

A higher proportion of confirmed BSE cases occurs in purchased cattle in beef than in dairy herds. This is because of the derivation of part of the beef suckler population from the dairy herd.

The following simplified explanation of the structure of the national beef suckler and dairy herds is given to indicate a principle and should not be construed to represent the situation in all herds. It applies predominantly to commercial, Holstein Friesian dairy herds. In such herds about 20% of adults are replaced by heifers annually. Thus, for example, in a 100 cow dairy herd 40 of the best milking cows will be put to a Holstein Friesian bull. On average 20 offspring will be heifer calves used for replacement. There will also be 20 bull calves which are reared

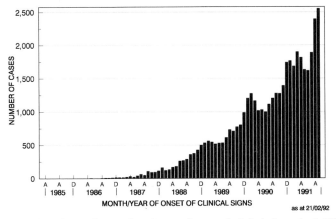

Fig. 5 Number of cases by month and year of onset of clinical signs. April 1985 – September 1991.

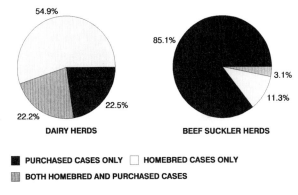

Fig. 6 Source of BSE cases in affected herds.

for beef and killed at 1–2 years of age. The remaining 60 cows are put to beef bulls and the resulting offspring often sold either for beef production or for eventual use as suckler cows. These young cattle contribute to a continuous replacement process of the national suckler herd, the backbone of which comprises beef breeds such as Aberdeen Angus, Galloway, Highland, Hereford or Charolais cattle. Within beef suckler herds BSE occurs predominantly in Holstein Friesian/beef breed crosses derived from the dairy herd and exposed to infection in feed when calves. This same herd structure also explains why, even if maternal transmission did occur in BSE (and there is little evidence for it) it could not support the one to one transmission ratio necessary to maintain the epidemic (*see* 'Maternal transmission' below).

Rendering of waste animal tissues and the meat and bone meal hypothesis

The data presented here resulted from a survey of all rendering plants in use in the Great Britain conducted during the Autumn of 1988.[14]

Two major changes occurred between 1970 and 1988 in the way waste tissues were rendered. The first was a change from batch to the more thermally efficient continuous processing. This was spread over a long period, starting in the early 1970's and was not temporally coincident with an increased effective exposure of cattle in 1981–1982 necessary to produce the first clinical cases in 1985–1986. Furthermore the different time and temperature combinations utilised in the different individual plants did not polarise with the 2 basic systems; plants utilising high and low temperatures were represented in each group. In any case the time/temperature combinations used in any plant were unlikely to have been capable of completely inactivating any scrapie-like agent that may have been present. The second change was a reduction in the use of hydrocarbon solvent to extract fat from the processed residue of rendering. The timing of a significant part of this reduction was coincident in broad measure with the time of increase in the effective exposure of cattle to a scrapie-like agent. Thus, unknowingly, rendering systems which used hydrocarbon solvents to extract additional fat appeared to have been better able to inactivate scrapie-like agents than others. Possible reasons for the more effective inactivation were the action of the hydrocarbon itself[17] and the use of a live steam stripping process to recover solvent for re-use. Wet heat is known to be more effective in reducing scrapie-like infectivity than dry heat[18] and it was employed on a product of low (approx. 1%) lipid content. In contrast, other methods produced MBM containing more lipid (7–14%) which may afford to micro-organisms greater protection from destruction by physical processes. It is clear that cattle have not changed, they have always been susceptible to scrapie-like agents but until 1981/1982 had not been sufficiently exposed. This is supported by the experimental studies reported by Gibbs et al.[19]

Though the findings of the rendering survey supported the MBM hypothesis a more vigourous and formal case control study was also undertaken.[20] This revealed that the feeding of proprietary concentrates containing MBM to calves during their first year of life was a statistically significant risk factor for the occurrence of BSE.

The geographical variation of risk from BSE

This can be considered from two angles – in the Great Britain and in other countries.

In the Great Britain the incidence of dairy herds in which a case of BSE has been confirmed shows a north to south gradient with a higher incidence in the south of England than in the north or in Scotland (Fig. 7). A variation is also apparent when examining the distribution of confirmed cases.

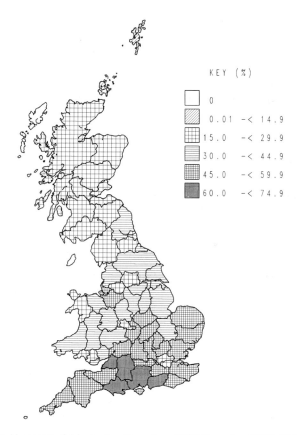

Fig. 7 Incidence (%) of dairy herds with confirmed BSE November 1986 to 30 July 1993.

The relatively low incidence in Scotland can be attributed to the retention of hydrocarbon solvent, lipid extraction systems in rendering plants there, to a greater use of reprocessed greaves[14] and the greater market share of compounders who used little or no MBM in cattle rations. The number of confirmed cases in Scotland would have been lower still had it not been for the movement into the country of already infected cattle from south of the border.

The epidemiology of BSE in Northern Ireland is similar to that in Great Britain but the peak annual incidence is much lower (2.3 confirmed cases per 10,000 animals in 1990,[21] compared with 1 per 100 adult cattle in Great Britain in 1993). As in Great Britain a food borne hypothesis is consistent with the epidemiological findings, but investigation of potential sources of infection including importation of MBM, protein supplements and compounded feed from Great Britain did not provide conclusive evidence.

BSE has been confirmed at a very low annual incidence in six other countries (Table 4), and cases are rumoured to have occurred without being reported, in some other countries. There are 3 main risk factors for the occurrence of BSE outside Great Britain:

- Importation of incubating cattle
- Importation of infected MBM (protein supplements or compounded feed) and feeding it to young cattle destined for breeding
- Feeding of MBM prepared from ruminant, especially sheep offals derived from indigenous sheep with a high incidence of scrapie. This risk would be enhanced if the ratio of total sheep to total cattle exceeded one. Furthermore the rendering systems in use must fail to inactivate the infectivity completely and there must be a high input feeding system using MBM and largely fed to calves destined for breeding.

Table 4 Countries in which BSE has been confirmed as at 18 June 1993

Great Britain •	97 968
Northern Ireland •	856
Republic of Ireland •	73
Oman †	2
Falkland Islands †	1
Switzerland •	37
France •	5
Denmark †	1

• Some or all cases in indigenous cattle; † Exported from UK.

The small number of cases in the Sultanate of Oman, Falkland Islands and Denmark occurred in cattle imported from and presumptively exposed in Great Britain. The same can be said of many of the rumoured cases.

Very few countries appear to fulfil the conditions necessary for an indigenous source of infection, but France and certain parts of the USA (which has not experienced a single case of BSE) might do so. However, in both countries steps have been taken to reduce any risk to a very low level. In France this has been done by instituting a ruminant protein feed ban for cattle and in the USA by preventing sheep heads, and adult or cull sheep from being rendered.

The confirmed cases of BSE reported in France and in Switzerland are all in indigenous cattle and in only once instance (in a case in Switzerland) has MBM been ruled out as a possible source of infection. In Switzerland almost all MBM associated with disease occurrence has been imported. In France there is a possible source from indigenous as well as imported meat and bone meal. The specific source of the Swiss and French cases is unlikely to be better defined in future.

Risk assessments for BSE have been conducted in the USA, Argentina and Spain.[22] No major risk at the national level has been identified for the occurrence of BSE from indigenous sources, and strict import controls now protect these countries from external risk. However, it is feasible that local conditions in a geographically restricted part of some countries could result in a local epidemic. Such local situations are monitored by surveillance schemes.

Recycling of infection in cattle in Great Britain

The detailed monitoring of the epidemic in Great Britain has revealed the importance of recycling infected bovine offals via MBM. This has been a major influence on the incidence of BSE. The first effects were seen in the second half of 1989, from which time a real and sustained, countrywide increased incidence of disease, best observed by reference to the epidemic curve (Fig. 5), has been apparent. The probable sequence of events was as follows; following the first effective exposure of cattle to a scrapie-like-agent there would be expected to be a sufficient titre of the agent in central nervous tissue in a significant proportion of the slaughter cattle population from 1984–1985 onwards. This presumes that BSE followed the natural scrapie model. In natural scrapie, lymphoreticular system (LRS) tissues from high risk individuals show increasing levels of infectivity from about 10 months of age, and infection is seen in the brain from 2.5 years of age, peaking at a titre greater than in the LRS when clinical signs develop.[23] In BSE, infectivity has so far only been found in brain and spinal cord of clinically affected animals (H Fraser, personal communication) though a full experimental pathogenesis study in cattle still in progress will reveal, as in Hadlow's study in sheep,[23] the range and titre of any infection in extraneural tissues.

Returning to the question of recycling, from 1984/1985 until 18 July 1988 infected bovine central nervous tissue would have been recycled via meat and bone meal to cattle. The Meat Products and Spreadable Fish Products Regulations[7] coincidentally limited human consumption of many lympho-reticular tissues, but full protection of human and other animal species was eventually provided by the specified bovine offals ban in 1989. This was extended to cover all animal species in 1990[8] (*see* 'Control' section below).

In the period 1984/1985 to July 1988 the amount of BSE infection being introduced into the rendering system, and thus MBM, would have increased continually as more and more cattle had become infected in the past. It is important to recognise that epidemiological monitoring has revealed that even at the time of maximum dietary infection in manufactured MBM destined for cattle (17 July 1988), the effective doses were likely to have been randomly distributed at a low level.

Since cattle exposed from this source would not be protected by a species barrier there was a possibility (which has so far proved to be unjustified) that the incubation period distribution might shift, resulting in one with a shorter mean and median in accordance with data derived from within species sub-passage of scrapie agent in mice and hamsters.[24] This could in turn accelerate the build-up of infection in cattle. The increasing probability of infection for cattle was due to increasing numbers of cattle incubating the disease which provided infected offals for rendering. Therefore as the prevalence of infected cattle increased so did the probability of exposure of cattle subsequently, and this would have supplemented exposure from sheep infected with scrapie. Also, as we now know, the ruminant feed ban, was not completely effective immediately. This means that cattle born in the year after the statutory ban was introduced were at greater risk of infection if fed MBM.

Newly reported spongiform encephalopathies in species other than cattle

Since 1985 spongiform encephalopathy has been identified in cattle, 5 species of captive wild *Bovidae*, 3 species of *Felidae* and moufflon (*Ovis musimon*) (Table 5). This last mentioned species presents like scrapie in sheep and goats and is presumptively acquired from them.[25] The first case in each of the 5 species of captive wild *Bovidae* had been fed the same type of diet, which included MBM, as cattle. Thus the origin of infection seems clear, though cannot be proven. The subsequent cases in greater kudu were not fed MBM. One was the offspring

Table 5 Naturally occurring transmissible spongiform encephalopathies reported from 1985 onwards

Host	Disease	First Report	Reported Distribution
Nyala	Spongiform encephalopathy (SE)	1987	England
Cattle	Bovine SE	1987	UK, Rep. of Ireland Oman*, Falkland Is.* Switzerland, France, Denmark*
Gemsbok †	SE	1988	England
Arabian Oryx †	SE	1989	England
Greater Kudu	SE	1989	England
Eland †	SE	1989	England
Cat	FSE	1990	UK
Moufflon †	Scrapie	1992	England
Puma †	FSE	1992	England
Cheetah †	FSE	1992	Australia*, UK

† Transmission not attempted; *Presumptively exposed in Great Britain.

of a confirmed case and thus may be a case of maternal or horizontal transmission though this cannot be confirmed either. It seems likely that direct transmission of disease may occur in this species as it does in sheep.

In May 1990 the first naturally occurring case of feline spongiform encephalopathy (FSE) was reported in a domestic cat in England.[26] To date (June 1993) 42 additional cases have been confirmed from widely geographically distributed areas of Great Britain, and one case occurred in Northern Ireland.

The domestic cat has long been known to be susceptible to CJD agent and has been used as an experimental animal.[27] The source of infection for the naturally occurring disease is not known. To date there is insufficient data to conduct an analytical epidemiological study. However the temporal occurrence and wide distribution of the disease suggest a source from BSE-infected feed though there is no proof. Any risk from commercial cat foods in Great Britain was eliminated by a voluntary ban on the inclusion of SBO in the summer of 1989 which was made compulsory in September 1990.

FSE has occurred in 2 captive cheetahs (born in the same British zoo) and in 1 captive puma. One of the cheetahs developed disease in Australia and was presumably in the incubating phase when imported from Great Britain. The most likely source of infection is presumed to be uncooked tissues including at least the spinal cord, from adult, fallen cattle and from animals affected with BSE before awareness of the clinical disease was complete and before the disease in cattle became notifiable.

For most of these species experimental transmissibility is assumed but has been proven for the cat disease (3 cases), and for the nyala and greater kudu[28] by successful transmission of SE to mice.

The characteristics of the mouse disease resulting from inoculation of brain from these species are very similar to those following experimental challenge of mice with brain from BSE-affected cattle.[29]

The age at onset of clinical signs (30–38 months) and the clinical duration (often only days) of disease in the captive wild *Bovidae* species are considerably shorter than in cattle (mean age of onset 60–62 months) and the incidence higher, suggesting that these species are more susceptible.

Other naturally occurring animal spongiform encephalopathies

Although wild and farmed deer (Family *Cervidae*) exist in Europe no case of spongiform encephalopathy has ever been suspected or diagnosed and no disease equivalent to chronic wasting disease of certain species of *Cervidae* has ever been seen outside of North America. Surveillance of deer for spongiform encephalopathy by the VIS is in progress in Great Britain to provide an added safeguard and early warning system.

Some captive deer in British zoological collections, like other ungulates,have received meat and bone meal in feed. The lack of cases could result from innate resistance or lack of exposure. In any event no exposure should have occurred after July 1988.

Mink are farmed in Europe, notably in Russia, Germany and Finland where TME has been identified in the past, and in Great Britain which has never had a case of the disease. Mink farmers are alert to both neurological diseases in general and to the potential sources of infection and the clinical signs. Investigation has indicated that the risk to mink in Great Britain from a feed-borne source has been minimal.

Experimental transmission of spongiform encephalopathy from cattle to domesticated species

Spongiform encephalopathy has been transmitted experimentally by parenteral exposure of sheep, goats[29] and pigs[30] but not so far (after 3 years from challenge) to chickens. It also been experimentally transmitted to sheep and goats by oral challenge[29] but not to pigs or poultry (M Dawson and GAH Wells, personal communication). Dogs, cats and horses have not been experimentally challenged.

These studies show only that sheep, goats and pigs are susceptible to spongiform encephalopathy (SE) when experimentally challenged with uncooked brain. They do not indicate susceptibility to infection or disease from MBM and do not provide epidemiological information to calculate the risk of SE developing naturally.

Maternal transmission

Maternal transmission is a factor in the transmission of scrapie between sheep. In this disease the vehicle of infection is probably the placenta. Pattison et al[31] showed that inoculation or feeding of placenta from Swaledale sheep with scrapie to uninfected sheep and goats resulted in disease transmission. Comparable studies in which native cattle have been oro-nasally challenged with placenta from cattle with confirmed BSE in their third trimester of pregnancy has not resulted in disease 3.5 years after challenge. In addition cattle killed at 2 years post-challenge showed no evidence of clinical disease or SE and tissues from them inoculated into mice have not transmitted SE so far. Furthermore oral or parenteral challenge of mice with placenta from cows with confirmed BSE in early and late pregnancy respectively has failed to reveal infectivity. The importance of placental infection in sheep is that this can be a source of infection for related and unrelated sheep, and for environmental contamination resulting in horizontal infection and therefore maintaining scrapie infection in a flock as an endemic disease. Only in SE of kudu and possibly CWD of deer is the disease apparently endemic though the means of transmission of infection is unknown. In kuru, TME and experimental CJD in mice[32] maternal transmission is not a feature.

The potential role and significance of maternal transmission alone in BSE was examined in modelling studies assuming that all offspring of BSE affected cows would become infective irrespective of the time in the incubation period that calves were born. The results indicated that the effective contact ratio was less than 1:1 without which infection cannot be maintained in the cattle population (Wilesmith and Ryan, unpublished findings – *see also* section on 'Purchased versus homebred cattle' above). On average not every infected cow will produce at least one female offspring which would survive to adulthood and produce a calf and so be able to perpetuate the chain *ad infinitum*. The result of any maternal transmission which did occur would therefore be to prolong the epidemic but not prevent its eradication.

Two important studies are in progress to determine whether or not maternal transmission is occurring. One is a cohort study of the incidence of BSE in the offspring of dams confirmed to have BSE and in control cattle. The other involves analysis of data from the monitoring of the epidemic.

In the cohort study 316 pairs of offspring are being studied for 7 years. One of each pair is the offspring of a case, the other the offspring of an unaffected dam over 6 years old, born in the same calving season and herd. By June 1993 most cattle were over 4 years old, some over 5. Less than 10 cases of BSE have been confirmed mostly in the oldest animals which also had opportunity for exposure via feed. The data so far do not give rise to concern in regard to maternal transmission, but since the study is being conducted as a double blind trial, interpretation is not possible until its conclusion when all animals have been killed, brains examined and the status of dams decoded.

In the second study a comparison is made of the observed annual incidence of BSE in the offspring of confirmed cases and the expected incidence from the feed-borne source alone (Fig. 8). In no year does the actual incidence exceed the expected incidence.

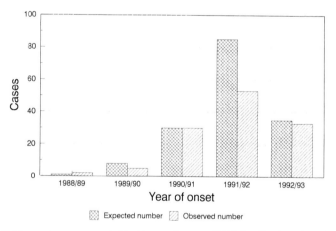

Fig. 8 Observed versus expected incidence of cases of BSE in offspring of confirmed cases.

Paternal transmission

Bioassay of semen from bulls clinically affected with confirmed BSE has not detected infectivity. The incidence of BSE in the progeny of the first 2 artificial insemination (AI) donor dairy bulls which were confirmed to have BSE has been compared with that in the progeny of 2 contemporaneously born dairy bulls whose semen was used in the same geographical areas (Table 6).

Table 6 The incidence of BSE in female offspring, born in 1986, of two bulls with confirmed BSE and of two bulls not affected by BSE as at April 1992

BSE status of bulls. Bull identification		Unaffected			Confirmed		
		BT	HM	Total	YC	PN	Total
BSE status of female offspring	Confirmed	2	2	4	2	1	3
	Unaffected	49	51	100	48	30	78
	Total	51	53	104	50	31	81

The results of the comparison did not reveal an excess of risk of BSE for offspring of affected bulls. The conclusion from these studies is that paternal transmission is a negligible factor in the transmission of BSE.

The decline of the BSE epidemic

The evidence so far accumulated supports the hypothesis of a feed origin for BSE with negligible evidence for paternal, maternal or horizontal transmission. At the very least a food origin is possible for all but 2 animals out of about 99,000 with confirmed disease in July 1993. A detailed investigation of the feeding of cattle born after the 18 July 1988 has eliminated, so far as is possible, a feed source of infection for 2 animals. As a result of the feed ban imposed in July 1988 a decline in incidence of disease, in successive age classes, (starting with 2 year olds then 3 years old followed by 4 and 5 year olds) in successive years would be expected (Fig. 9). This is in fact happening with a sustained decline in incidence in 2 and 3 year olds in 1992.

If horizontal transmission was a significant issue one would expect a high within-herd incidence in herds affected by BSE. The annual mean within-herd incidence has remained virtually constant during the course of the epidemic at approximately 2% of adult animals. This together with other relevant epidemiological findings suggests that horizontal transmission sufficient to maintain the epidemic is improbable.

Cattle born after 18 July 1988 should not develop BSE as a result of a food source yet to date (July 1993) nearly 2800 have done so. The greater majority of these were born before the end of January 1989 though some were born in 1989 and two in 1990. The occurrence of these upon further investigation can be attributed to the use of feed manufactured before 18 July 1988 but in the feed supply 'pipeline'. This effectively explains all the cases born in the latter half of 1988 and perhaps 1989. There should be no problem with feed prepared after September 1990 because the SBO ban introduced then would have 'double protected' cattle by preventing potentially infected bovine offals entering any animal feed from that date.

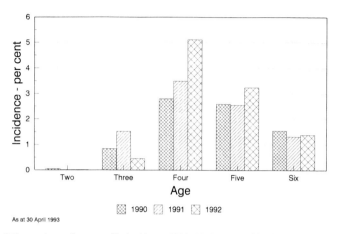

As at 30 April 1993

Fig. 9 Comparison of age-specific incidence 1990–1992 (cases with clinical onset January to June only).

To finally resolve whether other sources of infection than feed are significant a case control study has recently been initiated. This will provide comprehensive data from cases of BSE and age-matched controls born after 31 October 1988 for analysis.

The results to date from the monitoring of the epidemic and particularly the analyses of the age-specific incidences, show that the ruminant feed ban is effecting a decline in the epidemic as expected. If there is no other source of infection than feed, BSE will be eradicated.

CONTROL

Control of BSE is best examined via perceived risks and how to minimise them in respect of animal health and human health.[33] The first point to make is that a concept of zero risk is untenable. However, comprehensive examination of risk factors and selection of appropriate control measures can reduce any risk to a level which, on the basis of all our knowledge, would be most unlikely to initiate infection and lead to disease.

Human health controls

Theoretically there are 2 risks for man from BSE. The first relates to a possible increased exposure to the infectious agent compared with that experienced prior to the advent of BSE. To control this risk it is necessary to reduce the exposure of humans such that infection could not be established and disease would not result. This can be considered under 2 headings, short-term control and long-term control. The latter will ensue once the animal health controls referred to below begin to bite and will be ultimate when disease and infection (from cattle) are eliminated.

Of more immediate relevance is the short-term control. This is enforced by preventing suspect animals or milk derived from them from entering any food chain (except that milk from a suspect can be used to feed the dam's own calf) and by banning for consumption or any other use those offals, which in incubating animals and based on knowledge of scrapie, might carry infectivity.[8] The offals in question are brain, spinal cord, thymus, tonsil, spleen and intestine (from duodenum to rectum inclusive) from cattle over 6 months old.

The second potential risk for man arises from the possibility that the agent causing BSE is different from those strains of agent causing scrapie[33,34] (which on the basis of 250 years of experience is not a zoonosis). If the agent originated in sheep it might have altered on crossing the so-called species barrier between sheep and cattle in a way that could increase (or reduce) any pathogenicity for man. There is at present no way of telling whether or not this has happened, though the CJD surveillance programme set up by the Department of Health will eventually reveal any increased incidence provided the disease induced is similar to CJD. So far there is no evidence for this. This hypothetical scenario (a cattle strain of scrapie pathogenic for man) is equally well controlled by the measures mentioned above and there are currently no alternatives.

Summary of BSE public health controls (consumer protection)

- August 1988 – Carcasses of suspects destroyed
- December 1988 – Milk from suspects destroyed
- November 1989 – No specified bovine offal to humans

Animal health controls

The principle animal health control measure is the prohibition of feeding ruminant derived protein (other than milk or milk protein) to ruminant animals. This was implemented on 18 July 1988 and stemmed from the results of the epidemiological investigation. Its effects in reducing new exposures via feed, and thus the development of disease 4–5 years later, are now being observed. If the feed ban had not been introduced there would have been at least 20 000 more cases of BSE in 1992 than actually occurred.

Other control measures instituted to protect animal health

- June 1988 – Notifiable – Restrictions – Isolation
- July 1988 – No ruminant protein in ruminant feed
- September 1990 – No specified bovine offal to any species

From June 1988 the clinical suspicion of BSE became notifiable thus improving the ascertainment of disease. Suspect animals were not permitted to be moved from the premises but did not have to be isolated unless parturient. From 8 August 1988 clinical suspects believed to have BSE on inspection by a MAFF veterinary officer were slaughtered (with compensation) and the carcase was destroyed except, for the brain which was taken for microscopic examination to confirm the disease.

Because the placenta of sheep with scrapie is infective and, because in June 1988 it was assumed that in a worst scenario situation BSE would be similarly transmitted via the placenta, isolation of suspect parturient cows in approved premises was required. Such cows have to be kept isolated for 72 h after parturition and the placenta, discharges and bedding have to be destroyed and the isolation premises disinfected. Infectivity has not been found in placenta following bioassay in mice, or so far by bioassay in cattle, though this study is still in progress. Nevertheless the regulations stay in place.

Finally, following the successful experimental transmission of SE to a pig after parenteral challenge with pooled brain from cattle confirmed to have BSE, the SBO ban was extended to all species. The aim was primarily to prevent exposure of pigs to BSE, but it was considered wise to extend the ban to cover all animal and avian species.

A number of other control measures have been adopted by the UK authorities, by the EC and some other countries. The export of SBO or protein derived from them from Great Britain to any other country is prohibited. Such material must be destroyed and cannot even be used as a fertiliser. Safety guidelines have been provided for the biological industries directing them to source their bovine tissues from safe animals, herds and countries and specifying the methods of collection. Guidelines have also been provided for workers in at-risk occupations – such as veterinary surgeons, farmers, abattoir workers and those dealing with the transport and incineration of suspect animals. Improved record keeping systems have also been implemented for cattle and records must be kept for 10 years.

Outside the UK all countries with BSE have a complete or partial ban on feeding of ruminant derived protein, and Switzerland has an SBO ban similar to that in the UK.

The EC continuously reviews the BSE situation within Member States and decisions aimed at reducing or preventing any risk from cattle or cattle products that might carry infection have been taken. The UK is permitted to export calves under 6 months of age (which are slaughtered before they reach 6 months of age in the Member State of destination), provided the calves are not the offspring of a suspect or confirmed case, deboned and carcase beef and embryos subject to conditions and semen, hides, skins, milk and milk products which are perceived to present negligible risk unconditionally. However, certain non-food products destined for use in biological product manufacture are banned for export from the UK. These include SBO, bovine placenta, serum, endocrine organs and other lymphoid tissues.

All bovine carcases suspected to have BSE (which of course includes all those in which disease is finally confirmed – about 85% of the total on average) are now destroyed by incineration using a hearth temperature in excess of 750°C and a short after-burner temperature in excess of 1000°C. It is inconceivable that sufficient agent could survive such an environment in sufficient quantity to cause disease, even if the products of combustion could, in some unforeseen way contaminate grassland or cattle feed.

The chronology of introduction of the various control measures is shown in Table 7.

Table 7 Legislation in Great Britain — important dates

Notification	21 June 1988
Ruminant feed ban	18 July 1988
Slaughter and compensation (50%)	8 August 1988
Compensation increased (100%)	14 February 1990
Specified bovine offals (SBO) ban (man)	13 November 1989
SBO ban (all species)	25 September 1990
Prohibition on export of SBO to EC member states	25 September 1990
Prohibition on export of SBO (all countries)	10 July 1991
Prohibition on use of SBO in fertilisers	6 November 1991

CONCLUSION

It would seem that we are currently at a critical point in the epidemic with all the controls necessary to conclude it in place. It is hoped that the case control study of 'born after the ban' animals will confirm that there are no significant loopholes permitting further infections of the national cattle herd. Although some uncertainty remains the results of the monitoring of the epidemic auger well for its continued decline and eventual eradication. Even if this does not proceed as smoothly as is hoped comprehensive measures to protect public health are already in place and will be effective irrespective of the progress of the epidemic in cattle.

ACKNOWLEDGEMENTS

The authors thank many colleagues (too many to mention individually) but particularly those at the Central Veterinary Laboratory, Weybridge and at the Institute for Animal Health, AFRC/MRC Neuropathogenesis Unit in Edinburgh, for access to data. The secretarial support from Mrs W Bolton, the typing skills of Mrs E Davies and figure preparation by Mrs Y Spencer and Mrs C Humphries are also gratefully acknowledged. We appreciate comments on the script from Mr K C Taylor.

REFERENCES

1 Anon. Scrapie-like disease in a captive nyala. Animal Health 1986. Report of the Chief Veterinary Officer. London: HMSO, 1987; p.69.

2 Wells GAH, Scott AC, Johnson CT, et al. A novel progressive spongiform encephalopathy in cattle. Vet Rec 1987; 121: 419-420.

3 Hope J, Reekie LJD, Hunter N, et al. Fibrils from brains of cows with new cattle disease contain scrapie-associated protein. Nature 1988; 336: 390-392.

4 The Movement of Animals (Records) Order. Statutory Instrument 1960; No 105. London: HMSO, 1960.

5 The Tuberculosis (England and Wales) Order. Statutory Instrument 1984; No 1943. London: HMSO 1984.

6 The Tuberculosis (Scotland) Order. Statutory Instrument 1984; No 2063 (S.163) London: HMSO, 1984.

7 The Meat Products and Spreadable Fish Products Regulations. Schedule 2, Part I and Part II. Statutory Instruments 1984; No 1566. London:HMSO, 1984.

8 The Bovine Offal (Prohibition) Regulations. Statutory Instrument 1989; No. 2061. HMSO: London, 1989.

9 Cranwell MP, Hancock RD, Hudson JR, et al. Bovine spongiform encephalopathy. Vet Rec 1988; 122: 190.

10 Gilmour JS, Buxton D, Macleod, NSM, Brodie TA, Moore JB. Bovine spongiform encephalopathy. Vet Rec 1988; 122: 142.

11 Wells GAH, Hancock RD, Cooley WA, Richards MS, Higgins RJ, David GP. Bovine spongiform encephalopathy; diagnostic significance of vacuolar change in selected nuclei of the medulla oblongata. Vet Rec 1989; 125: 521-524.

12 Bradley R, Matthews D. Sub-acute, transmissible spongiform encephalopathies: current concepts and future needs. Rev sci tech Off int Epiz 1922; 11: 605-634.

13 Wilesmith JW, Wells GAH, Cranwell MP, Ryan JBM. Bovine spongiform encephalopathy: epidemiological studies. Vet Rec 1988; 123: 638-644.

14 Wilesmith JW, Ryan JBM, Atkinson MJ. Bovine spongiform encephalopathy: epidemiological studies on the origin. Vet Rec 1991; 128: 199-203.

15 Fraser H, McConnell I, Wells GAH, Dawson M. Transmission of bovine spongiform encephalopathy to mice. Vet Rec 1988; 123: 472.

16 Dawson M, Wells GAH, Parker BNJ. Preliminary evidence of the experimental transmissibility of bovine spongiform encephalopathy to cattle. Vet Rec 1990; 126: 112-113.

17 Mould DL, Dawson AM, Smith W. Scrapie in mice. The stability of the agent to various suspending media, pH and solvent extraction. Res Vet Sci 1965; 6: 151-154.

18 Brown P, Liberski PP, Wolff A, Gadjusek DC. Resistance of scrapie infectivity to steam autoclaving after formaldehyde fixation and limited survival after ashing at 360°C. Practical and theoretical implications. J Inf Dis 1990; 161: 467-472.

19 Gibbs Jr CJ, Safar J, Ceroni M, DiMartino A, Clark WW, Hourrigan JL. Experimental transmission of scrapie to cattle. Lancet 1990; 335: 1275.

20 Wilesmith JW, Ryan JBM, Hueston WD. Bovine spongiform encephalopathy: case control studies of calf feeding practices and meat and bone meal inclusion in proprietary concentrates. Res Vet Sci 1992; 52: 325-331.
21 Denny GO, Wilesmith JW, Clements RA, Hueston WD. Bovine spongiform encephalopathy in Northern Ireland: epidemiological observations 1988–1990. Vet Rec 1992; 130: 113-116.
22 Wilesmith JW. Bovine spongiform encephalopathy and related diseases: an epidemiological overview. NZ Vet J 1993 (In press).
23 Hadlow WJ, Kennedy RC, Race RE. Natural infection of sheep with scrapie virus. J Infect Dis 1982; 146: 657-664.
24 Kimberlin RH, Cole S, Walker CA. Temporary and permanent modifications to a single strain of mouse scrapie on transmission to rats and hamsters. J Gen Virol 1987; 68: 1875-1881.
25 Wood JLN, Lund LJ, Done SH. The natural occurrence of scrapie in moufflon. Vet Rec 1992; 130: 25-27.
26 Wyatt JM, Pearson GR, Smerdon T, Gruffydd-Jones TJ, Wells GAH. Spongiform encephalopathy in a cat. Vet Rec 1990; 126: 513.
27 Mitrova E, Mayer V. Neurohistology of early preclinical lesions in experimental subacute spongiform encephalopathy. Biologia (Bratislava) 1977; 32, 663-671.
28 Fraser H, Bruce ME, Chree A, McConnell I, Wells GAH. Transmission of bovine spongiform encephalopathy and scrapie to mice. J. Gen. Virol. 1992 73: 1891-1897.
29 Foster JD, Hope J, McConnell I, Fraser H. Slow infections of the central nervous system. Ann NY Acad Sci (In Press).
30 Dawson M, Wells GAH, Parker BNJ, Scott AC. Primary parenteral transmission of bovine spongiform encephalopathy to the pig. Vet Rec 1990; 127: 338.
31 Pattison IH, Hoare MN, Jebbett JN, Watson WA. Further observations on the introduction of scrapie in sheep by oral dosing with foetal membranes from scrapie-affected sheep. Br Vet J 1974; 130: LXV-LXVII.
32 Taguchi F, Tamai Y, Miura S. Experiments on maternal and paternal transmission of Creutzfeldt-Jakob disease in mice. Arch Virol 1993; 130: 219-224.
33 Taylor KC. The control of bovine spongiform encephalopathy in Great Britain. Vet Rec 1991; 129: 522-526.
34 Kimberlin RH. Bovine spongiform encephalopathy. FAO Animal Production and Health Paper 109, Rome: FAO; 1993.

British Medical Bulletin (1993) Vol. 49, No. 4, pp 960–970

Epidemiology of Creutzfeldt-Jakob disease

R G Will
National Creutzfeldt-Jakob Disease Surveillance Unit, Western General Hospital, Edinburgh, UK

Extensive information on the epidemiology of Creutzfeldt-Jakob Disease (CJD) has accumulated since the original transmission of CJD to primates in 1968. One aim of this research was to discover the mechanism of natural transmission of CJD but the epidemiological evidence virtually precludes case to case transmission as a causative mechanism, except in rare iatrogenic cases, and has provided little evidence to suggest an environmental 'source of infection'. An understanding of the few positive epidemiological findings such as the high incidence in Slovakia has depended on major advances in molecular biology rather than on epidemiological evidence. The occurrence of Bovine Spongiform Encephalopathy (BSE) has however reinforced the importance of having established the epidemiological characteristics of CJD and this information is an important background on which to evaluate the findings from basic scientific research.

INCIDENCE/GEOGRAPHICAL DISTRIBUTION OF CJD

The incidence of CJD is commonly quoted as 1 case per million per year. The basis for this figure is difficult to establish as systematic surveys have consistently documented an incidence of around 0.5 cases per million per annum.[1] The possibility of a true incidence rate that is significantly higher has arisen at least in part because of the reports from a number of countries of localised areas of high incidence. The rarity of CJD however may result in sampling error if incidence figures are based on the numbers of cases in a restricted area over a limited period of time. The geographical distribution of CJD in the United Kingdom over the past 20 years demonstrates no overall evidence of spatio-temporal aggregation of cases,[2] despite the occurrence of local areas of relatively high incidence over short periods.

Although contact between individual cases of CJD has been discovered this is exceptional and the absence of convincing evidence of aggregation of cases of CJD in any systematic survey indicates that CJD, as a rare and geographically widespread phenomenon, cannot be maintained by case to case transmission. The implication is that close contact with cases of CJD cannot be a risk factor for the development of disease. Spouses of sporadic cases do not have an increased incidence of disease[1] and in familial aggregates only those with a mutation of the 'prion protein gene' develop disease despite close contact between individual family members, often over decades.[3] Molecular biological evidence has also demonstrated that the 60–100 fold increase in incidence of CJD in Slovakia and Libyan born Israelis is related to a high frequency of PrP gene mutations and not to contact transmission or environmental risk factors.[4,5]

Following the original transmission of CJD, scrapie in sheep was considered as a candidate risk factor for CJD and dietary exposure to scrapie was originally proposed as an explanation for the high incidence of CJD in Libyan born Israelis.[6]

Scrapie is endemic in many countries, including the UK and France, and isolated scrapie outbreaks have been described in other countries previously thought to be free of scrapie including Japan, Sweden and probably Czechoslovakia. The absence of scrapie in any country is difficult to verify and depends on adequate veterinary surveillance but some countries are almost certainly free of scrapie including Australia and New Zealand. This contrasts with the distribution of CJD which has been identified in all developed countries, including Australia and New Zealand, and in an increasing number of countries with less well developed medical services. It is reasonable to presume that CJD occurs throughout the world[7] and furthermore available evidence suggests that the incidence in individual countries is independent either of the sheep population or the incidence of scrapie. Not only does this suggest that scrapie is unlikely to be causally related to CJD but also that any putative risk factor must be ubiquitous and independent of climatic, cultural or economic differences between countries. Evidence from co-purification studies and transgenic models provides powerful, if not conclusive, evidence that the transmissible agent is devoid of nucleic acid and may be a novel biological phenomenon in the form of a self-replicating protein.[8] It strains credibility to suggest that there is a ubiquitous environmental pool of such a protein and this has led to the proposition that sporadic cases of CJD may be due to spontaneous generation of a self-replicating protein, perhaps by somatic mutation.[9]

The presumed one-in-a-million chance of such a random event correlates broadly with the incidence of CJD and leads to the prediction that the incidence of CJD should increase linearly with age, as with other spontaneous mutations. Age specific incidence rates in CJD have however consistently shown a rapid decrease over the age of 70.[1,10]

Any hypothesis must also explain the marked clinico-pathological variation in CJD including cases with a diffuse cortical onset, those which are predominantly occipital or cerebellar and rare cases with a unilateral clinical and pathological pattern.[11] Epidemiological research has failed to establish the cause of CJD and the largely negative evidence has provided powerful support to the search for host determinants to the risk of disease. However the epidemiological features and clinico-pathological characteristics of CJD are now firmly established and must be accounted for by any new aetiological hypotheses.

RISK FACTORS FOR CJD

Familial incidence

The familial occurrence of CJD in 5–15% of cases with an apparently dominant pattern of inheritance has been recognized for decades.[7] Molecular biological research has now demonstrated that the familial occurrence of CJD is related to the presence of mutations of the prion protein (PrP) gene and not to contact transmission or vertical transmission of a viral-like agent.[3] The identification of affected families with branches in different countries with no possible contact between individual pedigrees provides powerful support to the view that PrP gene mutations are causative and not simply susceptibility genes. This molecular biological evidence has understandably prompted questions regarding the epidemiology of CJD, reinforced by the wide range of phenotypic expression in familial CJD and GSS.[12] Both within and between individual families there may be variation in clinical presentation and pathological features with a proportion of cases neither clinically nor pathologically typical of CJD. This raises the possibility that prion diseases might be more widespread than previously recognized, and indeed genetic screening of a range of familial neurodegenerative disorders has resulted in the identification of novel phenotypes including Fatal Familial Insomnia.[13] It has also been established that the high incidence of CJD in Slovakian and Libyan-born Israelis is related to a high frequency of the codon 200 mutation of the PrP gene and not due to other factors such as dietary exposure to scrapie. Although such discoveries are of crucial scientific importance, the relevance to the overall epidemiology of CJD remains unclear. Other than a slightly earlier average age of onset of disease, the clinical features in association with the codon 200 mutation are indistinguishable from CJD[14] and in families with other mutations, including those with multiple octopeptide repeats, the onset of progressive neuropsychiatric dysfunction at an early age is rare in general neurological practice. Extrapolating from this evidence, which is based on highly selected and atypical families, to the overall epidemiology is hardly scientific.[15] Preliminary evidence from screening studies in dementia[16] and from a group of cases of atypical dementia[17] suggests that PrP mutations in suspect Alzheimer's disease or unusual forms of sporadic dementia are likely to be discovered only exceptionally in these groups, if at all. Screening of a range of other neurodegenerative disorders, including Parkinson's disease, motor neurone disease and Pick's disease, for PrP gene mutations is surely in progress in centres throughout the world, but on current evidence the assertion that disorders associated with PrP gene mutations are likely to be common is unproven and unlikely.

The frequency of familial CJD, and by implication pedigrees associated with PrP gene mutations, ranges between 6–15% of cases of CJD in different studies.[1] This disparity is due to differing methodologies of ascertainment and also varying criteria for the definition of a familial case. Rigid criteria requiring the identification of definite or probable CJD in more than one family member will inevitably underestimate the true familial incidence. Criteria allowing any case of dementia in a relative of an index case to be classified as CJD will overestimate the familial incidence because of the inclusion of cases of more common forms of dementia such as Alzheimer's disease. The familial incidence of CJD is therefore likely to lie between the extremes at perhaps 10% of all cases. Therefore, even in the paradigm condition associated with PrP mutations, up to 90% of cases do not exhibit a mutation of the PrP gene. Synthesizing all this evidence, it is reasonable to conclude that despite the fact that molecular biological evidence has resolved some of the epidemiological paradoxes of CJD, the basic epidemiological parameters of CJD established by systematic and descriptive studies remain valid.

Iatrogenic transmission

The accidental transmission of CJD from person to person has depended on the direct inoculation of contaminated material either centrally or peripherally[18] (Table 1).

Central inoculation through neurosurgery, depth electrodes, corneal graft or dura mater graft results in disease after a mean incubation period of about 2 yr and a clinical presentation similar to sporadic CJD. Peripheral inoculation through human pituitary derived growth hormone (hGH) or pituitary derived gonadotrophin (hGnH) results in disease after an incubation period range from a minimum of 4 yr to a maximum of at least 30 yr with a mean of around 12 yr. The clinical presentation in

Table 1 Summary of Iatrogenic cases of Creutzfeldt-Jakob Disease (1992)

Mode of infection	Number of patients	Agent entry into brain	Mean incubation period (range)	Clinical presentation
Instrumentation				
Neurosurgery*	4	Intra-cerebral	22 months (18–28)	Dementia
Stereotactic EEG	2	Intra-cerebral	18 months (16–20)	Dementia
Tissue transfer				
Corneal transplant	1	Optic nerve	18 months	Dementia
Dura mater implant	6	Cerebral surface	42 months (19–84)	Dementia
*Tissue extract transfer***				
Growth hormone	21	Hematogenous	12 yr (4–30)	Cerebellar
Gonadotrophin	2	Hematogenous	13 yr (13–13)	Cerebellar

*Several additional CJD patients with preceding neurosurgery, but no proven link to CJD, are not tabulated. **Means calculated from the treatment mid-point to onset of symptomatic CJD in published and unpublished cases.

hGH and hGnH recipients is remarkably stereotyped with a progressive cerebellar syndrome and the development of cognitive impairment late, if at all. This closely parallels the clinical course in kuru and the likeliest explanation of the contrasting clinical presentation between central and peripheral inoculation is the route of inoculation of the agent. There is preliminary evidence of a genetic influence on susceptibility in hGH recipients with a relative excess of valine homozygosity at codon 129 of the PrP gene in individuals who have developed CJD after this therapy.[19] This contrasts with a relative excess of methionine homozygosity at codon 129 in cases of sporadic CJD[20] and in iatrogenic cases due to central contamination, therefore providing some support to the hypothesis that sporadic CJD may develop centrally and spontaneously rather than due to some external factor.

Some 1700 individuals in the UK and about 25,000 worldwide are at risk of developing CJD through prior treatment with hGH, but unfortunately genotyping at codon 129 is not sufficiently discriminating to allow identification of relative risk in the individual recipient. The risk in these individuals of developing CJD has been judged to be approximately 1 in 200 on the basis of epidemiological data[18] and laboratory studies of decontamination procedures.[21] Recently the increasing numbers of CJD affected hGH recipients in France has indicated that the relative risk may vary from country to country perhaps in relation to the level of contamination of source material.

The tragic occurrence of CJD in hGH recipients has led to difficult ethical dilemmas, for example whether at-risk individuals should be informed of this risk, and to a reassessment of measures to prevent

further episodes of accidental transmission. Contamination through neurosurgical procedures is now most unlikely to occur in the UK because
of improved standards of sterilisation and guidelines from the Department of Health which recommend destruction of any potentially contaminated neurosurgical instruments. The recommendation that corneas
should not be taken for transplantation from any demented patient is
clearly essential but the multiple contaminating events that must have
occurred in relation to both hGH and dura mater grafts suggest that
guidelines to ensure safe sourcing of human material cannot be fool-
proof. In combination with a latency of many years (at least 20 yr in
hGH) before the realisation of the risk of transmission of CJD, this
indicates that caution is essential in the use of human derived tissue
from the CNS or adjacent structures in the production of medicinal
products.

Dietary factors

The possibility that dietary contamination with the scrapie agent might
lead to CJD is a hypothesis that has been eroded by cumulative epidemiological and molecular biological evidence. The anecdotal reports
of CJD developing in individuals with dietary exposure to sheep brain[22]
or other potentially scrapie-infected material have been balanced by
reports of CJD in vegetarians.[23,24] Case-control studies have been mu-
tually contradictory and have revealed no consistent evidence of an
increase of incidence of CJD in relation to dietary factors. The increased
incidence in Libyan-born Israelis, already commented on, is now known
to be due to molecular biological factors rather than dietary factors, consistent with the previous case-control study which showed no difference
in dietary habits between affected and unaffected members in this ethnic
group.[25] In Iceland the distribution of scrapie has been under study for
many years and has established that scrapie is endemic in the north of
the island but not in the south. Despite the fact that scrapie-infected
material is known to have been consumed, including sheep brain, there
have been only two cases of CJD in Iceland in the past 35 yr, representing an incidence of 1 case per 3 million per annum, and both these
individuals were born and lived outside the scrapie endemic area.[26]

Together with the disparity between the worldwide distributions of
scrapie and CJD, available evidence suggests that scrapie cannot be
an important aetiological factor in CJD, although the possibility that
scrapie is causally linked to occasional cases of CJD cannot be completely excluded.

Occupation

Occupation as a risk factor for CJD was originally investigated because
of the possibility that occupational exposure to the scrapie agent might

result in an increased risk of developing CJD. Descriptive and analytic studies have failed to provide any convincing evidence of an increased risk in relation to occupation, although the small numbers of cases in at-risk occupational groups does 'not permit any meaningful conclusions to be drawn about relative risk, whatever statistical tests are used'.[1] For example, in France the annual mortality rate per million in shepherds of 3.81 cases has to be put in the context of the apparent 'elevated' mortality rate of 3.08 per million in the clerical profession.[1] The possibility that contact with cases of CJD might lead to increased risk led to careful analysis of the frequency of CJD in medical and paramedical staff. Although one early study showed an apparent increase of frequency of CJD within these groups,[7] no overall increased risk has been discovered from systematic surveys, including a case-control analysis of occupation throughout life.[2] This indicates that contact with individual patients suffering from CJD is unlikely to be a risk in itself and this is borne out by the epidemiological evidence which suggests that there is no significantly increased risk to spouses of affected patients.

There have been individual case reports of Creutzfeldt-Jakob disease developing in a neurosurgeon, a pathologist, 2 histology technicians and most recently in an individual who had processed human and sheep dura mater.[27,28]

Although the title of the latter article was 'Transmission of Creutzfeldt-Jakob disease by handling of dura mater', any causal link between these occupations and the development of Creutzfeldt-Jakob disease is hypothetical and must be judged on a background of the known epidemiology which has demonstrated no definite occupational links. This also applies to the recent description of CJD developing in an individual occupationally exposed to Bovine Spongiform Encephalopathy (BSE)[29] as every occupation will inevitably be represented if systematic epidemiological surveys are continued for long enough. Both farmers and shepherds have been identified in systematic surveys in the decades prior to the advent of BSE and in countries which were, or are, free of this condition. The current case-control study of occupation in the United Kingdom has shown no significant difference between cases and controls and in particular no difference in the frequency of various 'at-risk' occupations (such as abattoir workers, farmers or butchers) in which there is a potential occupational exposure to CNS tissue from BSE affected animals.

BOVINE SPONGIFORM ENCEPHALOPATHY

Following the occurrence of BSE in the United Kingdom, the South-wood Committee recommended the re-institution of epidemiological surveillance of CJD, although it was judged that the risk to the human population posed by BSE was likely to be remote.[30]

A prospective study of the epidemiology of CJD has been underway since May 1990 and a retrospective survey of CJD between 1985 and April 1990 has now been completed. Information is available from previous surveillance of CJD in England and Wales carried out by Professor WB Matthews of the University of Oxford which covered the years 1970–1984. There is therefore information available on the epidemiology and clinical features of CJD for the 15 years prior to BSE which will allow a comparison with similar parameters post 1985.

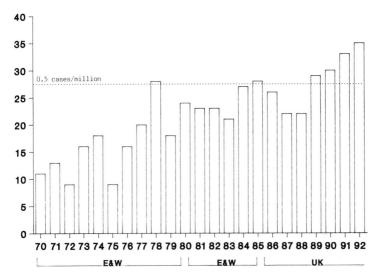

Fig. 1 Deaths from CJD (definite and probable cases) 1970-1992

Figure 1 shows the incidence of CJD from 1970 to 1992. Although there was an increase in incidence in Creutzfeldt-Jakob disease in England and Wales in the early 1970s, almost certainly due to increased case recognition with time as in France over the same period[1] (Fig. 2), there has been no significant overall change in the incidence of CJD since the mid 1970s. This is despite variations that might have occurred due to the different methodologies in the various study periods and the different population bases examined. Neither has there been a change in the clinical features or geographical distribution of Creutzfeldt-Jakob

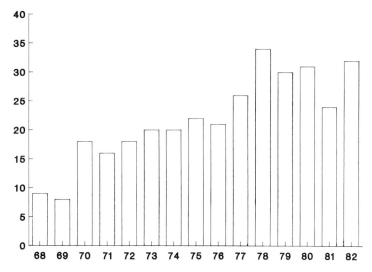

Fig. 2 Deaths from CJD in France 1968-1982.

disease pre- and post-BSE and the overall epidemiological picture indicates that there has been no change in Creutzfeldt-Jakob disease that can be attributable to BSE up to the present time. The incubation period in kuru and in iatrogenic CJD however indicate that it will be many years before any such change can be finally excluded. Although there is no consensus about the potential risk of BSE to the human population, assessment of available scientific evidence suggests that this risk is likely to be remote and that the surveillance programme will not demonstrate any change in the epidemiology of CJD in the future. Nonetheless the systematic accumulation of detailed information on incident cases of CJD will provide hard data on the natural disease which will be an important background on which to judge novel scientific hypotheses.

REFERENCES

1 Brown P, Cathala F, Raubertas RF, Gajdusek DC, Cataigne P. The epidemiology of Creutzfeldt-Jakob disease: Conclusion of a 15-year investigation in France and review of the world literature. Neurology 1987; 37: 895-904.
2 Harries-Jones R, Knight R, Will RG, Cousens S, Smith PG, Matthews WB. Creutzfeldt-Jakob disease in England and Wales, 1980–1984: a case-control study of potential risk factors. J Neurol Neurosurg Psych 1988; 51: 1113-1119.
3 Goldfarb LG, Brown P, Gajdusek DC. The molecular genetics of human transmissible spongiform encephalopathy. In: Prusiner SB, Collinge J, Powell J, Anderton B, eds. Prion Diseases of Humans and Animals. Ellis Horwood, 1992: 139-153.

4 Mitrova E, Bronis M. Clusters of CJD in Slovakia: the first statistically significant temporo-spatial accumulations of rural cases. Eur J Epidemiol 1991; 7(5): 450-456.
5 Hsiao K, Meiner Z, Kahana E, et al. Mutation of the prion protein in Libyan Jews with Creutzfeldt-Jakob disease. N Engl J Med 1991; 324: 1091-1097.
6 Alter M. Creutzfeldt-Jakob disease: hypothesis for high incidence in Libyan Jews in Israel. Science 1974; 186: 848.
7 Masters CL, Harris JO, Gajdusek DC, Gibbs CJ Jr, Bernoulli C, Asher DM. Creutzfeldt-Jakob disease: patterns of worldwide occurrence and the significance of familial and sporadic clustering. Ann Neurol 1979; 5: 177-188.
8 Prusiner SB. Molecular biology and transgenetics of prion diseases. Crit Rev Biochem Mol Biol 1991; 26(5/6): 397-438.
9 Hsiao K, Prusiner SB. Inherited human prion diseases. Neurology 1990; 40: 1820-1827.
10 Will RG, Matthews WB, Smith PG, Hudson C. A retrospective study of Creutzfeldt-Jakob disease in England and Wales 1970–1979 II: epidemiology. J Neurol Neurosurg Psych 1986; 49: 749-755.
11 Heye N, Cervos-Navarro J. Focal involvement and lateralization in Creutzfeldt-Jakob disease: correlation of clinical, electroencephalographic and neuropathological findings. Eur Neurol 1992; 32: 289-292.
12 Collinge J, Brown J, Hardy J, et al. Inherited prion disease with 144 base pair gene insertion. 2. Clinical and pathological features. Brain 1992; 115: 687-710.
13 Medori R, Tritschler HJ, LeBlanc A, et al. Fatal familial insomnia, a prion disease with a mutation at codon 178 of the prion protein gene. N Engl J Med 1992; 326: 444-449.
14 Brown P, Goldfarb L, Gibbs CJ, Gajdusek DC. The phenotypic expression of different mutations in transmissible familial Creutzfeldt-Jakob disease. Eur J Epidemiol 1991; 7: 469-476.
15 Will RG. Prion disease (Letter). Lancet 1990; 336: 369.
16 Schellenberg GD, Anderson L, O'Dahl S, et al. APP-717 APP-693 and PRIP gene mutations are rare in Alzheimer's disease. Am J Hum Genet 1991; 49(3): 511-517.
17 Brown P, Kaur P, Sulima MP, Goldfarb L, Gibbs CJ Jr, Gajdusek DC. Real and imagined clinicopathological limits of 'prion dementia'. Lancet 1993; 341: 127-129.
18 Brown P, Preece MA, Will RG. 'Friendly fire' in medicine: hormones, homografts, and Creutzfeldt-Jakob disease. Lancet 1992; 340: 24-27.
19 Collinge J, Palmer MS, Dryden AJ. Genetic predisposition to iatrogenic Creutzfeldt-Jakob disease. Lancet 1991; 337: 1441-1442.
20 Palmer MS, Dryden AJ, Hughes JT, Collinge J. Homozygous prion protein genotype predisposes to sporadic Creutzfeldt-Jakob disease. Nature 1991; 352: 340-341.
21 Pocchiari M, Peano S, Conz A, et al. Combination ultrafiltration and 6M-urea treatment of human growth hormone effectively minimizes risk from potential Creutzfeldt-Jakob disease virus contamination. Hormone Res 991; 35(3-4): 161-166.
22 Lo Russo F, Neri G, Figa-Talamanca L. Creutzfeldt-Jakob disease and sheep brain: a report from Central and Southern Italy. Ital J Neurol Sci 1980; 3: 171-174.
23 Matthews WB, Will RG. Creutzfeldt-Jakob disease in a lifelong vegetarian. Lancet 1981; ii: 937.
24 Singhal BS, Dastur DK. Creutzfeldt-Jakob disease in Western India. Neuroepidemiology 1983; 2: 93-100.
25 Goldberg H, Alter M, Kahana E. The Libyan Jewish focus of Creutzfeldt-Jakob disease: a search for the mode of natural transmission. In: Prusiner SB, Hadlow WJ, eds. Slow transmissible diseases of the nervous system. New York: Academic Press, 1979; 195-211.
26 Sigurdarson S. Epidemiology of scrapie in Iceland and experience with control measures. In: Bradley R, Savey M, Marchant B, eds. Sub-acute spongiform encephalopathies. London: Kluwer Academic, 1991: 233-242.
27 Berger JR, David NJ. Creutzfeldt-Jakob disease in a physician: review of the disorder in health care workers. Neurology 1993; 43: 205-206.

28 Weber T, Tumani H, Holdorff B, et al. Transmission of Creutzfeldt-Jakob disease by handling of dura mater. Lancet 1993; 341: 123-124.
29 Sawcer SJ, Yuill GM, Esmonde TFG, et al. Creutzfeldt-Jakob disease in an individual occupationally exposed to BSE. Lancet 1993; 341: 642.
30 Southwood Committee. Report of the Working Party on Bovine Spongiform Encephalopathy. London: Department of Health and Ministry of Agriculture, Fisheries and Food. 1989: ISBN 185197-405-9.

British Medical Bulletin (1993) Vol. 49, No. 4, pp. 971–979
©The British Council 1993

Developments in diagnosis for prion diseases

J Tateishi
T Kitamoto
Department of Neuropathology, Neurological Institute, Faculty of Medicine, Kyushu University, Fukuoka, Japan

The protease resistant isoform of prion protein (PrP) is a diagnostic marker of spongiform encephalopathies in humans and animals. Immunoblotting is a sensitive method but requires either fresh or frozen, unfixed materials. Immunohistochemistry using formalin-fixed, paraffin-embedded materials is now also considered to be sensitive and comparable to immunoblotting after various treatments, especially using the hydrolytic autoclaving method on tissue sections before staining. The advantage of this method is that it can be applied to routine pathology materials or long preserved materials. The kuru plaque-type deposition of PrP suggests abnormalities of the PrP gene, while synaptic-type deposition suggests either sporadic CJD or particular familial CJD. PrP gene abnormalities are thus related to PrP deposition and modify clinical symptoms and their progression. A PrP gene analysis can be done using either preclinical, clinical or post-mortem materials.

A protease resistant isoform (PrP^{CJD}, PrP^{Sc}) of the prion protein (PrP) has been exclusively detected in humans and animals with spongiform encephalopathies. Human and laboratory animal brains with either no disease or other diseases have never shown PrP^{CJD}, while those with PrP^{CJD} have often transmitted spongiform encephalopathies to laboratory animals, especially to mice in our laboratory. A cellular isoform (PrP^C) of the protein exists in normal cells, and can be eliminated by protease digestion and does not disturb the detection of PrP^{CJD} in our diagnostic procedures.

IMMUNOBLOTTING

We used various polyclonal antibodies raised against kuru plaque cores (KPC) purified from a patient with Gerstmann-Sträussler-Scheinker syndrome (GSS),[1] against amyloid fraction purified from CJD-infected mouse brains,[1] as well as against synthetic peptides with sequences identical to the 15 residues (138th–152nd amino acid)[1] corresponding to the putative cytoplasmic domain of human PrP[2], and 25 residues (25th–49th amino acid)[3] corresponding to the N-terminal domain (PrP-N) and against Fd-PrP fusion protein (Fd-PrP).[3]

Non-purified or a purified PrP fraction of tissue homogenates, were digested with proteinase K and applied on 15% polyacrylamide gel containing 0.1% sodium dodecyl sulphate (SDS). The proteins were electrophoretically transferred onto a Durapore membrane and labelled with anti-PrP.[3] All antibodies reacted similarly with 3 major bands of PrP^{CJD} at 27–31, 23–25 and 19–21 kDa. Without proteinase K digestion, 3 bands moved to 34–36, 29–33 and 24–27 kDa which shifted 5–6 kDa higher than digested PrP^{CJD}, keeping the N-terminal portion of the protein. With proteinase K digestion, PrP^{C} is completely hydrolyzed.

A semiquantitative blot analysis of PrP^{CJD} was done by applying diluted homogenates from both human and mouse tissues.[4] PrP^{CJD} is most abundant in the brains of patients and mice with CJD as in Table 1. A less dense PrP^{CJD} is found in the spinal cords but not in the peripheral nerves and visceral organs of CJD patients, while mice show a detectable amount of PrP^{CJD} in their lymphoreticular systems and intestine with a Peyer's patch. A biopsy on lymphoreticular tissues may also prove PrP^{CJD} in mice or PrP^{SC} in sheep.[5]

Table 1 Amount of tissue (mg) required PrP^{CJD}detection

Organ	CJD patients	Infected mice
Brain	0.3 – 1	0.3
Spinal cord	3 – 10	3
Spleen	ND	1–3
Lymph node	ND	3
Thymus		10
Intestine		10–30
Liver	ND	ND

ND: not detected

IMMUNOHISTOCHEMISTRY

Tissue specimens routinely fixed with formalin and embedded in paraffin are used to detect PrP^{CJD}. PrP^C is only detected by applying monoclonal antibodies on specially fixed tissues.[6,7] Tissues embedded in paraffin preserve immunoreactivity for a long period, while those kept in formalin gradually decrease in immunoreactivity. Paraffin blocks are cut into 7 μm sections which are then routinely mounted on slide glasses and kept warm for 10–20 min at a few degrees higher than the melting temperature of paraffin, in order not to be torn off from the glass slides during pretreatment. The sections are deparaffinized and blocked with 0.3% H_2O_2 in absolute methanol. To promote the binding of antibodies to the epitopes of PrP^{CJD} in the tissue specimens, various pretreatments were applied. We[8] and other groups[9] have reported that protein denaturants such as chaotropic salts, NaOH, heated SDS and formic acid could enhance the immunoreactivity. Among them, a 2 h treatment with 4–6 M guanidine-thiocyanate, 3 M trichloroacetate, and 80% phenol dissolved in ethanol was found to be almost equivalent to that of formic acid.[8] A few minutes treatment with 90–100% formic acid is the simple and most effective method to stain various amyloids, including PrP, β/A4, systemic amyloids: AA or AL, transthyretin (prealbumin), cystatin C (γ-trace) and others.[10] The method enabled us to identify diffuse, primitive and classical senile plaques in brains with Alzheimer's disease, kuru plaques in patients with GSS and small grains of PrP^{CJD} in CJD patients with a clinical course longer than 12 months, but not in patients with a shorter clinical course.[1,10]

A new pretreatment designated as 'hydrolytic autoclaving' revealed a punctuated deposition of PrP^{CJD} in the synaptic structures in almost all patients with CJD. Deparaffinized sections are autoclaved at 121°C for 10 min in a stainless-steel vessel filled with 1, 3, 10 or 30 mM HCl in distilled water to immerse the sections.[11] The longer the periods of formalin fixation, the higher the acidity needed to yield good staining. After the pressure in the autoclave has decreased to the atmospheric pressure, and the temperature drops to 60°C, the sections are taken out and washed with tap water and 50 mM Tris-HCl (pH 7.6).

The sections are incubated with antibodies diluted in TTBS (25 mM Tris-HCl (pH 7.6), 0.05% Tween 20, 0.5 M NaCl) containing 5% nonfat milk at 4°C over night. The following steps are performed with the biotin-streptavidin method (ICN Immunochemicals) or peroxidase-antiperoxidase method (Dakopatts) according to the manufacturer's instructions. Diaminobenzidine (DAB) is used to develop the colour. In case of a double immunostain, different antibodies are successively applied and a different colour is developed with DAB and cobalt chloride in the final step. Immunofluorescent stains are done in the same way using Texas Red or FITC.

Mice inoculated human CJD materials often survive for long periods and show only a mild spongiform change which is difficult to differentiate from that of physiological aging. The presence of PrP[CJD] in such animals can serve as a hallmark of a successful transmission.[1] After serial propagation, mouse-adapted pathogens cause distinct sponginess after short incubation periods around 120 days post i.c. inoculation. In such animals the distribution pattern of PrP[CJD] is different from that of mice in the first inoculation.[12]

In patient brains with GSS or GSS-like diseases with a long clinical course, kuru plaques are stained with anti-PrP[CJD]. Patients with kuru plaques usually possess PrP gene abnormalities to be stated separately, while sporadic CJD patients without gene abnormalities show diffuse gray matter staining corresponding to the synaptic structures.[11] If PrP[CJD] deposition cannot be proven in the brains of humans or animals, a diagnosis of either CJD or allied diseases is not likely.

PrP GENE ANALYSIS

High molecular weight DNA is prepared from either peripheral leukocytes or unfixed tissues as described by Sambrool et al.[13] The PrP coding region is amplified by the polymerase chain reaction (PCR) method as previously reported.[11,14] Each mutation or polymorphism is detected by dot differential hybridization using allele-specific oligonucleotides,[11,14] and by restriction fragment length polymorphism (RFLP) using various restriction enzymes as shown in Table 2. The PrP coding region is fully sequenced in some cases. Each abnormality influences the clinical signs and symptoms, the duration of illness and related pathological findings. Correlative studies of genotypes and phenotypes also have a diagnostic value.

CJD with wild type PrP gene (codon 129 Met/Met)

The majority of CJD patients shows neither heredity nor PrP gene mutation. The disease usually begins in either the presenile or senile ages with initial signs of dementia and then progresses rapidly to a devastated state, accompanied by myoclonus and a characteristic electroencephalogram (periodic synchronous discharge, PSD). Death usually occurs within 2 years. Pathology shows severe spongiform changes, as well as a loss of nerve cells and gliosis. PrP[CJD] deposits develop diffusely in the gray matter corresponding to the synaptic structures but do not form Congophilic amyloid plaques (kuru plaques).

Table 2 Changes in the PrP gene and the restriction enzymes used

Codon	Base	Amino acid	Enzyme used for RFL
51 – 91	Insertion 144, 168, 216 bp	48, 56, 72 residues	
102	CCG → CTG	Pro → Leu	Dde I
105	CCA → CTA	Pro → Leu	Alu I
117	GCA → GTG	Ala → Val	Pvu II
129	* ATG or GTG	Met or Val	Nsp I
145	TAT → TAG	Tyr → Stop	Mae I
178	GAC → AAC	Asp → Asn	Tth 111I
180	GTC → ATC	Val → Ile	Tth 111I
198	TTC → TCC	Phe → Ser	Hph I
200	GAG → AAG	Glu → Lys	BsmA I
217	CAG → CGG	Gln → Arg	Msp I
232	ATG → AGG	Met → Arg	Nla III

* normal variant modifying phenotype (see text).

CJD with a 168 bp insertion

After 7 years of progressive dementia and ataxic gait in the later stages, a 36-year-old Japanese woman died of subdural hematoma. Her brain showed mild atrophy, subcortical gliosis and loosely packed deposits of PrP[CJD], which were not stained with Congo red. The PCR products showed a 0.9 kbp large fragment in addition to an ordinary 0.74 kbp fragment. The sequence data revealed an additional 7 repeats of octapeptides (PHGGGWGQ) inserted between codon 51 and 91. Other insertions[15,16] or deletions[17] have also been reported in this proline-glycine rich domain. Patients with these genotypes mainly show dementia which is often difficult to differentiate from senile dementia.

GSS with Leu[102]

Proline to leucine substitution at codon 102 was first reported by Hsiao et al,[18] followed by detection in a descendant of the original case reported by Gerstmann, Sträussler and Scheinker.[19] Initial ataxic symptoms gradually progress like hereditary cerebellar degenerative diseases. Dementia appears in the later stages of a long clinical course of over several years. Myoclonus and PSD are not common. Pathologically, spongiform change, severe loss of nerve cells and gliosis are not common, but Congophilic kuru plaques are frequent. Immunostaining shows numerous and various types of PrP plaques[20] as well as synaptic type depositions to a milder degree.[11]

GSS with Val[117] and Val[129]

A missense mutation from alanine to valine at codon 117 combines with valine at codon 129 in one allele. This mutation was found in a large

Alsatian family[21] and in one USA family of German descent.[22] The predominant clinical picture was that of a triad of pyramidal, pseudobulbar syndrome and dementia. Multicentric PrP plaques were found but no synaptic-type diffuse gray matter stainings were observed.[11]

CJD with Val[129]

Codon 129 of the PrP gene has two variant alleles, one coding for methionine (Met[129]) and the other for valine (Val[129]) among the general population. Ethnic differences exist between the Japanese and UK populations as shown in Table 3. The frequency of the methionine allele is much higher among populations in Japan[14] than in the UK.[23] The ratio of the valine allele increases in CJD patients in Japan[24] and iatrogenic CJD patients in UK.[25] Val/Val[129] is often reported in iatrogenic CJD in the USA and in kuru in New Guinea.[26] This may be one of the reasons why many Japanese children receive growth hormone therapy but no CJD is reported among them and they also seldom have Val/Val[129].

Table 3 Incidence of polymorphism at codon 129

Genotype	Japan		UK		
	General population[14]	Sporadic CJD	General population[2]	Sporadic CJD[23]	Iatrogenic CJD**[25]
Met/Met	164(92)	50(82)	39(37)	16(73)	1(14)
Met/Val	15(8)	11(18)	54(51)	1(5)	2(29)
Val/Val	0	0	13(12)	5(23)	4(57)

( ) Percent. * CJD after treatment with pituitary-gland-derived products.

Val[129] often combines with other mutations such as Leu[102], Val[117], Asn[178], Ser[198], and Arg[217], and may modify each phenotype. Therefore, codon 129 polymorphism may be predisposed to sporadic and iatrogenic CJD, as well as modifying phenotypes of various type of CJD.

CJD with stop codon at 145

At codon 145, one point mutation from TAT to TAG stops any further translation. This mutation was found in one allele of a 59-year-old Japanese woman who suffered from progressive dementia since she was 38 years old. Her atrophied brain showed numerous kuru plaques and neurofibrillary tangles, but only mild spongiform changes. An antibody against the synthetic N-terminal domain of PrP did stain the plaques while that against the C-terminal domain (a gift of Dr Igarashi, Shionogi

Institute for Medical Science, Osaka 566, Japan) did not. This means that kuru plaques in this case are made exclusively from C-terminal truncated PrP, which was shown to be an extra-band of low molecular weight in a protein expression study.[27]

CJD with Asn[178]

Goldfarb et al[28] divided familial CJD with Asn[178] into 2 groups. One group showed untreatable insomnia, dysautonomia and selective atrophy of the thalamic nuclei. This group was named fatal familial insomnia (FFI),[29] and had methionine at codon 129 on the mutant allele with Asn[178]. Another group showed the phenotype of sporadic CJD, lacking insomnia and selective thalamic involvement. Spongiform changes were frequent and widely distributed. All members of this group had valine at codon 129 on the mutant Asn[178] allele.

Indiana kindred with Ser[198]

Autopsied members of this large family show numerous kuru plaques and neurofibrillary tangles. Of the 9 affected individuals, 3 had codon 129 Val/Val homozygotes while 6 had Met/Val heterozygotes. In all 6 doubly heterozygous cases, Ser[198] was in a coupling phase with Val[129].[30]

CJD with Lys[200]

This mutation was originally described in a sibling pair with CJD[31], and was also discovered in families in Slovakia, Libya[32] and Japan.[11] The rapidly progressive dementia, myoclonus and PSD in EEG resembled those of sporadic CJD. Severe spongiform change and a synaptic-type distribution of PrP[CJD] are also common in familial and sporadic CJD.

A Swedish family with Arg[217]

A Swedish patient showed a long clinical course of more than four years with progressive dementia, ataxia, and pathologically kuru plaques and neurofibrillary tangles.[33] This patient had 3 PrP variants: (a) GGC to GGG at codon 124 (no change in glycine); (b) ATG to GTG (methionine to valine) at codon 129; (c) CAG to CGG (glutamine to arginine) at codon 217. A precise correlation between PrP genotypes and disease phenotypes still remains to be established.

In conclusion, sporadic CJD without a PrP gene mutation and familial CJD with Lys[200] exclusively show a synaptic-type distribution of PrP[CJD], manifest severe and rapidly progressive dementia and normally cause death after a short clinical course. Other mutations or insertion cases, however, possess a plaque-type deposition of PrP[CJD] with either no deposits or only mild deposits in the synapses. This may be one of the reasons of slow progression of the disease symptoms. On the other hand, when plaque-type deposits are found by immunohistochemistry, PrP gene abnormalities are normally expected.

ADDENDUM

After submission of this manuscript, we have found 3 novel missense variants in PrP gene (Kitamoto T, et al Biochem Biophys Res Commun 1993; 191: 709).

The codon 105 point mutation (Pro to Leu) was found on the same allele with Val^{129} in 4 patients from 3 different Japanese families. Patients showed common clinical symptoms of spastic paraparesis and dementia for over 7 years, and numerous PrP plaques in the cerebrum. The codon 180 variant PrP (Val to Ile) was detected in 2 Japanese patients. The codon 232 mutation (Met to Arg) was found in 3 Japanese patients; 1 of them combined with Ile^{180} in the other allele. Patients with codon 180 and/or 232 variants showed similar clinico-pathological symptoms as seen in sporadic CJD.

REFERENCES

1 Kitamoto T, Tateishi J. Immunohistochemical confirmation of Creutzfeldt-Jakob disease with a long clinical course with amyloid plaque core antibodies. Am J Pathol 1988; 131: 435–443.

2 Kretzschmar HA, Stowring LE, Westaway D, Stubblebine WH, Prusiner SB, DeArmond SJ. Molecular cloning of a human prion protein cDNA. DNA 1986; 5: 315–324.

3 Kitamoto T, Muramoto T, Hilbich C, Beyreuther K, Tateishi J. N-terminal sequence of prion protein is also integrated into kuru plaques in patients with Gerstmann-Sträussler syndrome. Brain Res 1991; 545: 319–321.

4 Kitamoto T, Mohri S, Tateishi J. Organ distribution of proteinase-resistant prion protein in humans and mice with Creutzfeldt-Jakob disease. J Gen Virol 1989; 70: 3371–3379.

5 Shinagawa M, Munekata E, Doi S, Takahashi K, Goto H, Sato G. Immunoreactivity of a synthetic pentadecapeptide corresponding to the N-terminal region of the scrapie prion protein. J Gen Virol 1986; 67: 1745–1750.

6 DeArmond SJ, Mobley WC, Demott DL, Barry RA, Beckstead JH, Prusiner SB. Changes in the localization of brain prion proteins during scrapie infection. Neurology 1987; 37: 1271–1280.

7 Bendheim PE, Brown HR, Rudelli RD et al. Nearly ubiquitous tissue distribution of the scrapie agent precursor protein. Neurology 1992; 42: 149–156.

8 Doi-Yi R, Kitamoto T, Tateishi J. Immunoreactivity of cerebral amyloidosis is enhanced by protein denaturation treatments. Acta Neuropathol 1991; 82: 260–265.

9 Serban D, Taraboulos A, DeArmond SJ, Prusiner SB. Rapid detection of Creutzfeldt-Jakob disease and scrapie prion proteins. Neurology 1990; 40: 110–117.

10 Kitamoto T, Ogomori K, Tateishi J, Prusiner SB. Formic acid pretreatment enhances immunostaining of cerebral and systemic amyloids. Lab Invest 1987; 57: 230–236.

11 Kitamoto T, Doh-ura K, Muramoto T, Miyazono M, Tateishi J. The primary structure of the prion protein influences the distribution of abnormal prion protein in the central nervous system. Am J Pathol 1992; 141: 271–277.

12 Muramoto T, Kitamoto T, Tateishi J, Goto I. The sequential development of abnormal prion protein accumulation in mice with Creutzfeldt-Jakob disease. Am J Pathol 1992; 140: 1411–1420.

13 Sambrook J, Fritsch EF, Maniatis T. Molecular cloning: a laboratory manual. Cold Spring Harbor 1989.

14 Doh-ura K, Tateishi J, Sasaki H, Kitamoto T, Sakaki Y. Pro→Leu change at position 102 of prion protein is the most common but not sole mutation related to Gerstmann-Stäussler syndrome. Biochem Biophys Res Commun 1989; 163: 974–979.

15 Poulter M, Baker HF, Frith CD et al. Inherited prion disease with 144 base pair gene insertion. 1. Genealogical and molecular studies. Brain 1992; 115: 675–685.

16 Brown P, Goldfarb LG, Gajdusek DC. The new biology of spongiform encephalopathy: infectious amyloidoses with a genetic twist. Lancet 1991; 337: 1019–1022.

17 Bosque PJ, Vnencak-Jones CL, Johnson MD, Whitlock JA, Mclean MJ. A PrP gene codon 178 base substitution and a 24-bp interstitial deletion in familial Creutzfeldt-Jakob disease. Neurology 1992; 42: 1864–1870.

18 Hsiao K, Baker HF, Crow TJ et al. Linkage of a prion protein missense variant to Gerstmann-Stäussler syndrome. Nature 1989; 338: 342–345.

19 Kretzschmar HA, Honold G, Steitelberger F et al. Prion protein mutation in family first reported by Gerstmann, Sträussler, and Scheinker. Lancet 1991; 337: 1160.

20 Miyazono M, Kitamoto T, Doh-ura K, Iwaki T, Tateishi J. Creutzfeldt-Jakob disease with codon 129 polymorphism (Valine): a comparative study of patients with codon 102 point mutation or without mutations. Acta Neuropathol 1992; 84: 349–354.

21 Tranchant C, Doh-ura K, Warter JM et al. Gerstmann-Sträussler-Scheinker disease in an Alsatian family: clinical and genetic studies. J Neurol Neurosurg Psychiat 1992; 55: 185–187.

22 Hsiao KK, Cass C, Schellenberg GD et al. A prion protein variant in a family with the telencephalic form of Gerstmann-Sträussler-Scheinker syndrome. Neurology 1991; 41: 681–684.

23 Palmer MS, Dryden AJ, Hughes JT, Collinge J. Homozygous prion protein genotype predisposes to sporadic Creutzfeldt-Jakob disease. Nature 1991; 352: 340–342.

24 Doh-ura K, Kitamoto T, Sakaki Y, Tateishi J. CJD discrepancy. Nature 1991; 353: 801–802.

25 Collinge J, Palmer MS, Dryden AJ. Genetic predisposition to iatrogenic Creutzfeldt-Jakob disease. Lancet 1991; 337: 1441–1442.

26 Goldfarb LG, Brown P, Rubenstein R et al. Genetic characteristics of infectious forms of the transmissible spongiform encephalopathies. Ann Neurol 1992; 32: 233.

27 Kitamoto T, Iizuka R, Tateishi J. An amber mutation of prion protein in Gerstmann-Sträussler syndrome with mutant PrP plaques. Biochem Biophys Res Commun 1993; 191: 706–714.

28 Goldfarb LG, Petersen RB, Tabaton M et al. Fatal familial insomnia and familial Creutzfeldt-Jakob disease: Disease phenotype determined by a DNA polymorphism. Science 1992; 258: 806–808.

29 Medori R, Tretschler H-J, Blanc AL et al. Fatal familial insomnia, a prion disease with a mutation at codon 178 of the prion protein gene. N Engl J Med 1992; 326: 444–449.

30 Dlouhy SR, Hsiao K, Farlow MR et al. Linkage of the Indiana kindred of Gerstmann-Sträussler-Scheinker disease to the prion protein gene. Nature Genet 1992; 1: 64–67.

31 Goldgaber D, Goldfarb LG, Brown P et al. Mutations in familial Creutzfeldt-Jakob disease and Gerstmann-Sträussler-Scheinker's syndrome. Exp Neurol 1989; 106: 204–206.

32 Goldfarb LG, Korczyn AD, Brown P, Chapman J, Gajdusek DC. Mutation in codon 200 of scrapie amyloid precursor gene linked to Creutzfeldt-Jakob disease in Sephardic Jews of Libyan and non-Libyan origin. Lancet 1990; 336: 637.

33 Hsiao K, Dlouhy SR, Farlow MR et al. Mutant prion proteins in Gerstmann-Sträussler-Scheinker disease with neurofibillary tangles. Nature Genet 1992; 1: 68–71.

British Medical Bulletin (1993) Vol. 49, No. 4, pp 980–994
©The British Council 1993

Fatal familial insomnia and the widening spectrum of prion diseases

P Gambetti, R Petersen, L Monari, M Tabaton,
L Autilio-Gambetti
Division of Neuropathology, Institute of Pathology, Case Western Reserve University,
Cleveland, OH, USA

P Cortelli, P Montagna, E Lugaresi
Neurological Institute, University of Bologna, Italy

The history of the diseases known as spongiform encephalopathies or prion diseases is fascinating and still unfolding. The events that brought these diseases together, despite their apparent diversity, and the pathogenic mechanism which they apparently share are equally compelling.

The first spongiform encephalopathy was Creutzfeldt-Jakob disease (CJD), described in 1921, as a rapidly progressive dementia of less than 1 year duration with pyramidal and extrapyramidal signs, and myoclonus.[1] Next came the description of Gerstmann-Sträussler-Scheinker syndrome (GSS) in 1928[2] as a slowly progressive ataxia of 2–10 year duration with various degrees of mental deterioration. A series of twisted events eventually brought these 2 diseases together 50 years later.[3] The missing link was provided when Gajdusek and his collaborators described kuru, a disease of 1 year duration characterized by severe cerebellar ataxia.[3,4] Subsequently, Hadlow emphasized the similarity of kuru to scrapie, whose infectivity was already known, and suggested that transmission of kuru be attempted.[5] Finally, in a series of studies, Gajdusek and collaborators proved that kuru, CJD and GSS were all transmissible.[6,7] Thus, these 3 diseases came to be grouped together under the label of transmissible spongiform encephalopathies.

Interest in spongiform encephalopathies was further heightened by the more recent discovery of the prion protein (PrP).[8,9] Prusiner, along with others, showed that an abnormal isoform of PrP plays an important role in the pathogenesis and transmissibility of all the spongiform encephalopathies. Thus, transmissible spongiform encephalopathies also became known as prion diseases.[10]

For many years CJD, kuru and GSS were the only known human prion diseases. The cloning of the PrP gene (PRNP) and availability of sensitive methods to detect PrP opened the way to the identification of novel familial and non-familial forms of prion diseases.[10] As a result, this group of diseases now includes a larger number of genotypically distinct familial forms as well as sporadic and iatrogenic forms which cover a wide spectrum of clinical and pathological phenotypes (Table 1).

Table 1 Prion diseases – familial forms

PRNP genotype	Phenotype				
	Designation	Onset[†]	Duration[†]	Clinical Features	Pathology
INSERTIONS					
120 bp[(40)]	120 Ins. subtype	31–45yr	5–15yr	Dementia, abnormal behaviour, myoclonus	Spongiosis, gliosis, neuronal loss (2)[*]
144 bp[(41,42)]	144 Ins. subtype	22–53yr	1–13yr	Slow personality changes followed by dementia, ataxia, pyramidal and extrapyramidal signs, myoclonus	Marked, widespread atrophy and PrP plaques, or no changes (47)
168 bp[(40,43)]	168 Ins. subtype	23–35yr	10–> 13yr	Clinically as 144 ins. subtype	Widespread atrophy and spongiosis (3)
196 bp[(40,44)]	196 Ins. subtype	35–54yr	3 months –13yr	Ataxia, abnormal behaviour, pyramidal signs, mutism, myoclonus	Widespread atrophy, mild spongiosis, PrP plaques in cerebral cortex and cerebellum (6)
216 bp[(45)]	216 Ins. subtype	55yr	> 2yr	Ataxia, abnormal behaviour, dementia, myoclonus	N/A [§](1)
POINT MUTATIONS					
102[Leu(2,10,32)]	120 GSS subtype	15–40yr	2–10yr	Cerebellar syndrome pyramidial and extrapyramidial signs, late dementia	Cerebral and cerebellar atrophy and PrP plaques
117[Val(10,36)]	117 GSS subtype	20–64yr	1–> 11yr	Dementia, parkinsonism, pyramidal and extrapyramidal. Occasional cerebellar signs, amyotrophy	Atrophy and PrP plaques in cerebrum
198[Ser(2)]	198 GSS subtype	34–71yr	3–11yr	As 102 mutation	As 102 GSS subtype but NFT in cerebral cortex (16)
217[Arg(38,39)]	217 GSS subtype	67–79yr	1–5yr	Ataxia, dementia	As 198 GSS subtype with more prominent subcortical spongiosis (2)
200[Lys(26–30)]	200 CJD subtype	35–66yr	2–41 months	As CJD sporadic form	As CJD sporadic form (19)
178[Asn], 129[Val(16,25)]	178 CJD subtype	26–56yr	9–51 months	Dementia, ataxia, myoclonus, extrapyramidal and pyramidal signs. Slowing EEG	Widespread spongiosis(15)
178[Asn], 129[Met (11–16)]	FFI	20–71yr	6–32 months	Sleep disorder, ataxia, myoclonus, dysautonomia, pyramidal and extrapyramidal signs	Preferential thalamic atrophy (26)
No mutation					
		40–57yr	2–18yr	Spastic paraparesis, dementia, ataxia	Cerebral PrP angiopathy, PrP plaques, NFT (10)

[†]Range; [§]NA: not available; [*]Number of patients examined clinically.

A prerequisite to establishing a clear classification of prion diseases is the availability of a detailed clinical, pathological and genotypic characterization of each disease so that they can be diagnosed and their individuality established. We have tried to follow these principles with Fatal Familial Insomnia (FFI), a novel prion disease that we recently described and characterized.[11-16] In this chapter we provide a detailed description of FFI and a summary of clinical, pathological and genotypic features of other recently characterized prion diseases.

FATAL FAMILIAL INSOMNIA

Patient population

At this time 5 families have been shown to have members affected by FFI.[12,13,15,16] Of these 2 are Italian, 1 is French, and 2 are American (of whom 1 is of British and the other of German extraction). A total of 24 members are very likely to be affected on the basis of detailed clinical charts or have been shown to be affected by histopathological examination.

Clinical characteristics

The clinical features result from the impairment of several systems or functions listed in Table 2, along with the age of onset and duration of the disease.

Typically, FFI begins between 40 and 60 years of age and has a duration of 7–18 months. There are 3 different presentations: (a) sleep disturbances that are commonly reported as insomnia, agitation during sleep, and dreams that are often enacted; (b) motor signs such as dysarthria and ataxia; and (c) memory impairment. As the disease progresses, the full array of symptoms develops with involvement of motor, endocrine and autonomic systems along with the sleep disorders and cognitive deficits reported in Table 2. Important clinical tests are polysomnography, which shows a marked reduction or loss of EEG sleep patterns, and positron emission tomography (PET) scanning that shows preferential hypometabolism in the thalamic region.

Histopathology

The histopathology is dominated by thalamic atrophy[11,14] (Table 3). The anterior-ventral and medial dorsal thalamic nuclei are consistently and severely affected. The centromedian and pulvinar nuclei are frequently affected while involvement of other thalamic nuclei is variable and less consistent. The cortex usually shows minimal to moderate astrogliosis, that especially involves the deep layers and extends to the superficial white matter. Widespread spongiosis was only found in two

Table 2 FFI: clinical characteristics

AGE OF ONSET, DURATION

Age of onset (yr)   Mean: 51 (20–71 range; 40–60 in 73%)
Duration (months)   Mean: 14 (6–32 range; 7–18 in 84%)

SYSTEMS PREFERENTIALLY AFFECTED

I. Sleep and Vigilance

Progressive insomnia, proven by polysomnography or overnight EEG recording
in eight subjects from four families,[11,13,14,15]resistant to diazepam
and barbiturates[11]; progressive dream states and hallucinations followed
by stupor and coma in the terminal stages.

II. Cognitive Functions

Impairement of working memory, attention and visumotor performances;
preservation of global intelligence.[11]

III. Autonomic System

Hyperhidrosis, tachycardia, pyrexia, blood hypertension, irregular
breathing.[11,14,15]

IV. Motor System

Dysarthia progressing to anarthria, dysphagia, ataxia, spontaneous and evoked
myoclonus, hyperreflexia, Babinski sign.

V. Endocrine System

Decreased ACTH and increased cortisol and catecholamine levels, abnormal
circadian rhythms of GH, prolactin and melatonin.[11,14,15]

VI. EEG

During sleep: Decrease to complete loss of delta activity, sleep spindles,
K complexes; abnormal REM phase.[11,14,15]
During wakefulness: Progressive and flattening of background activity; slowing;
inability to generate drug-induced sleep activities (periodic spike activity
was seen in only two of seven subjects examined. These two subjects had the
longest course, 25 and 32 months, and widespread spongiosis of the cerebral
cortex.)

VII. PET Scanning (carried out in four subjects)

Hypometabolism (-36%) virtually limited to the anterior thalamus in two
subjects; hypometabolism present also in the cerebral cortex, especially
frontal and parietal lobes (-40%), in hippocampus basal ganglia and cerebellum
but always more severe in the thalamus, in the other two subjects.[17]

subjects who had a disease duration of 25 and 32 months. (These sub-

jects also had a periodic EEG). Focal spongiosis limited to the subicu-
lum was seen in one subject with a 13 week course.[15] Severe atrophy
of the inferior olive is common while atrophy of the cerebellar cortex
is minimal to moderate. Other regions are generally normal. Minimal
gliosis of the basal ganglia was seen in 4 of the 14 cases examined
while in one case there was moderate gliosis of the superior colliculus.

Table 3 FFI: Histopathology

Thalamus	
Loss of neurons and gliosis	15/15
Spongiosis	0/15
Cerebral Cortex	
Gliosis[1]	4/14
Spongiosis[2]	2/14
Cerebellum	
Loss of neurons and gliosis	7/12
'Torpedo' formation	9/12
Inferior Olive	
Loss of neurons and gliosis	11/14

[1]Refers to moderate or severe. [2]Refers to widespread spongiosis; focal spongiosis was
present in one case.

Protease resistant PrP

The presence of proteinase K-resistant PrP (PrP^{Res}) was demonstrated
in 4 of the 5 subjects analyzed.[12,18] Proteinase K treatment generates
2 major PrP^{Res} fragments of 29 and 27 kDa.[12] This is at variance with
the 3 major species of 29, 25 and 21 kDa we consistently generated
from sporadic CJD. Whether the pattern of PrP^{Res} in FFI also differs
from that of other familial forms of prion diseases, and hence is unique
to FFI, remains to be established. The amount of PrP^{Res} appears to
correlate with the duration of the disease but not with the severity of
the lesions in the various brain regions, since the amount of PrP^{Res} was
not notably high in the thalamus of FFI cases but was substantial in the
basal ganglia of one subject in the absence of histological lesions in
this region.[12,18]

PRNP gene analyses

17 affected members from 5 unrelated FFI families were shown to
have a mutation at codon 178 of PRNP resulting in the substitution of
asparagine for aspartic acid (178^{Asn}).[12,13,15] A combined lod score of
6.5 was obtained that indicates strong linkage between the 178^{Asn} mu-

tation and FFI.[15] In addition, the distribution of the methionine/valine (Met/Val) polymorphism at PRNP codon 129 was markedly skewed in FFI-affected subjects. The distribution of this polymorphism in the normal Caucasian population is 0.37 Met/Met, 0.51 Met/Val and 0.12 Val/Val whereas in FFI cases it was 0.82 Met/Met, 0.18 Met/Val and no Val/Val.[16] Further analysis showed that codon 129 in the mutant allele specified methionine in all 17 FFI-affected subjects from the 5 kindreds examined to date.[16] We concluded that FFI is linked to the 129Met, 178Asn haplotype.[16]

Diagnostic criteria

The characteristics needed to establish a probable diagnosis and those required for a definitive diagnosis of FFI are:

1. Autosomal dominant disease, onset at adult age, and duration of 6–32 months.
2. Presence of untreatable insomnia, dysautonomia, memory impairment, ataxia and/or myoclonus, pyramidal and extrapyramidal signs.
3. Decrease or loss of sleep-related EEG activities.
4. Preferential hypometabolism in the thalamic region using [18F]PET.
5. Preferential thalamic atrophy.
6. 129Met, 178Asn haplotype.

Any combination of criteria 1–5 makes the diagnosis of FFI highly probable. Criterion 6 in combination with any one of the other criteria makes the diagnosis definitive.

Families with a variant of FFI

Recently, Bosque et al reported a family with a 24 bp interstitial deletion between codons 82 and 91, 129Met and 178Asn all on the mutated PRNP allele.[19] Thus, the mutated haplotype of this family corresponds to that of FFI but has, in addition, a 24 bp deletion. Unfortunately, the disease phenotype expressed in this family is unclear. Insomnia was reported in 3 of the 5 affected but was not assessed by polysomnography. [18F]FDG showed slightly more severe hypometabolism in the cerebral cortex than in the thalamus. In accordance with this finding, the histopathological lesions were apparently more severe in the cerebral cortex than in the thalamus, although the medial dorsal nucleus was not examined.

Is there a sporadic form of fatal insomnia?

Mizusawa et al published a study on a 37-year-old man who died following a 30-month history of insomnia, dementia, myoclonus, ataxia, nocturnal agitation and dysautonomia.[20] Histopathological examination revealed severe atrophy of anterior dorsal, mediodorsal, lateral dorsal and pulvinar nuclei of the thalamus. The cerebral cortex had mild spongiosis; scattered 'torpedoes' were present in the cerebellar cortex while the olives had severe neuronal loss. Thus, both the clinical and pathological phenotype of this case corresponds to that of FFI. Moreover, a recent study of this case (Tateishi & Gambetti, unpublished data) demonstrated the presence of PrP[Res] and no mutations in PRNP. Thus, the case by Mizusawa et al can be considered as a sporadic form of fatal insomnia. Other cases that may also be sporadic fatal insomnia are those published under the label of selective thalamic atrophy or the thalamic form of CJD.[21–24]

Conclusions

The study of 5 unrelated families establishes FFI as a well defined disease entity with distinct phenotype and genotype. Interfamilial variability of the disease phenotype is minimal (Table 4) especially when those subjects with identical PRNP genotype, i.e. homozygous for methionine at codon 129, are compared. However, it is likely that phenotypes similar to FFI may also be found in association with similar but distinct genotypes. An example of this may be the family studied by Bosque et al.[19]

Table 4 Interfamilial variability in FFI families

Family	1	2	3	4	5
Onset (Mean, yr)	52.5	52.5	49	51	46 (48)
Duration (Mean; months)	16 (12.2)	8	10	11	16 (15)
Insomnia	9/9	2/2	2/2	2/2	2/3
Dysautonomia	8/9 (6/6)	2/2	1/1	1/1	NR
Myoclonus	9/9	2/2	2/2	2/2	3/3
Ataxia	6/8 (4/5)	1/2	2/2	2/2	2/3
Preferential thalamic atrophy	7/7	1/1	2/2	2/2	2/2
Widespread spongiosis	2/7 (0/5)	0/1	0/2	0/2	0/2

NR: Not reported. In parenthesis: values after exclusion of the subjects heterozygous at PRNP codon 129.

OTHER SUBTYPES OF INHERITED PRION DISEASE

With the advent of genetic analysis (i.e. PCR), the number of subtypes of familial prion diseases has increased considerably (Table 1). The phenotypes of the various familial subtypes are described in detail in other parts of this book. Here, they will be discussed briefly to put into perspective their differences and to demonstrate the widening spectrum of prion diseases.

178[Asn] CJD subtype

The phenotype of the 178[Asn] CJD subtype is similar to but distinct from that of FFI.[16,25] The 178[Asn] CJD subtype apparently lacks progressive untreatable insomnia, the clinical hallmark of FFI. Insomnia has not been reported in any of the 15 cases examined and polysomnography, carried out in one subject at an advanced stage of the disease, was unremarkable[16 and Haltia, personal communication] The major differences between the FFI phenotype and that of the 178[Asn] CJD subtype, however, lay in the topography and type of the histopathological lesions. All 17 cases of 178[Asn] CJD subtype examined histologically to date had cerebral cortex spongiosis. Examination of the thalamus in 11 affected members revealed moderate to minimal spongiosis, some neuronal loss and gliosis but not the severe neuronal loss, gliosis and lack of spongiosis characteristic of FFI. No cases of the 178[Asn] CJD subtype has had a PET scan, that is likely to provide a topography of the hypometabolism different from that of FFI and therefore this could be a useful test in differentiating the two diseases. The puzzle presented by two phenotypically distinct diseases linked to the same mutation has been at least partly clarified by the finding that they do indeed have different genotypes. The 178[Asn] CJD subtype segregates with the 178[Asn], 129[Val] while, as mentioned above, FFI segregates with the 178[Asn], 129[Met] haplotype.[16]

200[Lys] CJD subtype

Detailed studies of this disease phenotype in the individual affected families are lacking. A review of published cases shows that the mean age of onset is approximately 10 years later than that of FFI and the 178[Asn] CJD subtype, and the duration, approximately 6 months, is much shorter.[25–31] Clinical signs appear to be very similar to those of the 178[Asn] CJD subtype except that they frequently include EEG periodic sharp wave complexes that are absent in the latter. The histopathological features are dominated by spongiosis which, in the few cases with detailed examination, seem to extend more to the deep brain nuclei, cerebellum and brain stem than in the 178[Asn] CJD subtype.

GSS subtypes

A 102[Leu] mutation has been found in the original GSS family.[2] However, the mutations at codons 117, 198, and 217 of PRNP also result in disease phenotypes similar to the original GSS phenotypes as to age of onset, duration, and presence of PrP plaques, justifying their classification as subtypes of GSS.[2,10,32–39]

The phenotypic differences between these subtypes, inferred from the few families examined to date, relate largely to the distribution of PrP plaques and the presence or absence of neurofibrillary tangles (NFT). Thus, while the 102 and 198 subtypes have PrP plaques in cerebral and cerebellar cortices, as well as in the white matter of the basal ganglia and thalamus, those of the 117 subtype have no plaques in the cerebellum.[2,33,34,36] The 198 subtype has NFT, that also have been observed in the 217 subtype, although insufficient information is available to characterize the phenotype associated with this mutation.[2,37,38,39] The phenotypes of the 102[Leu], 117[Val], and 198[Ser] have been identified also as ataxic, telencephalic, and NFT forms of GSS, respectively.[32]

Prion diseases associated with PRNP insertions

A more challenging problem concerning phenotypic characterization is presented by the prion diseases associated with octapeptide repeat insertions between codons 51 and 91 in PRNP.[40–45] In at least two of these forms, the 144 bp and 216 bp insertions, methionine has been shown to be specified at codon 129 of the mutated allele.[41,45]

The phenotype linked to the **144 bp insertion** has been reported and examined in detail in one large family.[41, 42] The only consistent clinical feature is the long-standing personality disorders leading to cognitive deficit. Age of onset, although variable, is comparable to that of the GSS subtypes while the duration is longer (> 8 years in 60% of the subjects). Histopathological examination in 4 subjects has revealed a profound variability in the severity and distribution of the lesions. Severe neuronal loss, astrocytosis, spongiosis, PrP plaques and plaques of Alzheimer type were present in 2 subjects, while the other 2 subjects had virtually no histological lesions. The 2 subjects with histopathological lesions had valine specified at codon 129 of the normal allele, whereas the 2 subjects lacking the lesions were homozygous for methionine at that codon. A similar situation was observed in FFI. Widespread spongiosis was present only when valine was specified at codon 129 of the normal allele. Whether the presence of valine at codon 129 of the normal allele always influences the pathological features and, therefore, contributes to phenotypic variability, remains to be seen.

Other insertions of 120, 168, 196, and 216 bp (always between codons 51 and 91) have also been reported.[40,43–45] The clinical features common to all the phenotypes associated with these insertions are the early age of onset and the relatively long duration of the disease which is over 10 years in the majority of individuals. The pathological features vary, but seem to reflect the size of the inserts: widespread spongiosis without PrP plaques in the family with 120 bp repeat; variable histopathological features including spongiosis, atrophy, PrP plaques or minimal or no changes in families with 144 and 168 bp insertions; spongiosis and PrP plaques in the family with the 196 bp insertion. No histopathological data are available for the family with the 216 bp insertion.[45]

Inherited prion diseases without PRNP mutations

The presence of cerebral PrP plaques, PrP angiopathy, and NFT has been reported in an extended family with an autosomal dominant disease clinically characterized by progressive spastic paraparesis followed by dementia, cerebellar ataxia and dysarthria.[46,47] Sequencing of the PRNP open reading frame revealed no mutation. This observation, presented as an abstract, would be the first example of a familial prion disease lacking a mutation in the coding region of the PRNP.[47]

NON-FAMILIAL FORMS

The number of phenotypes of non-familial forms may also increase when more sensitive methods of PrP^{Res} detection and characterization become available and will allow us to establish whether the subtypes of CJD already known, such as the Heideneim form, and the sporadic cases of GSS indeed deserve to be grouped separately.[2,48,49] The beginning of this trend is exemplified by the possible identification of a sporadic case of fatal insomnia which seems to coincide with the thalamic form of CJD.

Iatrogenic forms

The spectrum of the non-familial forms has been further widened with the appearance of forms acquired either by tissue transplant, use of contaminated instruments or systemic administration of contaminated bioproducts.[49] The large scale administration of growth hormone (GH) has resulted in a relatively large number of individuals who have developed a prion disease.[50] Detailed study of 4 such cases has revealed a disease duration between 1 and 2 years.[50] T Billette De Villemeur, personal communication Presentation is characterized by cerebellar ataxia with late appearance of severe mental deterioration. The histopathology consists of spongiosis and gliosis that is marked in frontal cortex, basal ganglia and pontine nuclei and is less severe in the cortex of other lobes, thalamus and cerebellum; severe neuronal loss in cerebral and cerebellar cortices and marked gliosis of the white matter are also present. In addition, PrP plaques of the kuru type are observed in the subcortical white matter of the frontal lobe. Thus, the phenotype of the form acquired through the administration of contaminated GH is different from the classical forms of CJD, GSS and kuru as for duration, and type and distribution of the lesions.

CONCLUSION

Prion diseases exhibit a much greater phenotypic heterogeneity than it was thought when 'typical' CJD and GSS were the only known prion diseases. This has heightened the interest in this group of diseases, but at the same time has raised questions related not only to the terminology, but also to our understanding of these diseases. The phenotypic differences among the various subtypes relate to clinical features, such as age of onset and duration of the disease, as well as to pathological characteristics such as topographic distribution and types of lesions.

Phenotypic differences have also been found in experimental scrapie and are related to either the scrapie isolate or the host genotype.[51–53] Injection of different scrapie prion isolates to a single animal strain, results in markedly different incubation times and disease durations while the lesions differ both in type and topography. For example, one prion isolate has been shown to produce severe spongiosis of the cerebral cortex, basal ganglia, and cerebellum, while the spongiosis produced by another isolate is minimal and limited to the cortex. Moreover, the distribution of PrP[Res] also varies. Following administration of one prion isolate, PrP[Res] was present throughout the entire cerebral cortex while with another prion isolate, it was confined to thalamic and mesencephalic structures.[51] The distinct pathologic properties associated with different scrapie prion isolates have been ascribed to conformational characteristics of PrP which in turn determine a tropism for, and 'replication' in, specific cell types. The influence of genotype has also been clearly shown. Following administration of the same prion isolate to hamsters from two strains that differed in three amino acids between residues 102 and 109, animals from both strains developed disease, but only those from one of the strains developed PrP plaques.[53] Therefore, it is not surprising that the various mutant PrPs in the inherited prion diseases are associated with different clinical and pathological phenotypes.

Similar arguments can be applied to the phenotypic differences found in non-familial forms of prion diseases. The sporadic (non-iatrogenic) forms are not believed to result from infection, since they have both uniform and worldwide distribution, but rather from somatic mutation in PRNP or post-translational modifications of PrP that triggers the conversion into PrP[Res].[55] Different PrP[Res] are likely to be generated by this process leading to different phenotypes. Phenotypic differences are also to be expected between the sporadic and the iatrogenic forms since the mechanism of conversion of PrP into PrP[Res] is different in the two forms. Among the iatrogenic cases, phenotypic expression may vary according to the route of infection, for example intracerebral as opposed to systemic administration. Thus, the spectrum of the non-familial forms of prion disease will expand as new cases are discovered.

Another challenging issue is phenotypic heterogeneity among different families, as well as among affected members of the same family, linked to identical PRNP mutations. Striking examples of this heterogeneity are FFI and the 178^{Asn} CJD subtype, which have distinct clinical and histopathological features but share the 178^{Asn} mutation. In a recent study of 30 affected members from 5 FFI and 6 178^{Asn} CJD subtype families, the polymorphism at PRNP codon 129 was implicated in determining both clinico-pathological features and severity of either disease.[16] As mentioned above, 129^{Met}/178^{Asn} was found in all FFI subjects while 129^{Val}/178^{Asn} was present in all subjects of the 178^{Asn} CJD subtype. The phenotypic heterogeneity of the 2 diseases could be explained by a difference in the interaction of asparagine at position 178 with methionine or valine at position 129 resulting in different conformations of the mutant PrP.[16] Moreover, we observed that in both diseases, affected subjects that were homozygous at codon 129 had an earlier onset and a more severe clinical picture. An increase in the severity of, or susceptibility to, prion diseases in subjects homozygous at codon 129 has been reported previously and was attributed to a higher rate of conversion of PrP to PrP^{Res} in the homozygous subjects.[55] In familial forms in which the 129 polymorphism has been studied, when 129^{Met} is present in the mutant allele, such as FFI[16] and 144 bp insertion subtype[42], valine at codon 129 of the normal allele seems to determine the presence of spongiosis, although the number of subjects is too low to reach definitive conclusions. Thus, the polymorphism at codon 129 provides a major element of heterogeneity in prion diseases.

The synergistic interaction of a mutation and a common polymorphism resulting in distinct disease phenotypes represents a recent advance in clarifying the phenotypic variability associated with mutations. Other mechanisms of phenotypic variability are genomic imprinting, which differentially affects the level of expression of parental genes, environmental factors, and 'modifying' genes which influence the expression of an inherited mutation.[55] Prion diseases, however, are especially prone to heterogeneity because of the apparent importance of PrP conformation in the pathogenesis of the disease. In contrast to diseases due to an inherited enzyme defect, in which heterogeneity is dictated only by the degree of impairment and the cellular requirement for that particular enzyme, the phenotypic heterogeneity of prion diseases may stem from a myriad of interdependent conditions. The different conformation of PrP molecules from different genetic backgrounds would dictate different rates of conversion from normal to PrP^{Res}, different rates of propagation from one brain region to the other, and different modes of aggregation, the net effect of which is different and selective cell damage. In a phenotypic context, this would translate into different ages of onset and durations of the disease as well as different distribution and types of structural lesions.

The situation may be even more complex in the subtypes resulting from octapeptide insertions in which subjects with widespread histopathological changes have been reported along with others lacking structural lesions. In these forms, subtle genetic differences (perhaps polymorphisms) might result in deposition of PrP^{Res} leading to structural lesions in some subjects, while in others the mutant PrP might only alter neuronal function without any structural damage. In view of the complexity of prion diseases, their heterogeneity is understandable and a further widening of the spectrum of these diseases is foreseeable.

REFERENCES

1 Kirschbaum WR. Jakob-Creutzfeldt disease. Amsterdam: Elsevier, 1968: 1-251.

2 Farlow MR, Tagliavini F, Bugiani O, Ghetti B. Gerstmann-Sträussler-Scheinker disease. In: Handbook of clinical neurology. Amsterdam: Elsevier, 1991: 619-633.

3 Ceroni M, Simonetti F, Karau J, Pergami P, Savoldi EF. Storia, clinica e nuove acquisizioni in tema di malattia di Creutzfeldt-Jakob. In: XI Corso Di Aggiornamento della Societa' Italiana Di Neurologica, Monduzzi Editore, Bergamo, 20-23 October, 1992: 317-326.

4 Klatzo I, Gajdusek DC, Zigas V. Pathology of kuru. Lab Invest 1959; 8: 799-847.

5 Hadlow WJ. Scrapie and kuru. Lancet 1959; 2: 289-290.

6 Gajdusek DC, Gibbs CJJ, Alpers M. Experimental transmission of a kuru-like syndrome in chimpanzees. Nature 1966; 209: 794-796.

7 Gibbs CJJ, Gajdusek DC, Asher DM. Creutzfeldt-Jakob disease (subacute spongiform encephalopathy): transmission to the chimpanzee. Science 1968; 161: 388-389.

8 Aiken JM, Marsh RF. The search for scrapie agent nucleic acid. Microbiol Rev 1990; 54: 242-246.

9 Alper T. In: Prusiner SB, McKinley MP, eds. Prions – Novel infectious pathogens causing scrapie and Creutzfeldt-Jakob disease. Orlando: Academic Press, 1987: 113-148.

10 Prusiner SB. Chemistry and biology of prions. In: Biochemistry. 1992: 12277-12288.

11 Lugaresi E, Medori R, Montagna P et al. Fatal familial insomnia and dysautonomia with selective degeneration of thalamic nuclei. N Engl J Med 1986; 315: 997-1003.

12 Medori R, Tritschler HJ, LeBlanc A et al. Fatal familial insomnia, a prion disease with a mutation at codon 178 of the prion protein gene. N Engl J Med 1992; 326: 444-449.

13 Medori R, Montagna P, Tritschler HJ et al. Fatal familial insomnia: A second kindred with mutation of prion gene at codon 178. Neurology 1992; 42: 669-670.

14 Manetto V, Medori R, Cortelli P et al. Fatal familial insomnia: Clinical and pathologic study of five new cases. Neurology 1992; 42: 312-319.

15 Petersen RB, Tabaton M, Berg L et al. Analysis of the prion gene in thalamic dementia. Neurology 1992; 42: 1859-1863.

16 Goldfarb LG, Petersen RB, Tabaton M et al. Fatal familial insomnia and familial Creutzfeldt-Jakob disease: disease phenotype determined by a DNA polymorphism. Science 1992; 258: 806-808.

17 Perani D, Cortelli P, Lucignani, Montagna P et al. [^{18}F] FDG PET in fatal familial insomnia: the functional effects of thalamic lesions (submitted).

18 Gambetti P. Insomnia familiare fatale. Istopatologia, biologia molecolare, nosografia. In: XI Corso Di Aggiornamento della Societa' Italiana Di Neurologia. Monduzzi Editore, Bergamo, 20-23 October, 1992: 359-369.

19 Bosque PJ, Vnencak-Jones CL, Johnson MD, Whitlock JA, McLean MJ. A PrP gene codon 178 base substitution and a 24-bp interstitial deletion in familial Creutzfeldt-Jakob disease. Neurology 1992; 42: 1864-1870.

20 Mizusawa H, Ohkoshi N, Sasaki H et al. Degeneration of the thalamus and inferior olives associated with spongiform encephalopathy of the cerebral cortex. Clin Neuropathol 1988; 7: 81-86.

21 Stern K. Severe dementia associated with bilateral symmetrical degeneration of the thalamus. Brain 1939; 62: 157-171.

22 Schulman S. Bilateral symmetrical degeneration of the thalamus. J Neuropathol Exp Neurol 1957; 16: 446-470.

23 Garcin R, Brion S, Khochneviss AA. Le syndrome de Creutzfeldt-Jakob et les syndromes corticotries du presenium (a l'occasion de 5 observations anatomo-cliniques). Rev Neurol (Paris) 1963; 109: 419-441.

24 Martin JJ. Thalamic degeneration. In: Vinken PY, Bruyn GW, eds. Handbook of Clinical Neurology, Vol. 21, Amsterdam, North-Holland, 1975: 587-604.

25 Brown P, Goldfarb LG, Kovanen J et al. Phenotypic characteristics of familial Creutzfeldt-Jakob disease associated with the codon 178Asn PRNP mutation. Ann Neurol 1992; 31: 282-285.

26 Bertoni JM, Label LS, Sackelleres C, Hicks SP. Supranuclear gaze palsy in familial Creutzfeldt-Jakob disease. Arch Neurol 1983; 40: 618-622.

27 Bertoni JM, Brown P, Goldfarb LG, Rubenstein R, Gajdusek DC. Familial Creutzfeldt-Jakob disease (codon 200 mutation) with supranuclear palsy. J Am Med Assoc 1992; 268: 2413-2415.

28 Korczyn AD, Chapman J, Goldfarb Lg, Brown P, Gajdusek DC. A mutation in the prion protein gene in Creutzfeldt-Jakob disease in Jewish patients of Libyan, Greek and Tunisian origin. Ann N Y Acad Sci USA 1991; 640: 171-176.

29 Hsiao K, Meiner Z, Kahana E et al. Mutation of the prion protein in Libyan Jews with Creutzfeldt-Jakob disease. N Engl J Med 1991; 324: 1091-1097.

30 Brown P. Neurological Progress: The phenotypic expression of different mutations in transmissible human spongiform encephalopathy. Rev Neurol (Paris) 1992; 148(5): 317-327.

31 Brown P, Goldfarb LG, Cathala F et al. The molecular genetics of familial Creutzfeldt-Jakob disease in France. J Neurol Sci 1991; 105: 240-246.

32 Hsiao K, Cass C, Schellenberg GD et al. A prion protein variant in a family with the telencephalic form of Gerstmann-Sträussler-Scheinker syndrome. Neurology 1991; 41: 681-684.

33 Kretzschmar HA, Honold G, Seitelberger F et al. Prion protein mutation at codon 102 in an Italian family with Gerstmann-Sträussler-Scheinker syndrome. Neurology 1992; 42: 809-810.

34 Genthon R, Gray G, Salama J et al. Maladie de Gerstmann-Sträussler-Scheinker etude pathologique et genealogique. Rev Neurol (Paris) 1992; 148(5): 335-342.

35 Laplanche J, Chatelain J, Beaudry P et al. La Revue a requ la lettre suivante. Rev Neurol 1992; 10: 646.

36 Tranchant C, Doh-ura K, Warter JM et al. Gerstmann-Sträussler-Scheinker disease in an Alsatian family: clinical and genetic studies. J Neurol Neurosurg Psychiat 1992; 55: 185-187.

37 Dloughy SR, Hsiao K, Farlow MR et al. Linkage of the Indiana kindred of Gerstmann-Sträussler-Scheinker disease to the prion protein gene. Nature Genet 1992; 1: 64-67.

38 Ikeda S, Yanagisawa N, Allsop D, Glenner GG. A variant of Gerstmann-Sträussler-Scheinker disease with β-protein epitopes and dystrophic neurites in the peripheral regions of PrP-immunoreactive amyloid plaques. In: Amyloid and Amyloidosis 1990. Kluwer Academic, 1991: 737-740.

994 FATAL FAMILIAL INSOMNIA

39 Hsiao K, Dloughy SR, Farlow MR et al. Mutant prion proteins in Gerstmann-Sträussler-Scheinker disease with neurofibrillary tangles. Nature Genet 1992; 1: 68-71.
40 Goldfarb LG, Brown P, McCombie WR et al. Transmissible familial Creutzfeldt-Jakob disease associated with five, seven and eight extra octapeptide coding repeats in the PRNP gene. Proc Natl Acad Sci USA 1991; 88: 10926-10930.
41 Poulter M, Baker HF, Frith CD et al. Inherited prion disease with 144 base pair gene insertion. Brain 1992; 115: 675-685.
42 Collinge J, Brown J, Hardy J et al. Inherited prion disease with 144 base pair gene insertion. Brain 1992; 115: 687-710.
43 Brown P, Goldfarb LG, McCombie WR et al. Atypical Creutzfeldt-Jakob disease in an American family with an insert mutation in the PRNP amyloid precursor gene. Neurology 1992; 42: 442-427.
44 Goldfarb LG, Brown P, Vrbovska A et al. An insert mutation in the chromosome 20 amyloid precursor gene in a Gerstmann-Sträussler-Scheinker family. J Neurol Sci 1992; 111: 89-194.
45 Owen F, Poulter M, Collinge J et al. A dementing illness associated with a novel insertion in the prion protein gene. Mol Brain Res 1992; 13: 155-157.
46 Wroster-Drought C, Greenfield J, McMenemey W. A form of familial presenile dementia with spastic paralysis (including the pathological examination of a case). Brain 1940; 63: 237-254.
47 Palmer MS, Sidle KCL, Campbell TA et al. Absence of PrP gene mutation in patient showing PrP-immunostaining. In: Third International Conference on Alzheimer's Disease. New York: Pergamon Press, 1992; S94: No. 371.
48. Meyer A, Leigh D, Bagg CE. A rare presenile dementia associated with cortical blindness (Heidenhain's syndrome). J Neurol Neurosurg Psychiat 1954; 17: 129-133.
49 Brown P, Preece MA, Will RG. 'Friendly fire' in medicine: hormones, homografts, and Creutzfeldt-Jakob disease. Lancet 1992; 340: 24-27.
50 Billette de Villeneur T, Gourmelen M, Beauvais P et al. Maladie de Creutzfeldt-Jakob chez quatre enfants traites par hormone de croissance. Rev Neurol (Paris) 1992; 148(5): 328-334.
51 Hecker R, Taraboulos A, Scott M et al. Replication of distinct scrapie prion isolates is region specific in brains of transgenic mice and hamsters. Genes & Develop 1992; 6: 1213-1228.
52 Beesen RA, Marsh RF. Biochemical and physical properties of the prion protein from two strains of the transmissible mink encephalopathy agent. J Virol 1992; 66: 2096-2101.
53 Lowenstein DH, Butler DA, Westaway D et al. Three hamster species with different scrapie incubation times and neuropathological features encode distinct prion proteins. Mol Cell Biol 1990; 10: 1153-1163.
54 Palmer MS, Collinge J. Human prion diseases. Curr Opin Neurol Neurosurg 1992; 5: 895-901.
55 Steel M. Genetics: Polymorphism, proteins and phenotypes. Lancet 1993; 341: 212-213.
56 Brown P, Cathala F, Castaigne P, Gajdusek DC. Creutzfeldt-Jakob disease: clinical analysis of a consecutive series of 230 neuropathological verified cases. Ann Neurol 1986; 20: 597-602.
57 Gajdusek DC. Unconventional viruses and the origin and disappearance of Kuru. Science 1977; 197: 943-960.
58 Boudoureques J, Toga M, Khalil R, Chérif AA, Pellissier JF, Gosset A. Dégénérescence spino-cérébelleuse tardive avec amyotrophies, comportant une atteinte pallido-luysienne sévère et des lésions histologiques diffuses de sénilité. Rev Neurol (Paris) 1976; 132: 623-637.

British Medical Bulletin (1993) Vol. 49, No. 4, pp. 995–1011
©The British Council 1993

Role of PrP in prion diseases

C Weissmann, H Büeler, A Sailer,
M Fischer, M Aguet,
Institut für Molekularbiologie I, Universität Zürich, Zürich, Switzerland
A Aguzzi
Institut für Neuropathologie, Universitätsspital, Zürich, Switzerland

Scrapie, the prototype of a group of diseases designated as transmissible spongiform encephalopathies (TSEs) or prion diseases, is a naturally occurring affliction of sheep which was recognized more than 250 years ago. Characteristically, affected animals present with twitching, excitability, intense itching and finally paralysis and death. Transmission of the disease by inoculation of healthy sheep and goats with lumbar cord of diseased animals was first demonstrated in 1936[1] and soon confirmed by Gordon.[2] This led to the recognition of the unusual properties of the pathogenic agent (later designated as 'prion'[3], such as the extremely long incubation periods, exceeding 1 year, and resistance to high temperatures, formaldehyde treatment and UV irradiation.[2,4,5]

In a separate development, Creutzfeld-Jakob disease (CJD), Gerstmann-Sträussler-Scheinker disease (GSS) and kuru were characterized as slow degenerative diseases of the central nervous system. The suggestion by Hadlow[6] that these diseases might be the counterpart of scrapie in humans was followed by long-term inoculation studies by Gajdusek and his colleagues which resulted in the transmission, first of kuru[7], then of CJD[8] to chimpanzees. Later, GSS was also transmitted to the chimpanzee[9] and to the mouse.[10] Recently we have witnessed the emergence of a new form of a prion disease, namely bovine spongiform encephalopathy (BSE), which is attributed to the feeding of cattle with meat and bone meal supplements derived from scrapie-contaminated sheep and then cattle offal.[11,12]

The overall properties of the prion differ from those of any known virus or viroid[2–4,13] and early on gave rise to speculations that it might be devoid of both nucleic acid and protein,[14] consist of protein only[15–17] or be a polysaccharide[17a] or a membrane fragment.[18] In this article we review the current hypotheses regarding the pathogenesis of

Note added in proof: Unheated brain extracts of PrP[0/0] mice 25, 33 and 48 weeks after inoculation with scrapie prions show no scrapie infectivity. Thus, the positive result for the 20-week PrP[0/0] mouse (Table) is likely accidental.

this class of diseases (for recent reviews, *see* Refs 19–24), in particular the so-called 'protein only' hypothesis and the major lines of evidence in its support, and describe experiments carried out in our laboratory demonstrating the essential role of the host gene *Prn-p* in the pathogenesis of scrapie.[25]

THE 'PROTEIN ONLY' HYPOTHESIS

Prusiner has suggested that the prion is devoid of nucleic acid and identical with PrP[Sc], a modified form of PrP[C] (the 'protein only' hypothesis).[26] PrP[C] is a normal host protein[27–29] encoded within a single exon of a single copy gene[30] and is found predominantly on the outer surface of neurons, attached by a glycosyl phosphatidyl inositol anchor[19,26,31,32] but also in a variety of other tissues, both in the embryonic and the adult mouse.[33,34]

PrP[Sc] is defined as a largely protease-resistant form of PrP[C] which readily forms aggregates after treatment with detergents and protease.[27, 35–37] It accumulates intracellularly, in cytoplasmic vesicles[38,39] and is the major component of the extracellular amyloid plaques characteristic for some forms of prion diseases. No chemical differences have so far been detected between PrP[Sc] and PrP[C19,40,41], however, it must be stressed that the ratio of infectious units to PrP[Sc] molecules is in the order of 1:100 000,[42] so that if the infectious entity were a subspecies of PrP[Sc] or a different modification of PrP altogether a chemical difference between PrP[C] and the infectious subspecies could be analytically undetectable.

Prusiner proposed that PrP[Sc], when introduced into a normal cell, causes the conversion of PrP[C] or its precursor into PrP[Sc19,27,43,45–46] (Fig. 1A). The nature of the conversion is unknown and could be due to a chemical or conformational modification, during or after its synthesis. However, the existence of many different strains of scrapie which can be propagated in one and the same inbred mouse line, and the apparent mutability of the agent[21–23] are cited in support of the virino hypothesis (Fig. 1B), which holds that the infectious agent consists of a nucleic acid genome and the host-derived PrP, which is recruited as some sort of coat.[27,48] No credible evidence for such a nucleic acid has yet been forthcoming.[22,43,44,48] Finally, the possibility that the infectious agent is a virus with unusual properties is still upheld by some.[24,49]

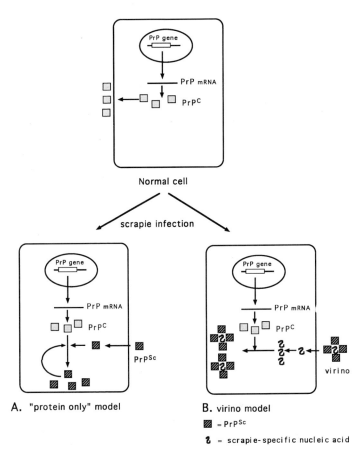

Fig. 1 Models for the propagation of the scrapie agent (prion). (**A**) The 'protein only' model assumes that the prion is identical with PrPSc. Exogenous PrPSc causes the conversion of the normal cellular protein PrPC into PrPSc. (**B**) The 'virino hypothesis' assumes that the infectious agent consists of a scrapie-specific nucleic acid associated with or packaged in PrPSc. The 'scrapie specific nucleic acid' (to date never found) is replicated in the cell and recruits PrPC into association with it. Strain specificity would be mediated by the nucleic acid.

PREVIOUS EVIDENCE BEARING ON THE RELATIONSHIP OF PrP TO TRANSMISSIBLE SPONGIFORM ENCEPHALOPATHIES

Scrapie infectivity is associated with PrPSc

Purification of scrapie infectivity results in a preparation highly enriched with regard to PrPSc.[35,50,51] Conversely, purification of PrPSc by affinity chromatography on an anti-PrP antibody column leads to enrichment of infectivity.[52]

A nucleic acid larger than about 100 nucleotides is not essential for infectivity of scrapie prion preparations

This claim is based on: (a) the unusually small target size of scrapie infectivity for UV and ionizing radiation[16,53,54]; (b) the low ratio of nucleic acids to infectious units in highly purified prion preparations[44] and the failure to find scrapie-specific nucleic acid in prion preparations or scrapie-infected brain tissue[22,43,55]; (c) resistance of infectivity to treatment with agents modifying or damaging nucleic acids.[3] Collectively, these data suggest that a nucleic acid of more than 50–100 nucleotides is not required for infectivity (but *see* Ref. 56 for a different conclusion).

The susceptibility of a host to scrapie infection is co-determined by the prion inoculum and the PrP gene

The significance of the host PrP genotype for the susceptibility to scrapie infection and the course of the disease is revealed by two sets of findings. First, the incubation time for one and the same prion isolate may be different in distinct mouse strains, and is determined predominantly by *Sinc*[57,58] or *Prn*-i[59,60] which is very closely linked to or coincident with *Prn-p*, the gene encoding PrP.[59–63] Second, when prions are transmitted from one animal species to another, disease often develops only after a very long incubation period, if at all. However, upon serial passaging in the new species, the incubation time may decrease dramatically and then stabilize. At least in the case of hamster and mouse, this so-called species barrier[64] can be overcome by introducing into the recipient host the PrP transgene from the prion donor.[45,65] Moreover, prion preparations from mice carrying hamster PrP-transgenes and inoculated with hamster scrapie prions are highly infectious to the hamster but not to the mouse. The same transgenic mouse strain, infected with mouse-derived prions, yields preparations highly infectious for mice but not for hamsters.[45] Within the framework of the 'protein only' hypothesis this means that hamster PrP^C, but not murine PrP^C, is a suitable substrate for conversion to hamster PrP^{Sc} by hamster prions and vice versa.

Hereditary forms of spongiform encephalopathies are linked to mutations of the PrP gene

The human prion diseases, Creutzfeldt-Jakob (CJD) and Gerstmann-Sträussler-Scheinker disease (GSS), are very rare in the overall population, but also occur as a familial form.[8,9,66,67] Hsiao et al[68] found that in two apparently unrelated GSS families the disease is tightly linked to a proline-to-leucine change in codon 102 of one of the *Prn-p* alleles. Subsequently other GSS and CJD families were identified, carrying the

102 mutation or one of a number of other mutations in the PrP gene (for a review see Ref. 69). Prusiner[26] proposed that the mutations allow spontaneous conversion of PrP^C into PrP^{Sc} with a frequency sufficient to allow the disease to be expressed within the lifetime of the individual. Sporadic CJD would be attributable to a somatic mutation in the *Prn-p* gene or to rare instances of spontaneous conversion of PrP^C into PrP^{Sc} (Fig. 2A).

Hsiao et al.[70] showed that mice carrying a murine PrP transgene with the pro→leu mutation corresponding to the human GSS mutation at position 102 spontaneously come down with a lethal scrapie-like disease. However, it has not yet been reported whether or not the brains of these animals contain prions.

SUSCEPTIBILITY TO SCRAPIE OF MICE DEVOID OF PrP^C

The 'protein only' hypothesis predicts that in the absence of PrP^C, mice should be resistant to scrapie infection, both with regard to symptoms and to propagation of the infectious agent.

Generation and properties of *Prn-p$^{0/0}$* mice

Mice devoid of PrP[71] were generated by the general approach described by others.[72–75] In short, one *Prn-p* allele of murine embryonic stem (ES) cells was disrupted (Fig. 2A) by homologous recombination with a 4.8 kb DNA fragment in which codons 4–187 of the 254-codon open reading frame, which is located within a single exon, were replaced by a neomycin phosphotransferase (*neo*) gene under the control of the HSV TK promoter (Fig. 2B). In the resulting construction (Fig. 2C) the first 3 *Prn-p* codons, the *neo* encoding sequence and the residual 67 *Prn-p* codons were fused in frame, with one nonsense codon interposed between the initial *Prn-p* codons and the *neo* sequence and two nonsense codons between the latter and the residual *Prn-p* sequence (Fig. 2D). Thus, the synthesis of PrP or any fragment thereof is precluded. Blastocysts from black mice were injected with *agouti* ES cells carrying the disrupted *Prn-p* gene and implanted into foster mothers. Chimeric males (showing *agouti* patches) were mated with wild type black mice and *agouti* offspring carrying the disrupted gene were identified by PCR analysis. *Prn-p$^{0/+}$* heterozygotes were mated and 176 superficially indistinguishable offspring analyzed by PCR. Of these, 24% were homozygous for the disrupted *Prn-p* gene.

As shown by Northern analysis, normal PrP mRNA was not detectable in brain from *Prn-p$^{0/0}$* homozygotes, however substantial quantities of a fused mRNA containing the *neo* and the residual *Prn-p* sequence were present. Western analysis of brain proteins showed that

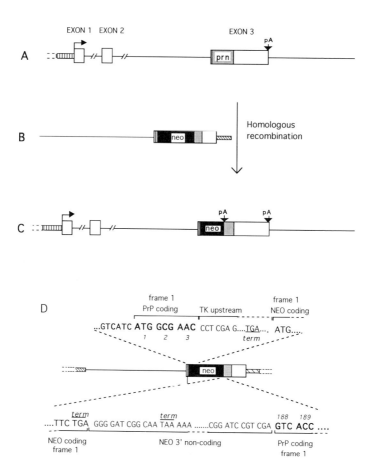

Fig. 2 Construction of the PrP targeting vector. (**A**) Map of the murine PrP gene.[88] (**B**) The targeting vector was constructed by replacing 552 bp of the *Prn-p* coding region (extending from position 10–562) by a 1.1 kb cassette containing the HSV thymidine kinase promoter followed by the *neo* gene. (**C**) The disrupted PrP gene. (**D**) The first 3 *Prn-p* codons, the *neo* coding sequence and the residual 67 *Prn-p* codons were fused in frame, with one nonsense codon interposed between the initial *Prn-p* codons and the *neo* sequence and two nonsense codons between the latter and the residual *Prn-p* sequence.

PrP was undetectable in *Prn-p[0/0]* samples and present at about half the normal level in *Prn-p[0/+]* samples.

No gross abnormalities were noted in *Prn-p[0/0]* mice at the macroscopic or microscopic level, in particular of the brain, skeletal muscle and visceral organs.[71,76] Disruption of the *Prn-p* gene had no detectable effect on the normal maturation of the lymphocyte subsets. No significant difference in the response of splenocytes from *Prn-p[0/0]* and *Prn-p[+/+]* mice to activation by concanavalin A was detected.[71]

Because PrP^C is a predominantly neuronal protein and present in a high proportion of hippocampal neurons, the learning ability of *Prn-p$^{0/0}$*, *Prn-p$^{+/+}$* and *Prn-p$^{0/+}$* mice, all derived from the mating of the first generation of heterozygotes, was compared. Three tests, the **swimming navigation test**,[77] the **Y-maze discrimination** test[78] and the **two-way avoidance (shuttlebox)** test[79] revealed no differences between the three groups of mice.

Homozygous *Prn-p$^{0/0}$* mice are fertile and normal progeny result from homozygous *Prn-p$^{0/0}$* breeding pairs. No abnormalities of homozygotes were recorded during 18 months of observation. It is surprising that a protein expressed in many areas of the brain and in other tissues and whose gene has been found in mammals, birds and fish can be ablated without apparent detrimental effects. It is possible that its function is too subtle to be detected under laboratory conditions, or that it can be replaced by some other gene product(s), particularly if adaptive processes are facilitated during development.

Challenge of *Prn-p$^{0/0}$* and *Prn-p$^{0/+}$* mice with scrapie prions

Mice devoid of PrP were challenged with mouse prions and proved to be completely protected against scrapie disease, at least up to 14 months after inoculation (Fig. 3). Moreover, even heterozygous *Prn-p$^{0/+}$* mice proved to be partially protected, inasmuch as scrapie-inoculated animals showed signs of scrapie only **253-337** days after inoculation but are still alive after 380 days, while all *Prn-p$^{+/+}$* controls died within about 180 days. Moreover, disease progression in *Prn-p$^{0/+}$* mice is distinctly slower than in *Prn-p$^{+/+}$* mice, the interval between first symptoms and death being 13 days in the case of *Prn-p$^{+/+}$* mice while no *Prn-p$^{0/+}$* mice have died to date, about 3 months after the appearance of scrapie symptoms (Büeler and Weissmann, unpublished results).

We conclude that development of scrapie symptoms and pathology is strictly dependent on the presence of PrP and that incubation time and disease progression are inversely related to the level of PrP. It has previously been found that the length of the scrapie incubation time for hamster-derived prions in mice expressing SHaPrP genes was inversely related to the level of SHaPrP.[45]

Are prions propagated in *Prn-p$^{0/0}$* mice?

It was shown that if infectious agent is propagated in *Prn-p$^{0/0}$* mice, this would be at a level about five orders of magnitude lower than that in *Prn-p$^{+/+}$* animals.[25] Scrapie prion titers were determined by preparing tissue extracts at various times after inoculation, heating them for 20 min at 80°C to destroy any adventitious conventional pathogens and inoculating them into wild type indicator mice. In scrapie-

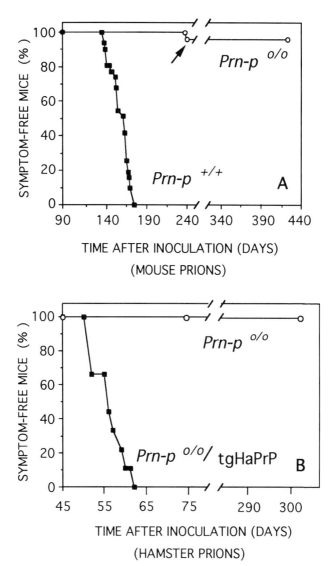

Fig. 3 Susceptibility of mice with various PrP genotypes to inoculation with scrapie prions. Mice were inoculated intracerebrally and the percentage of mice remaining free of scrapie symptoms was plotted as a function of time. (**A**) *Prn-p^0/0* and *Prn-p^+/+* mice were inoculated with mouse prions. One *Prn-p^0/0* mouse (arrow) showed ataxic gait and was sacrificed at 240 days: it showed no histopathological changes typical for scrapie and brain homogenate from this mouse did not transmit scrapie to CD-1 indicator mice after more than 170 days. (**B**) *Prn-p^0/0* and *Prn-p^0/0*/tgHaPrP mice (*Prn-p^0/0* mice carrying Syrian hamster transgenes) were inoculated with hamster scrapie prions.

inoculated *Prn-p^+/+* animals, infectious agent was detected in the brain at 8 weeks and increased to about 8.6 log LD_{50} units/ml by 20 weeks after inoculation (Table). No infectious agent was detected in Prn-$p^{0/0}$ animals 25 weeks after inoculation, the latest time point for which data are presently available. However, in a parallel assay using unheated samples, a low level of infectivity, about 3.2 log LD_{50} units/ml, was found in the 20 week sample from Prn-$p^{0/0}$ animals. Because only one Prn-$p^{0/0}$ brain sample in the entire experiment was positive, accidental contamination of the homogenate or infectivity due to residual traces of inoculum in the occasional mouse cannot be excluded. However, the possibility must be considered that the infectious agent is something other than PrP[Sc], and that in the absence of PrP[Sc] in the host it is much less infectious than in its presence. This question can only be resolved by further experiments, which are now underway.

Table Prion titers in brain and spleen of Prn-$p^{+/+}$ and Prn-$p^{0/0}$ mice[a]

Time after inoculation	Brain (heated)		Brain (not heated)		Spleen (heated)	
	$PrP^{+/+}$	$PrP^{0/0}$	$PrP^{+/+}$	$PrP^{0/0}$	$PrP^{+/+}$	$PrP^{0/0}$
4 days	< 1.5	2.0[b]	n.d.	n.d.	5.7 ± 0.9	2.3[c]
2 weeks	< 1.5	< 1.5	n.d.	n.d.	6.2 ± 0.8	< 1.5
8 weeks	5.4	< 1.5	7.7 ± 0.6	< 1.5	6.9 ± 1.0	< 1.5
12 weeks	6.8	< 1.5	7.1 ± 1.6	< 1.5	5.9 ± 0.6	< 1.5
20 weeks	8.6	< 1.5	7.7 ± 1.1	3.2 ± 1.4[d]	6.9 ± 0.6	< 1.5
23/25 weeks	8.1 ± 0.8	< 1.5	n.d.	n.d.	n.d.	< 1.5

[a]The samples designated 'heated' were kept 20 min at 80°C prior to inoculation. The titers of brain homogenates recovered at 8, 12 and 20 weeks after inoculation and of the Chandler-derived mouse prion inoculum 'RML' (8.5 log LD_{50} units/ml) were determined by end point dilution. The titers of the other samples were determined by the incubation time assay (Ref. 25) [b]1/6 mice died after inoculation with 10^{-1} diluted homogenate. [c]2/6 mice died after inoculation with 10^{-1} diluted homogenate [d]6/6 mice died after inoculation with 10^{-1} diluted homogenate

Restoration of susceptibility to scrapie by introduction of PrP transgenes.

When ablation of a gene product gives rise to a specific phenotype, in this case resistance to scrapie, it is desirable to demonstrate that reinstatement of the gene restores the original phenotype. Indeed, insertion of mouse PrP genes rendered Prn-$p^{0/0}$ mice susceptible to mouse prions (Fischer and Weissmann, unpublished data). More interestingly, introduction of hamster PrP transgenes into Prn-$p^{0/0}$ mice rendered them very susceptible to hamster-derived prions (56 ± 3 days incubation time) but much less so (303 ± 19 days) to mouse-derived prions, demonstrating the requirement of a homotypic relationship between incoming prion and resident PrP protein for prion propagation and development of pathology, as foreshadowed by the results of Prusiner et al.[45]

IMPLICATIONS AND OUTLOOK

Both the biochemical and genetic data discussed in this review support the proposal that the prion is composed partly or entirely of a PrP isoform (either PrP^{Sc} or a subfraction of it), and that protein-encoding nucleic acid is not an essential component. Other explanations of the data, such as that PrP^C is or contributes to a receptor for the scrapie agent, while less likely, are not yet formally excluded.

How is PrP^C converted to PrP^{Sc}?

No chemical differences between PrP^C and PrP^{Sc} have been detected, however, as pointed out above, the ratio of infectious units to PrP^{Sc} molecules is about 1:10^5. Therefore, chemical analyses may not bear on the structure of a conjectural minor component responsible for the infectivity. Nonetheless, this minor component is likely PrP^C-derived, as indicated by the genetic evidence, and is as resistant to proteinase digestion as PrP^{Sc}.[80]

Prusiner postulated that the difference between PrP^C and PrP^{Sc} is conformational. In Figure 4A it is suggested that a molecule of PrP^{Sc} binds to PrP^C and thereby imposes its conformation upon it. The species barrier is explained by the assumption that heterologous PrP species interact poorly and/or that the conversion only occurs rarely. Mutations of the Gerstmann-Sträussler and CJD type would allow spontaneous, albeit very rare conversion events, yielding PrP^{Sc} that can then act catalytically (Fig. 4B). Sporadic cases of CJD could be attributed to even rarer cases of spontaneous conversion of wild type PrP^C or of a somatically mutated PrP^C.

It has so far not been possible to denature infectious preparations containing PrP^{Sc} and renature them to regain infectivity and/or protease resistance[81] contrary to previous reports,[82,83] nor has it been possible to convert PrP^C into PrP^{Sc} in a cell free system.[84] In addition, PrP^C does not, or only in the rarest of cases, spontaneously convert to PrP^{Sc} in vivo, despite the inordinate stability of PrP^{Sc}. To explain these findings within the framework of the 'protein only' model, Figure 4C suggests that the PrP^{Sc} state is separated from that of PrP^C and of a random coil by very high activation energy barriers, while the PrP state is separated from the random coil state by a far lower barrier. Thus, the only way PrP^C can convert to PrP^{Sc} is by 'tunnelling' through the activation energy barrier by a catalyzed, probably energy-dependent process which might involve chaperonins.

THE "PROTEIN ONLY" HYPOTHESIS"

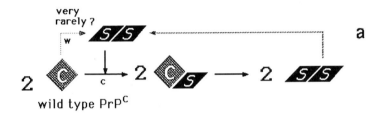

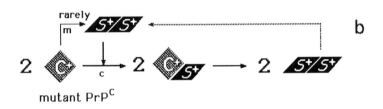

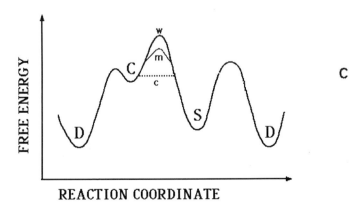

Fig. 4 Model for the catalyzed conformational conversion of PrP[C] to an infectious PrP form. (**A**) Following a proposal by Prusiner[45] PrP[C] (C) is converted to the conformer PrP[Sc] (S) via dimers formed with exogenously introduced PrP[Sc]. This results in an exponential cascade of conversion. Sporadic forms of prion disease (such as sporadic CJD) may come about when an extremely rare event (w) leads to spontaneous conversion of PrP[C] to PrP[Sc] and gives rise to a conversion cascade. (**B**) In the case of certain mutations in PrP[C] (C+) spontaneous conversion (m) to PrP[Sc] may occur about a million times more frequently than in the case of the wild type protein, but still remains a rare event, explaining why familial forms of prion diseases arise only late in life. (**C**) Postulated energy diagram for different forms of PrP. The PrP[C] conformation (C) is separated from the PrP[Sc] conformation (S) by a high activation energy barrier, and from the denatured state (D) by a low activation energy barrier. Thus a spontaneous conformational change from PrP[C] to PrP[Sc] (pathway w) will be extremely rare. Interaction of PrP[C] with PrP[Sc] facilitates the conversion (pathway c) by lowering the activation energy for the transition. In the case of certain mutations in PrP[C] the activation energy for the conversion (pathway m) is lowered, increasing the probability of the spontaneous conformational change to PrP[Sc].

Scrapie strains

As mentioned above, the finding that there are many distinct strains of scrapie prions which can be propagated in one and the same mouse strain (homozygous with regard to its PrP gene) is not readily explained by the 'protein only' hypothesis (for a review, see Ref 23) because it implies that an incoming PrP[Sc] strain can convert one and the same PrP precursor into a likeness of itself, and that this can happen for several if not many different strains. Two subsidiary hypotheses have been suggested to circumvent this difficulty. The 'unified theory'[85] proposes that PrP[Sc] is associated with a small host-derived nucleic acid which is not required for infectivity but determines the characteristic phenotype of the strain. This nucleic acid would be replicated by host cell enzymes and then associate with newly formed PrP[Sc] leading to preservation of the prion's phenotype. The 'targeting theory'[86] (and KH Meyer, personal communication 1991) proposes that PrP[Sc] carries a variable modification, for example carbohydrate residues, which target it to a specific subset of cells. These cells would impart the same modification to the newly formed PrP[Sc] molecules. Different strains would thus be targeted to different subsets of cells and retain their specific modification (Fig. 5). This hypothesis is supported by the observation that different hamster prion strains[86] or mouse prion strains[87] give rise to different patterns of PrP[Sc] deposition in the brain. It predicts that if two different prion strains are propagated through a singular cellular species they should emerge with identical properties.

PRACTICAL IMPLICATIONS OF PRION RESEARCH

The results of Büeler et al[25,71] show that it is possible to generate normal mice which are resistant to scrapie by knocking out their PrP genes.

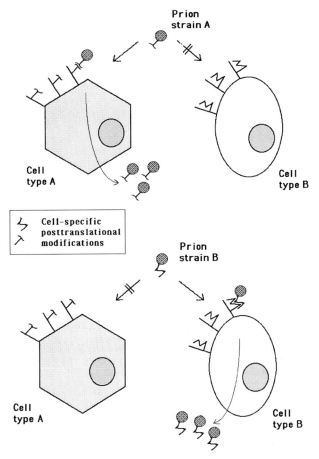

Fig. 5 The 'targeting model' to explain prion strain specificity. It is assumed that strain specificity of the prion is imparted by a cell specific post-translational modification which targets the prion to the same type of cell as the one in which it was synthesized. A possible modification would be glycosylation.

In principle it should thus be possible to breed sheep or cattle resistant to this disease, either by PrP gene disruption or by the introduction of transgenes expressing PrP antisense RNA. Moreover, the fact that $Prn-p^{0/+}$ heterozygous mice show much longer scrapie incubation times than their wild type counterparts argues that disease progression may be rate-limited by the PrP^C concentration. This conclusion is consistent with the observation that in several mouse lines containing hamster PrP transgenes the incubation time for hamster prion-induced scrapie is a function of the hamster PrP expression level.[45] A practical implication of this conclusion is that a moderate reduction of PrP^C synthesis, such as might eventually be achieved by antisense oligonucleotide therapy, could substantially mitigate disease progression in incipient cases of spongiform encephalopathies.

ACKNOWLEDGEMENTS

This work was supported by the Erziehungsdirektion of the Kanton of Zürich and grants of the Schweizerische Nationalfonds to CW. We thank Dr S Prusiner for advice and discussions.

REFERENCES

1 Cuille J, Chelle PL. Experimental transmission of trembling to the goat. C R Seances Acad Sci 1939; 208: 1058-1160.

2 Gordon WS. Vet Rec 1946; 58: 516.

3 Prusiner SB. Novel proteinaceous infectious particles cause scrapie. Science 1982; 216: 136-144.

4 Pattison IH. Resistance of the scrapie agent to formalin. J Comp Pathol 1965; 75: 159-164.

5 Alper T, Haig DA, Clarke MC. The exceptionally small size of the scrapie agent. Biochem Biophys Res Commun 1966; 22: 278-284.

6 Hadlow WJ. Scrapie and kuru. Lancet 1959; 2: 289-290.

7 Gajdusek DC, Gibbs CJ Jr, Alpers M. Experimental transmission of a Kuru-like syndrome to chimpanzees. Nature 1966; 209: 794-796.

8 Gibbs CJ Jr, Gajdusek DC, Asher DM et al. Creutzfeldt-Jakob disease (spongiform encephalopathy); Transmission to the chimpanzee. Science 1968; 161: 388-389.

9 Masters CL, Gajdusek DC, Gibbs CJ Jr. Creutzfeldt-Jakob disease virus isolations from the Gerstmann-Sträussler syndrome. Brain 1981; 104: 559-588.

10 Tateishi J, Ohta M, Koga M, Sato Y. Transmission of chronic spongiform encephalopathy with kuru plaques from humans to small rodents. Ann Neurol 1979; 5: 581-584.

11 Wells GAH, Scott AC, Johnson CT et al. A novel progressive spongiform encephalopathy in cattle. Vet Rec 1993; 121: 419-420.

12 Wilesmith JW, Ryan JB, Hueston WD, Hoinville LJ. Bovine spongiform encephalopathy: epidemiological features 1985 to 1990. Vet Rec 1992; 130: 90-94.

13 Brown P, Liberski PP, Wolff A, Gajdusek DC. Resistance of scrapie infectivity to steam autoclaving after formaldehyde fixation and limited survival after ashing at 360 degrees C: practical and theoretical implications. J Infect Dis 1990; 161: 467-472.

14 Stamp JT, Brotherston JG, Zlotnik I, Mackay JM, Smith W. Further studies on scrapie. J Comp Pathol 1959; 69: 268-280.

15 Griffith JS. Self-replication and scrapie. Nature 1967; 215: 1043-1044.

16 Alper T, Cramp WA, Haig DA, Clarke MC. Does the agent of scrapie replicate without nucleic acid? Nature 1967; 214: 764-766.

17 Pattison IH, Jones KM. The possible nature of the transmissible agent of scrapie. Vet Rec 1967; 80: 2-9.

18 Gibbons RA, Hunter GD. Nature of scrapie agent. Nature 1967; 215: 1041-1043.

19 Prusiner SB. Molecular biology of prion diseases. Science 1991; 252: 1515-1522.

20 Weissmann C. Spongiform encephalopathies. The prion's progress (news). Nature 1991; 349: 569-571.

21 Kimberlin RH. Scrapie and possible relationship with viroids. Semin Virol 1990; 1: 153-162.

22 Aiken JM, Marsh RF. The search for scrapie agent nucleic acid. Microbiol Rev 1990; 54: 242-246.

23 Bruce ME, Fraser H. Scrapie strain variation and its implications. Curr Top Microbiol Immunol 1991; 172: 125-138.

24 Rohwer RG. The scrapie agent: 'a virus by any other name'. Curr Top Microbiol Immunol 1991; 172: 195-232.
25 Büeler H, Aguzzi A, Sailer A, Greiner R-A, Autenried P, Aguet M. Mice devoid of PrP are resistant to scrapie. Cell 1993; 73: 1339-1347.
26 Prusiner SB. Scrapie prions. Annu Rev Microbiol 1989; 43: 345-374.
27 Oesch B, Westaway D, Walchli M et al. A cellular gene encodes scrapie PrP 27–30 protein. Cell 1985; 40: 735-746.
28 Chesebro B, Race R, Wehrly K et al. Identification of scrapie prion protein-specific messenger RNA in scrapie-infected and uninfected brain. Nature 1985; 315: 331-333.
29 Hope J, Morton LJ, Farquhar CF, Multhaup G, Beyreuther K, Kimberlin RH. The major polypeptide of scrapie-associated fibrils (SAF) has the same size, charge distribution and N-terminal protein sequence as predicted for the normal brain protein (PrP). EMBO J 1986; 5: 2591-2597.
30 Basler K, Oesch B, Scott M et al. Scrapie and cellular PrP isoforms are encoded by the same chromosomal gene. Cell 1986; 46: 417-428.
31 Prusiner SB, DeArmond SJ. Prion diseases of the central nervous system. Monogr Pathol 1990; 32: 86-122.
32 Stahl N, Borchelt DR, Hsiao K, Prusiner SB. Scrapie prion protein contains a phosphatidylinositol glycolipid. Cell 1987; 51: 229-240.
33 Manson J, West JD, Thomson V, Mcbride P, Kaufman MH, Hope J. The prion protein gene a role in mouse embryogenesis? Development Camb 1992; 115: 117-122.
34 Bendheim PE, Brown HR, Rudelli RD et al. Nearly ubiquitous tissue distribution of the scrapie agent precursor protein. Neurology 1992; 42: 149-156.
35 Prusiner SB, Bolton DC, Groth DF, Bowman KA, Cochran SP, McKinley MP. Further purification and characterization of scrapie prions. Biochemistry 1982; 21: 6942-6950.
36 Prusiner SB, McKinley MP, Bowman KA et al. Scrapie prions aggregate to form amyloid-like birefringent rods. Cell 1983; 35: 349-358.
37 McKinley MP, Meyer RK, Kenaga L et al. Scrapie prion rod formation in vitro requires both detergent extraction and limited proteolysis. J Virol 1991; 65: 1340-1351.
38 Taraboulos A, Serban D, Prusiner SB. Scrapie prion proteins accumulate in the cytoplasm of persistently infected cultured cells. J Cell Biol 1990; 110: 2117-2132.
39 McKinley MP, Taraboulos A, Kenaga L et al. Ultrastructural localization of scrapie prion proteins in secondary lysosomes of infected cultured cells. J Cell Biol 1990; 111(5, Part 2): 316a.
40 Turk E, Teplow DB, Hood LE, Prusiner SB. Purification and properties of the cellular and scrapie hamster prion proteins. Eur J Biochem 1988; 176: 21-30.
41 Stahl N, Baldwin MA, Hecker R, Pan K-M, Burlingame, AL, Prusiner SB. Glycosylinositol phospholipid anchors of the scrapie and cellular prion proteins contain sialic acid. Biochemistry 1992; 31: 5043-5053.
42 Bolton DC, Rudelli RD, Currie JR, Bendheim PE. Copurification of Sp33–37 and scrapie agent from hamster brain prior to detectable histopathology and clinical disease. J Gen Virol 1991; 72: 2905-2913.
43 Oesch B, Groth DF, Prusiner SB, Weissmann C. Search for a scrapie-specific nucleic acid: a progress report. Ciba Found Symp 1988; 135: 209-223.
44 Kellings K, Meyer N, Mirenda C, Prusiner SB, Riesner D. Further analysis of nucleic acids in purified scrapie prion preparations by improved return refocusing gel electrophoresis. J Gen Virol 1992; 73: 1025-1029.
45 Prusiner SB, Scott M, Foster D et al. Transgenetic studies implicate interactions between homologous PrP isoforms in scrapie prion replication. Cell 1990; 63: 673-686.
46 Bolton DC, Bendheim PE. In: Bock G, Marsh J, eds. Novel infectious agents and the central nervous system. Chichester: John Wiley, 1988: 164-177.
47 Dickinson AG, Outram GW. Genetic aspects of unconventional virus infections: the basis of the virino hypothesis. Ciba Found Symp 1988; 135: 63-83.
48 Meyer N, Rosenbaum V, Schmidt B et al. Search for a putative scrapie genome in purified prion fractions reveals a paucity of nucleic acids. J Gen Virol 1991; 72: 37-49.

49 Diringer H. Transmissible spongiform encephalopathies (TSE) virus-induced amyloidoses of the central nervous system (CNS). Eur J Epidemiol 1991; 7: 562-566.

50 Bolton DC, McKinley MP, Prusiner SB. Identification of a protein that purifies with the scrapie prion. Science 1982; 218: 1309-1311.

51 Diringer H, Gelderblom H, Hilmert H, Ozel M, Edelbluth C, Kimberlin RH. Scrapie infectivity, fibrils and low molecular weight protein. Nature 1983; 306: 476-478.

52 Gabizon R, McKinley MP, Groth D, Prusiner SB. Immunoaffinity purification and neutralization of scrapie prion infectivity. Proc Natl Acad Sci USA 1988; 85: 6617-6621.

53 Latarjet R, Muel B, Haig DA, Clarke MC, Alper T. Inactivation of the scrapie agent by near monochromatic ultraviolet light. Nature 1970; 227: 1341-1343.

54 Bellinger-Kawahara CG, Kempner E, Groth D, Gabizon R, Prusiner SB. Scrapie prion liposomes and rods exhibit target sizes of 55 000 Da. Virology 1988; 164: 537-541.

55 Diedrich J, Wietgrefe S, Zupancic M et al. The molecular pathogenesis of astrogliosis in scrapie and Alzheimer's disease. Microb Pathol 1987; 2/6: 435-442.

56 Sklaviadis T, Akowitz A, Manuelidis EE, Manuelidis L. Nuclease treatment results in high specific purification of Creutzfeldt-Jakob disease infectivity with a density characteristic of nucleic acid-protein complexes. Arch Virol 1990; 112, 215-228.

57 Dickinson AG, Meikle VM, Fraser H. Identification of a gene which controls the incubation period of some strains of scrapie agent in mice. J Comp Pathol 1968; 78: 293-299.

58 Bruce ME, Dickinson AG. Biological evidence that scrapie agent has an independent genome. J Gen Virol 1987; 68: 79-89.

59 Carlson GA, Kingsbury DT, Goodman PA et al. Linkage of prion protein and scrapie incubation time genes. Cell 1986; 46: 503-511.

60 Hunter N, Hope J, McConnell I, Dickinson AG. Linkage of the scrapie-associated fibril protein (PrP) gene and Sinc using congenic mice and restriction fragment length polymorphism analysis. J Gen Virol 1987; 68: 2711-2716.

61 Carlson GA, Goodman PA, Lovett M et al. Genetics and polymorphism of the mouse prion gene complex control of scrapie incubation time. Mol Cell Biol 1988; 8: 5528-5540.

62 Carlson GA, Westaway D, DeArmond SJ, Peterson Torchia M, Prusiner SB. Primary structure of prion protein may modify scrapie isolate properties. Proc Natl Acad Sci USA 1989; 86: 7475-7479.

63 Race RE, Graham K, Ernst D, Caughey B, Chesebro B. Analysis of linkage between scrapie incubation period and the prion protein gene in mice. J Gen Virol 1990; 71: 493-497.

64 Pattison IH. The relative susceptibility of sheep, goats and mice to two types of the goat scrapie agent. Res Vet Sci 1966; 7: 207-212.

65 Scott M, Foster D, Mirenda C et al. Transgenic mice expressing hamster prion protein produce species-specific scrapie infectivity and amyloid plaques. Cell 1989; 59: 847-857.

66 Gajdusek DC. Unconventional viruses and the origin and disappearance of kuru. Science 1977; 197: 943-960.

67 Masters CL, Gajdusek DC, Gibbs CJ Jr. The familial occurrence of Creutzfeldt-Jakob disease and Alzheimer's disease. Brain 1981; 104: 535-558.

68 Hsiao K, Baker HF, Crow TJ et al. Linkage of a prion protein missense variant to Gerstmann-Sträussler syndrome. Nature 1989; 338: 342-345.

69 Baker HF, Ridley RM. The genetics and transmissibility of human spongiform encephalopathy. Neurodegeneration 1992; 1: 3-16.

70 Hsiao KK, Scott M, Foster D, Groth DF, DeArmond SJ, Prusiner SB. Spontaneous neurodegeneration in transgenic mice with mutant prion protein. Science 1990; 250: 1587-1590.

71 Büeler H, Fischer M, Lang Y et al. Normal development and behaviour of mice lacking the neuronal cell-surface PrP protein (see comments). Nature 1992; 356: 577-582.

72 Hooper ML, Hardy K, Handyside A, Hunter S, Monk M. HPRT-deficient (Lesh-Nyhan) mouse embryos derived from germline colonization by cultured cells. Nature 1987; 326: 292-295.

73 Doetschman T, Maeda N, Smithies O. Targeted mutation of the *Hprt* gene in mouse embryonic stem cells. Proc Natl Acad Sci USA 1988; 85: 8583-8587.

74 Bradley A. In: Robertson EJ, ed. Teratocarcinomas and embryonic stem cells: a practical approach. Oxford: IRL Press, 1987: 113-151.

75 Capecchi MR. The new mouse genetics: altering the genome by gene targeting. Trends Genet 1989; 5: 70-76.

76 Brenner HR, Herczeg A, Oesch B. Normal development of nerve-muscle synapses in mice lacking the prion protein gene. Proc R Soc Lond B 1992; 250: 151-155.

77 Morris RGM. Development of a water-maze procedure for studying spatial learning in the rat. J Neurosci Meth 1984; 11: 47-60.

78 Lipp H-P, Van der Loos H. A computer-controlled Y-maze for testing vibrisso-tactile discrimination learning in mice. Behav Brain Res 1991; 45: 135-145.

79 Anisman H. In: Anisman H, Bignami G, eds. The psychopharmacology of aversively motivated behavior. New York: Plenum Press, 1978: 1-62.

80 McKinley MP, Bolton DC, Prusiner SB. A protease-resistant protein is a structural component of the scrapie prion. Cell 1983; 35: 57-62.

81 Prusiner SB, Groth D, Serban A, Stahl N, Gabizon R. Attempts to restore scrapie prion infectivity after exposure to protein denaturants. Proc Natl Acad Sci USA 1993; 90: 2793-2797.

82 Brown P, Liberski PP, Wolff A, Gajdusek DC. Conservation of infectivity in purified fibrillary extracts of scrapie-infected hamster brain after sequential enzymatic digestion or polyacrylamide gel electrophoresis. Proc Natl Acad Sci USA 1990; 87: 7240-7244.

83 Safar J, Wang W, Padgett MP et al. Molecular mass, biochemical composition, and physicochemical behavior of the infectious form of the scrapie precursor protein monomer. Proc Natl Acad Sci USA 1990; 87: 6373-6377.

84 Raeber A, Borchelt DR, Scott M, Prusiner SB. Attempts to convert the cellular prion protein into the scrapie prion isoform in cell-free systems. J Virol 1992; 66: 6155-6163.

85 Weissmann C. A 'unified theory' of prion propagation. Nature 1991; 352: 679-683.

86 Hecker R, Taraboulos A, Scott M, et al. Replication of distinct scrapie prion isolates is region specific in brains of transgenic mice and hamsters. Genes Dev 1992; 6: 1213-1228.

87 Manson J, Mcbride P, Hope J. Expression of the PrP gene in the brain of sinc congenic mice and its relationship to the development of scrapie. Neurodegeneration 1992; 1: 45-52.

88 Westaway D, Goodman PA, Mirenda CA, McKinley MP, Carlson GA, Prusiner SB. Distinct prion proteins in short and long scrapie incubation period mice. Cell 1987; 51: 651-662.

Index Vol. 49 No. 4